Localization in Neuropsychology

Localization in Neuropsychology

EDITED BY

ANDREW KERTESZ

Department of Clinical Neurological Sciences
University of Western Ontario
St. Joseph's Hospital
London, Ontario, Canada

1983

ACADEMIC PRESS

A Subsidiary of Harcourt Brace Jovanovich, Publishers

New York   London

Paris   San Diego   San Francisco   São Paulo   Sydney   Tokyo   Toronto

ACADEMIC PRESS, INC.
111 Fifth Avenue, New York, New York 10003

United Kingdom Edition published by
ACADEMIC PRESS, INC. (LONDON) LTD.
24/28 Oval Road, London NW1 7DX

Library of Congress Cataloging in Publication Data

Main entry under title:

Localization in neuropsychology.

    Includes bibliographical references and index.
    1. Brain--Diseases. 2. Neuropsychology.
3. Brain--Localization of functions. I. Kertesz,
Andrew. [DNLM: 1. Brain mapping. 2. Brain
injuries--Diagnosis. 3. Language disorders--Diagnosis.
4. Agnosia--Diagnosis. WL 354 L811]
RC386.2.L63 1983   616.8   83-2537
ISBN 0-12-405050-6

PRINTED IN THE UNITED STATES OF AMERICA

83 84 85 86   9 8 7 6 5 4 3 2 1

Contents

**3. CT Scan Lesion Size and Lesion Locus
in Cortical and Subcortical Aphasias**

Margaret A. Naeser

**4. Positron-Computed Tomography
in Neurobehavioral Problems**

*D. Frank Benson, E. Jeffrey Metter, David E. Kuhl,
and Michael E. Phelps*

**5. Localization of Cognitive Function
with Cerebral Blood Flow**

Niels A. Lassen and Per E. Roland

**6. Localization of Language and Visuospatial Functions
by Electrical Stimulation**

Catherine A. Mateer

7. Localization of Lesions in Broca's Motor Aphasia

David N. Levine and Eric Sweet

8. Localization of Lesions in Wernicke's Aphasia

Andrew Kertesz

9. Localization of Lesions in Conduction Aphasia

Hanna Damasio and Antonio R. Damasio

10. The Localization of Lesions in Transcortical Aphasias

Alan B. Rubens and Andrew Kertesz

Contributors $\times$

Numbers in parentheses indicate the pages on which the authors' contributions begin.

Martin L. Albert (393), Aphasia/Behavioral Neurology Unit of the Boston Veterans Administration Medical Center, and Department of Neurology, Boston University School of Medicine, Boston, Massachusetts 02130

Michael P. Alexander (393), Aphasia/Behavioral Neurology Unit of the Boston Veterans Administration Medical Center, and Department of Neurology, Boston University School of Medicine, Boston, Massachusetts 02130

D. Frank Benson (121, 429), Department of Neurology, Reed Neurological Research Center, UCLA School of Medicine, Los Angeles, California 90024

Antonio R. Damasio (231, 417, 471), Department of Neurology (Division of Behavioral Neurology), University of Iowa College of Medicine, Iowa City, Iowa 52242

Hanna Damasio (231, 417), Department of Neurology, University of Iowa College of Medicine, Iowa City, Iowa 52242

Albert M. Galaburda (21), Department of Neurology, Harvard University Medical School, Beth Israel Hospital, Boston, Massachusetts 02215

Norman Geschwind (295), Department of Neurology, Harvard University, Beth Israel Hospital, Boston, Massachusetts 02215

Samuel H. Greenblatt (323), Department of Neurosciences, Medical College of Ohio, Toledo, Ohio 43699

Kenneth M. Heilman (371, 471), Department of Neurology, University of Florida, J. Hillis Miller Health Center, Gainesville, Florida 32610

Andrew Kertesz (1, 209, 245, 371, 455, 509), Department of Clinical Neurological Sciences, University of Western Ontario, St. Joseph's Hospital, London, Ontario, N6A 4V2, Canada

David E. Kuhl (121), Division of Nuclear Medicine, UCLA School of Medicine, Los Angeles, California 90024

Niels A. Lassen (141), Department of Clinical Physiology, Bispebjerg Hospital, DK 2400 N.V. Copenhagen, Denmark

David N. Levine (185), Department of Neurology, Harvard University Medical School, Massachusetts General Hospital, Boston, Massachusetts 02114

Catherine A. Mateer (153), Departments of Neurological Surgery and Speech and Hearing Sciences, University of Washington, Seattle, Washington 98195

Marek-Marsel Mesulam (21), Neurology Unit, Beth Israel Hospital, Boston, Massachusetts 02215

E. Jeffrey Metter (121), Department of Neurology, VA Medical Center, Sepulveda, California 91343, and UCLA School of Medicine, Los Angeles, California 90024

J. P. Mohr[1] (269), Department of Neurology, University of South Alabama, Mobile, Alabama 36617

Margaret A. Naeser (63), Department of Neurology, Boston University School of Medicine and Aphasia Research Center, Boston Veterans Administration Medical Center, Boston, Massachusetts 02130

Michael E. Phelps (121), Division of Nuclear Medicine, UCLA School of Medicine, Los Angeles, California 90024

Per E. Roland (141), Department of Neurology, Bispebjerg Hospital, DK 2400 N.V. Copenhagen, Denmark

Elliot D. Ross (493), Department of Neurology, University of Texas Southwestern Medical School, Dallas, Texas 75235

Leslie Rothi (371), Department of Neurology, University of Florida, Gainesville, Florida 32610

[1] Present address: College of Physicians and Surgeons, Columbia University, New York Neurological Institute, New York, New York 10032.

Alan B. Rubens (245), Hennepin County Medical Center, Minneapolis, Minnesota 55415

Richard L. Strub (295), Department of Neurology, Louisiana State University Medical Center, New Orleans, Louisiana 70112

D. T. Stuss (429), Schools of Medicine (Neurology) and Psychology, University of Ottawa, Ottawa General Hospital, Ottawa, Ontario K1H 8L6, Canada

Eric Sweet (185), Neurology Service, Massachusetts General Hospital, Boston, Massachusetts 02114

Edward Valenstein (471), Department of Neurology, University of Florida College of Medicine, J. Hillis Miller Health Center, Gainesville, Florida 32610

Luigi A. Vignolo (357), Clinica Neurologica, Universita di Milano, 20122 Milan, Italy

Robert T. Watson (471), Department of Neurology, University of Florida College of Medicine, J. Hillis Miller Medical Center, Gainesville, Florida 32610

Preface

The challenge of integrating function with structure is nowhere as great as in the central nervous system. The complexity of the issue is multiplied exponentially when cognitive behavior and language are examined. In this volume, we rise to meet this challenge and to summarize current knowledge in this area.

This is a book by clinicians whose training and perspective are basically anatomical and structuralist. Although the majority of authors are practicing neurologists, contributors also include speech pathologists, psychologists, and physiologists. Interdisciplinary boundaries are not as clear as they used to be, and the anatomical–mosaicist thinking in neurology has evolved toward a functional integration of behavior and lesions. The gaps in knowledge are still large, but the recent advances associated with *in vivo* localization techniques are summarized in this volume. Hughlings Jackson's century-old warning must be kept in mind when interpreting these lesion localization studies: "To locate the damage which destroys speech and to localize speech are two different things."

This warning, of course, should not deter attempts to correlate function with structure. The many complexities of this correlation cannot be simplified into a short aphorism. We hope that this volume will serve not only as a reference and guide to a significant part of our current knowledge, but also as an inspiration for the vast amount of research that remains to be done.

This volume consists of five major sections, each representing an area of research and methodology. Chapters 1–6 introduce the field and summarize recent knowledge in the various techniques of localization such as postmortem examination, computerized tomographic (CT) scanning, positron-emission tomography, cerebral blood flow, and direct electrical stimulation of the cortex. Each of these reviews provides specific examples and new data in its field, in addition to providing an insight into the methodology. Chapters 7–10 provide an up-to-date review of modern localization in the left-hemisphere syndromes whose primary manifestation is a language disturbance. Chapters 11 and 18, and to some extent 21, use an anatomical area as the point of departure to correlate behavior with lesions. Chapters 13–17 deal primarily with modality-based symptoms and syndromes. Finally, Chapters 19–21 deal with the so-called right-hemisphere syndromes.

I owe a great deal to my colleagues and co-workers, who are too numerous to list here. I will, however, mention Bonita Caddel and Jackie Robertson, who tirelessly and skillfully typed and retyped manuscripts, and my wife Ann, who helped by proofreading and smoothing my writing style. Dr. José Ferro read many of the chapters and provided valuable comments, and the thoroughness and organizing ability of Debbie Willsie greatly eased the birth pangs of the last few months.

While the volume was being prepared, support was received from the Ontario Ministry of Health (grant PR969) and the Medical Research Council of Canada (grant MA-7698).

1

Issues in Localization

Andrew Kertesz

Introduction

The issues in localization in neuropsychology have undergone a substantial evolution in the last decade partly because of our increasing sophistication in neuropsychological methods and concepts and partly because of a revolution in anatomical imaging techniques, especially computerized tomography (CT).

The belief in a unitary function of the cerebrum culminated in the idea of the "sensorium commune" of the nineteenth and the "black box" approach of the twentieth century. This holistic view was contradicted by the nineteenth-century anatomists who observed the gyri and their connections and began to assign function to them, at times in a speculative fashion. An absurd outgrowth of a mosaicist view of cerebral function was phrenology. The greatest scientific support for the localization of function came from the clinicians and physiologists of the second half of the nineteenth century who ob-

LOCALIZATION
IN NEUROPSYCHOLOGY

served the close relationship of stimulation of cortical points with movements in animals (Fritsch & Hitzig, 1870), extirpation of occipital cortex with loss of vision (Munk, 1881), and language impairment with the left periSylvian brain lesion (Broca, 1861).

Associationist psychology, reflex physiology, and the method of clinicopathologic correlation are responsible for the theoretical background of localization of function. However, the idea of cerebral centers of language (and other cognitive functions interconnected by a complicated neural pathway) has been under attack ever since diagrams of various processes and their interconnections have been superimposed on drawings of brains. Since Henry Head (1926) decried the diagram-makers, they have practically disappeared from the neurological literature. However, the so-called processing diagrams flourish in cognitive psychology, and the terminology used is interchanged from computer and linguistic sciences. These diagrams often bear resemblance to those created after clinicopathologic correlations in the last century. Since then, the study of clinicoanatomical correlation has been continued and elaborated. The aim of this book is to summarize the current advances related to higher cerebral functions.

Is Function Localizable?

The first and foremost issue is the extent to which function is localizable in the brain. There is relatively little argument concerning localization of certain functions, although much of their cortical mechanisms remains under intense scrutiny. These commonly are associated with primary sensory and motor areas, including the cortical areas for special senses such as hearing and vision. Head (1926) emphasized the distinction between the localizable function of motion, sensation, and vision and "disorders of speech or similar higher grade functions . . . in that there is no such relation to parts of the body or their projection in space." The sophisticated correlation of the columnar organization of visual cortex with visual feature analysis by Hubel & Wiesel (1965) is a prime example of our recent level of neurophysiological knowledge of primary and secondary neocortex.

Localization of function in the secondary association areas connected with the primary areas is more complicated, and large areas of the brain, commonly called "tertiary association areas," remain the subject of intense controversy concerning function. The unique role of the left hemisphere in language is a well-established doctrine since Broca, but there is some recent evidence for oral and visual comprehension of concrete nouns and even some automatic speech output in the right hemisphere, which may not be as speechless as was formerly thought. This knowledge obtained from hemisphe-rectomies and corpus callosum sections has been reviewed exten-sively elsewhere and is not detailed in this book.

The left-hemisphere tertiary areas are of special interest to neu-rologists studying aphasias. The initial enthusiasm that greeted Broca's discovery was dampened somewhat by Jackson's (1878) warning that only lesions but not functions can be localized. Never-theless, the observation that lesions in the same location were as-sociated with the same deficit encouraged many to draw conclusions about how the brain functions. This principle receives further sup-port by modern investigators who combine lesion experiments with histochemical and physiological techniques.

The antilocalizationists have pointed out the numerous difficul-ties with the concept of centers of function, and the evidence for widespread cerebral activation in higher functions has been accu-mulating physiologically and anatomically. The alerting role of the reticular activating system, the ubiquitous thalamocortical projec-tions, and the multiplicity and redundancy of limbic and cortical connections serve notice that central nervous system activity is complex and much of our brain may be activated even for simpler acts of cognition. These physiological notions recently have been confirmed by the multiple areas that are shown to be activated on the cerebral blood flow technique in reasonably well-defined stages of the mental activity (see Chapter 5 by Lassen). Indirect measures of function such as electroencephalogram, and evoked, event-re-lated, averaged responses, or the distribution of neurotransmitters also underline the diffuse and complex nature of cerebral activity.

The definition of what constitutes a function is arbitrary at the best of times and clinicians, physiologists, and psychologists have different concepts about the same behavior. Often complex alter-native theories are offered regarding how a function should be in-terpreted (Caplan, 1981). Reduction of a complex behavior to its components is fraught with the hazard of losing the meaning and biological significance to the organism. On the other hand, more complex behaviors are likely to have widespread input and will be affected by lesions in many areas (see chapter on the constructional apraxia and spatial deficit). Some psychological concepts of function may not be appropriate to describe actual brain function or connectivity. On the other hand, anatomy and physiology alone do not provide even the questions, let alone the answers, about behavior.

The functional analysis of normal cognitive systems may not supply enough background to test the damaged or reorganized functions in patients. The behavior observed after the lesion may not be analyzable in terms of normal function. These discrepancies often prevent any direct conclusion about normal mechanisms based on pathological observations. This is not to deny the usefulness of theoretical constructs based on normative data. As long as caution is used in the interpretation of pathological behavior as a model of brain function, the gap can be bridged with some extrapolation.

The analysis of behavior after a lesion should be supplanted by studies in normals to confirm conclusions about the function of an organism. A detailed analysis of a function is necessary to the understanding of complex ways a lesion can affect it; even then, there is no guarantee that the lesion localizations will provide the correct interpretation.

Lesions versus Functions

A major theoretical issue in localization is whether the performance observed should be attributed to the damaged area that functions without some of its lost components or to other functionally related or even unrelated structures which take over from the damaged one. An example of this would be the difficulty in constructional tasks observed in right-hemisphere lesions. One cannot be certain whether this is related to a poor performance of the damaged right hemisphere, or to the "normal performance" of the left hemisphere alone, without the usual right-sided input for the task. At times after a lesion, not only are deficit or negative symptoms observed, but new behavior or positive symptoms also appear. Positive symptoms may represent elements of neural activity that had been controlled or suppressed by the structure destroyed by the lesion.

It is an often-voiced argument confronting localizationists that the new performance observed after a lesion has little to do with the function of the lesioned area, but it is, in fact, the function of a new combination of the remaining structures. This criticism of localization can be applied to other methods such as electrical stimulation of the brain, the local application of neurotransmitters or recording from single units, as they are connected to the whole system (Glassman, 1978). To a certain extent, this consideration is useful for the interpretation of any method, but it does not justify the elimination of any approach from the search for causality, an important principle in science.

Some functions such as word retrieval or the phonemic assembly (that may be the normal function impaired with phonemic paraphasias) may be distributed in a diffuse fashion through the language area as they seem to be affected by lesions from many locations. Similarly widespread distribution of certain cognitive functions, such as visuospatial ability, directed attention, memory, and judgment, defy efforts to localize them. Large neuronal networks are obviously necessary in much of the performance of complex cognitive tasks and even those who are interested in functional–anatomical correlations stay away from the concept of pinpoint or even gyral centers of function.

The network approach to functional localization was applied to the conceptualization of directed attention by Mesulam (1981). He summarized several general principles applicable to the clinicopathologic correlation of complex functions:

> (1) Components of a single complex function are represented within distinct but interconnected sites which collectively constitute an integrated network for that function; (2) individual cortical areas contain the neural substrate for components of several complex functions and may therefore belong to several partially overlapping networks; (3) lesions confined to a single cortical region are likely to result in multiple deficits; (4) severe and lasting impairments of an individual complex function usually require the simultaneous involvement of several components in the relevant network; and (5) the same complex function may be impaired as a consequence of a lesion in one of several cortical areas, each of which is a component of an integrated network for that function.

These principles are general enough to explain many of the findings in localization studies, and are particularly applicable to the stimulation studies summarized in Chapter 3.

Behaviorism, Dualism, and Anatomy

As a backlash against localization, a large number of psychologists followed Lashley's (1938) rallying cry of equipotentiality and considered the brain a black box which consisted of more or less equipotential components, none indispensable for higher cortical function. This provided the excuse to ignore anatomy and study behavior only. Behavioral psychology, although trying to follow a strict scientific method, often remains too narrow in its outlook and misses important avenues of knowledge and information by neglecting the role of anatomy or pathology in the observed behavior. At least behaviorists do not deny the connection between the brain and behavior but some express disinterest in brain structure.

An even worse form of denial is that of the mentalist or dualist who considers the mental process to be independent from brain activity. The makers of modern diagrams and the information process modelers tend, to some extent, to fall into the same trap. To them, the functional modeling assumes a much greater importance than the "hardware" of brain tissue and its connections. The importance of structure only lies in the connections of processes, not in the actual reality of carrying out these processes. The issue is then raised whether anatomy can contribute at all to the knowledge of mental processes. Although some deny this, anatomy can, in fact, even on a superficial inspection, provide important knowledge as to the limitation and possibilities of various thought processes. The extent of interconnection between localizable cerebral processes is important to our knowledge of predicting these processes and their possible theoretical connections. One cannot proceed without the other as one cannot be understood without the other. It is this correlation of brain and behavior that is the subject of this book.

Human Complexities

Animal experimenters have the advantage of controlling lesion size and location in addition to other factors. This is not available, of course, to human neuropsychologists and since this book deals with localization in humans only, the biological implications of human pathology need to be considered in their own right. The complexity of human behavior perhaps is matched only by the complexity of the human brain. Many investigators have tried to cope with the resulting difficulties by constraining themselves to hemispheric asymmetries for the last 25 years.

Studies of hemispheric function have been largely based on injury which is restricted to one side or the other. Many of these studies have suffered from the difficulty that, when a task is examined in right- and left-hemisphere damaged patients, other biological factors such as age, sex, location, size of injury, and etiology are difficult to match. The location and the size of the lesions are rarely, if ever, considered, and often right- and left-hemisphere patients are compared without controlling these parameters.

The vast literature on hemispheric asymmetries and cerebral dominance, reinforced by studies of hemispherectomies and callosal-sectioned patients, resulted in postulated differences of hemispheric styles in cognition such as the analytical versus the global processing by the left and right hemisphere. Chapter 20 (constructional and visuospatial function) touches on this issue of cognitive differences between the human hemispheres (so far not established in animals), indicating that the right side of the brain may well be more diffusely organized than the left. The thrust of the information in this book however goes beyond hemispheric asymmetries into lesion–behavior correlation.

The issue of generalizing from single case reports for or against localizing certain functions must be kept in mind in all circumstances. The human brain is complex, not only functionally but also in terms of individual variability in many biological factors. There are many cases in the literature when a single case or a few cases are documented to show that a lesion in a certain location does not produce the symptoms expected. Often the conclusion is then drawn that function is not related to that area. However, often important biological factors, such as the time elapsed from the injury, for example, are ignored or inadequately considered in the interpretation of the behavior observed. Since an experimental series of lesions is often not available to investigate the function of an area, single, well-documented case reports that are followed with several examinations and that have good lesion localization can be very informative.

Variability of Deficit following Similar Lesions

THE EFFECT OF RECOVERY

Deficits caused by a lesion are often recoverable. The early deficit that may be related to edema, cellular reaction, transient ischemia, and so forth is followed by a great deal of early spontaneous recovery. The chronic deficit is related not only to a loss of function, but to compensatory changes by the whole brain, or homologous areas, or neighboring areas during subsequent stages of recovery. The deficit with acute lesion cannot be considered in the same category as the recovered state, although the lesion persists. These two instances lead to conflicting conclusions about localization. There-fore, in every attempt to correlate deficit with lesions, the time from onset is crucial. Failure to consider this variable is a major source of confusion in this field.

The extent of substitution and reorganization in the central nerv-ous system appears considerable, far beyond what can be attributed to anatomical regeneration. To some extent, this complicates the ef-forts to localize function in any one part of the nervous system. Any logical scheme of conditions such as the one, for example, by Klein (1978), postulating that a loss of a functional component results in a certain pathological behavior, falls down if the extent of recovery is not accounted for in the structural correlation.

THE EFFECT OF ETIOLOGY

The sudden removal of large areas of functioning brain in stroke or experimental lesions may produce distance effect in functionally connected neural structures. This is also known as "diaschisis" after von Monakow (1914). Slowly growing tumors, on the other hand, often displace tissues with relatively little functional deficit. Rap-idly expanding tumors produce distant effects by edema, hemor-rhage, and vascular occlusion. Therefore, in many instances, lesions of the same size or location will not produce the same deficit unless the study is strictly controlled for etiology. Unfortunately, this is still not done in many areas of research in neuropsychology.

Occasionally, different etiologies produce the same deficit but with different localization. An example of this is the appearance of transcortical sensory aphasia and even Wernicke's aphasia in cases of Alzheimer's disease with diffuse neuronal degeneration (at least not localizable with our present methods to the same extent as a focal infarct). The same clinical syndrome can appear then in the course of deterioration of one kind of disease process (Alzheimer's disease) and in the course of recovery of another (cerebral infarc-tion).

AGE, SEX, AND HANDEDNESS

There are other biological factors, some more recently empha-sized, that interfere with the expectation of similar lesions produc-ing similar deficits. A major difference is the age of the organism.

When a child sustains brain damage, the plasticity of the brain allows for compensation by the homologous hemisphere or other structures. Hemispherectomy in a young child (Basser, 1962) or damage to the prepubertal brain results in almost complete recovery, indicating the possibility of hormonal influence on plasticity. Certain aphasic syndromes such as fluent Wernicke's aphasia appear to be more frequent with older age. Whether this is related to anatomical differences in the vasculature affected or to continuing functional lateralization remains controversial.

Sex differences in cerebral organizations are considered to be significant by some studies. It is assumed that language may be more bilaterally distributed in women; therefore, lesions may have different effects in different sexes. Recent epidemiological studies of aphasia tend not to support this contention (Kertesz & Sheppard, 1981). This is not to deny that there may be important psychological sex differences, but there has been no convincing evidence from lesion studies that the resulting deficit is influenced by sex.

Handedness is considered an important factor in cerebral dominance for certain functions. Everyone agrees that left-handers have somewhat different cerebral organization, not just mirroring right-handers but also important qualitative differences which may result in certain lesions producing different deficits in left- than in right-handers (Kertesz, 1979). Gloning, Gloning, Haube and Quatember (1969) suspected that lefthanders are likely to become aphasic regardless of which hemisphere is damaged, but we found fewer left-handers among our aphasics than expected from the general population even in the acute stage. In the chronic stage, one would expect to see fewer left-handed aphasics because of the suggested better recovery from the deficit (Gloning, Gloning, Haube & Quatember, 1969).

ANATOMICAL VARIATIONS

Anatomical differences between individuals are often observable but are difficult to quantitate. Some follow a pattern such as the 65:15 ratio of larger planum temporale on the left versus on the right (Geschwind & Levitsky, 1968). Perhaps this accounts for the variable extent superior temporal lobe lesions affect behavior. Chapter 3 of this book deals with a similar asymmetry in the occipital volume as seen on the CT scans that may account for the variation in hemispheric dominance for language.

Hemispheric anatomical asymmetries are just a beginning in our exploration of the anatomical variables in localization. The complex gyral pattern of the human brain shows a great deal of individual variation. The importance of this variation becomes evident when a neurosurgeon is called upon to describe the area he starts to stimulate or excise. There are two chapters in this volume concerned with cortical anatomy specifically: Chapter 2 provides some insight into the cytoarchitectonic divisions of normal gyral patterns and the possible delineation of speech and other association areas. Chapter 6 deals with the method of stimulating the surface of the exposed brain in an attempt to achieve functional localization during removal of brain tissue for epilepsy or brain tumor. In studies such as this, the anatomical variation of gyri and sulci becomes a crucial factor.

In a complex nervous system, alternative ways of explaining a phenomenon should be considered carefully. Even an anatomical issue—for instance, whether a target organ is actually damaged or only passing fibers are disconnected by a lesion—may be a source of alternative solution in localization. On the behavioral side of the same issue is the consideration of a disturbed function as an effect of the whole system or only of a component of it with the same result, provided that the impaired component is crucial enough in the performance of a function. The difference, however, could mean that the same phenomenon is observed from lesions at different locations. The possibility of the organism using alternate structures for a function or the "redundancy" of organization would also account for variously located lesions producing the same deficit. That the same function is represented at various levels of the nervous system is the well-known principle of "hierarchial" representation. It probably accounts for some of the recovery or reorganization seen after lesions of the central nervous system (CNS) rather than the "taking over" by completely unrelated structures or "vicarious functioning."

The Measurement of Behavior

STANDARDIZATION FOR COMPARISON

The measurement of deficit is an essential prerequisite for meaningful localization. This has been a weak point in many localization reports. Even the localization of motor functions in the pre-Rolandic cortex has been the subject of a great deal of argument, especially concerning the extent to which a part of a movement or the actual whole can be localized. Stimulation and ablation studies indicated that fairly complex functional units seem to be affected together (Zulch, Creutzfeldt, & Galbraith, 1975). Much of the clinicopathologic literature is handicapped by a rudimentary description of the psychologic and language deficits. Although Henschen (1920–1922) collected a monumental number of autopsied cases in the early decades of this century, they suffer from an uneven degree of description and lack of standardized examination. It is very difficult to know what each author means by "word deafness" and criteria used to establish a certain diagnosis. In fact, a careful study of the descriptions reveals that the terminology covers contradictory clinical pictures. A few attempts at quantitation are unstandardized and impossible to reproduce. Many have attempted to test aphasia in a comprehensive fashion, but language testing tended to remain unstandardized. Some investigations tested aphasics in great detail, exploring language modalities in addition to the available intelligence tests. However, the procedures were lengthy and rarely applied in a consistent fashion. Standardized, practical, and consistently used aphasia tests have not been utilized in localization until recently. Without a standardized measure of any deficit, it is impossible to establish a reliable taxonomy and without such taxonomy, localization can be misleading. The lack of standardized examination prevents the comparison of cases. Even more current terminologies are controversial and are dependent on the tests used. However, as long as these differences are recognized and the measures comprehensive enough to cover the behavior in question, a comparison can be made between various studies.

Symptoms or Syndromes

The syndrome approach versus the analytical examination of isolated behavior has been advocated at one time or other in functional localization. Clinicians generally attempt to deal with syndromes as they are presented to them by the patient and draw conclusions from the lesions causing these deficits. Chapters 7–12 are examples of this approach, although the symptom analysis often goes far beyond the syndromes themselves. Pure psychological phenomena are difficult to find or test and even more difficult to localize. Chapters 13–16 examine more isolated phenomena, although it is often impossible to draw the line between a pure function and a syndrome of related functions. The reverse paradigm in localization is to start with lesions in a common location and determine the deficit related to them. Chapters 18–20 make use of this method, analyzing certain functions in a selective fashion when specific areas of the brain are affected.

The syndrome versus function controversy is best exemplified by a series of articles on the Gerstmann syndrome (Benton, 1977). The combination of agraphia, acalculia, finger agnosia, and right–left confusion has caught on among clinicians as a useful syndrome (see Chapter 12). The rationale and justification as well as its appropriateness have been questioned and the discussion which resulted can be applied to other syndromes in localization studies. Intuitive clinical taxonomy can and should be re-examined with modern statistical methods. The clinical taxonomy of aphasias also has been attacked for being arbitrary and based on a prejudicial conceptual framework, but numerical taxonomy or cluster analysis has shown that grouping of patients based on performance scores is not only clinically but statistically valid (Kertesz, 1979). Different taxonomies have been used for clinical localization than for behavioral analysis, but to increase our knowledge about the brain and its function, integration of the two levels is most desirable.

TAXONOMY AND LOCALIZATION

The taxonomy issue is a crucial one in many aspects of localization. Many discrepancies are simply related to the same terminology applied to different behaviors such as the different definitions of transcortical motor aphasia in two subsequent chapters. Sometimes, the opposite occurs and the similar behaviors are grouped differently—therefore, the conclusions are contradictory. An example of this is the use of the term "jargon" for the stereotypies of global aphasia instead of restricting it to fluent Wernicke's aphasia. These disagreements may come about because the phenomenon is poorly defined and only described qualitatively. Researchers have been reluctant to use standardized examinations, fearing the restrictions and rigidity that such efforts may incur. Even when standardized tests are used, classifications differ because the criteria for each group are different.

Some investigators prefer to use exclusive limits that allow one to classify everyone in a population of aphasics (Kertesz, 1979). Some prefer to draw typical syndrome profiles (Goodglass & Kaplan, 1972), and consider those who do not fall within these limits as "mixed" aphasics. The former method may result in a number of similar individuals being placed in different groups; this may blur some distinctions in localization. The latter system results in a high proportion of unclassifiable patients who are often deleted from population studies, thereby jeopardizing the validity of localization by using selected individuals only. Despite some of these differences, as long as the behavior criteria are clearly defined on the basis of standardized measurement, various groups can be compared with reasonable efficiency, and correlation with lesion sites can be successful and convincingly consistent for many syndromes of higher cerebral function.

Objectivity, Accuracy, and Approaches in Localization

AUTOPSY CORRELATIONS

The issue of the objectivity of localization is closely tied in with technical aspects of localization. Until recently, much of our knowledge came from autopsies, surgical resection, and stimulation and post-traumatic skull defects. Although postmortem examination can provide very fine anatomical detail that continues to be the gold standard of localization, recent developments in imaging *in vivo* (especially CT) allow us unparalleled opportunity to reopen many of the issues in topography.

Autopsy correlations have been important to neurologists for more than a century. The development of anatomical techniques such as myelin- and cellular staining and improved methods of fixation and photography allow certain accuracy in the description of the involved structures as well as the description of interconnecting pathways.

Clinicopathologic correlation, although providing the most detailed anatomical information, is burdened by several inherent difficulties. One of the problems is the considerable interval between testing and the death of the patient during which time other stroke lesions, or extension of the original lesion, or just an aging process takes place. Tumors grow and, by the time they are autopsied, they occupy a larger area than that responsible for causing the deficit at the time of testing. They also exert distant effects by compression, edema, and endocrine and vascular changes.

Strokes are more stable but, frequently, there is a repeated vascular accident, and it is difficult to interpret the interaction of multiple lesions and the oft-associated atrophy in that age group. Recovery and the functional result from two lesions is different from a single one as it was observed by Ades and Raab (1946), who found smaller deficit from serial lesions than an equivalent single one in animals. The serial lesion, in fact, may be one of the mechanisms by which slowly growing tumors may produce smaller deficits than strokes, besides the obvious effect of displacement instead of destruction.

Another drawback to autopsy studies is the unavailability of autopsy, when some well-studied cases may be lost to follow-up, or conversely, when autopsied cases do not have the appropriate clinical or behavioral studies in life. Improvement in this situation may be expected with systematic surveys of stroke populations and the advancing technology in the anatomical examination of the brain such as improved methods of cytoarchitectonics and pathology.

The difficulties of localization by tracing the skull defects in traumatic injuries are well known even though some of the basic studies in localizations were done in post-traumatic populations, examining head-injured soldiers after both world wars. Penetrating injury often creates deep, distant destruction, not evident from the skull defect. Minor head injuries, on the other hand, recover quite fast, and this produced some negative conclusions.

THE TOPOGRAPHY OF ARTERIAL OCCLUSIONS

The localization and size of lesions in strokes is determined by the arterial distribution and the frequency with which these arteries are affected. The incidence of certain lesion location in some behavior deficit will be influenced by the frequency of infarcts in that area. There could be more than one reason why a behavior is found more frequently with lesions in one location than in another. This may be related to the higher frequency of lesion in that area in addition to the relationship between the topography and behavior. Even tumors do not occur randomly and show predilection to one region or another, apart from the great handicap of their distance effects, poorly defined borders, and rapid growth. Certain "crucial" or controversial locations such as the angular gyrus or Broca's area are rarely affected in isolation by strokes or tumors; therefore, the arguments about their uniqueness or specificity go on interminably.

Many composite maps of lesions based on one behavior deficit closely resemble other maps in association with another behavior. This could be interpreted that the two behaviors are functionally or anatomically related, or both. However, another and equally plausible explanation—even though not necessarily compatible with the previous ones—is available. The maps are close to each other in size and location because that is where the lesions occur, due to pathophysiological constraints, and the coincidence is not caused by a functional relationship. Nevertheless, there is enough variability in the distribution of arterial occlusions that, given a large enough number of cases, valid conclusions can be drawn about differences in location and size. Statistical comparisons of lesion size and location remain difficult and the high incidence of large, central-middle cerebral arterial infarcts dominate most series of stroke localizations, confounding anatomical landmarks, lobar boundaries, and simple concepts of connectionisms. It is possible that, in the future, well-defined stroke lesions—eventually matched in size and incidence of location—can be compared in respect to certain individual and associated deficits (or syndromes).

FROM LESIONS TO BEHAVIOR OR FROM BEHAVIOR TO LESIONS

In certain studies, the area that is common to a series of patients exhibiting a certain change of behavior is taken to indicate a relationship. This "overlap" technique has been used successfully in skull defect localization (Schiller, 1947), isotope localization (Kertesz, Lesk, & McCabe, 1977), and CT localization (several chapters in this book). How the overlap is chosen is arbitrary to some extent, although a priori criteria such as taking 75–80% of the overlapping lesions could provide increased objectivity in the selection of critical areas. Paradoxically, the more lesions are included, the smaller the 100% overlap becomes; sooner or later, the odd lesion will fall outside the previous overlap entirely. Too few lesions result in mis-leadingly large areas considered to be significant.

The lesions can be correlated with behavior in several ways. One can define the behavioral syndrome or symptom and then overlap the lesions to see which is the common area that correlates best with the behavior. This has the disadvantages already discussed. The second method overlaps the lesions that involve certain anatomical areas, and then determines the behavioral deficit occurring with these areas. An example of this technique is in Chapter 19 of this volume on right hemisphere localization of lesions with construc-tional apraxia and visuospatial deficits. A third method uses a checklist of predetermined anatomical structures and calculates the extent of involvement for each syndrome or symptom or for indi-vidual patients. This is similar to the second method in that the ba-sis for grouping the individual subjects is the lesion and not the functional deficit. It has the effect of blurring the distinctions be-tween the behaviors, but it is most suitable when syndrome com-plexes are not available or when the investigator wants to avoid them. The combined use of several of these methods may result in more informative correlations than just one or the other.

ADVANCES IN IMAGING

Significant advances in technology allow us to examine the extent, nature, and location of lesions *in vivo*, and often achieve the indirect localization of the lesion at the time of the examination. These in-novations are the isotope brain scan (BS), computerized tomography (CT), positron emission tomography (PET), and nuclear magnetic resonance (NMR). Each one of these produces images and measures some parameters of the lesion. Isotope uptake occurs in the brain whenever a lesion is vascular or the so-called blood brain barrier is breached as in tumors and in the acute stages of stroke. CT scans show decreased densities in infarcts rather early, becoming well-defined and sharper-edged with time, allowing us to localize lesions occurring in the past or present. The increased densities distin-guished hemorrhages from tumors. At our present state of knowl-edge, it is the best available imaging for lesion localization *in vivo*. Many of the chapters in the book utilize CT information.

NMR is the latest of the imaging techniques with an intriguing promise of visualizing functional changes in the brain. The recent images available indicate gray matter–white matter discrimination exceeding that of CT. The method shows promise in the investigation of cancer and demyelinating lesions beyond anything seen previously. It has the advantage over other methods in that it avoids the use of ionizing radiation, making prolonged and repeated examinations possible without any known biohazard. Whole-volume data or sagittal, coronal, and horizontal slices can be collected simultaneously. Bone interference is eliminated. The possibility of defining the biochemistry in association with anatomy is the most attractive feature. Many researchers feel that the method has more potential than any other in existence.

Figures 1 and 2 show the author's cranial contents in the sagittal and oblique horizontal views on a prototype Technicare NMR imager. The three-dimensional data set was acquired in 20 minutes, using a saturated recovery procedure and back projection to a 256 × 256 matrix in 1.5 mm slices.

PET scanning studies *in vivo* metabolism, indirectly provides images of lesions or the effects of lesion, but it requires expensive technology not yet widely available. Chapter 4 gives the reader insight into the technique as well as new information concerning functional localization in dementia and aphasia.

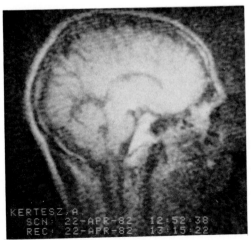

Figure 1. NMR lateral image 1 cm to the left of the midline outlining the ventricles, the cerebellum, and the pituitary. The scalp is light and the underlying bone is dark.

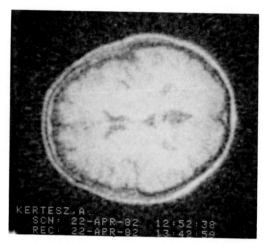

Figure 2. NMR horizontal oblique image indicating ventricles in a cut similar to CT.

Requirements for Functional Correlation

Some of the principles of the acceptability of lesion evidence in localization of function may be summarized. The function of an area may be related to the lesion if:

1. The same functional deficit always follows the lesion.
2. The same deficit is not produced by other, independent lesions.
3. The deficit is measured according to standardized and meaningful methods.
4. The lesion location is determined objectively and accurately.
5. Biological variables such as time from onset, age, etiology, and so forth are controlled.

These idealized situations—practically never satisfied—should be the goals. The difficulties in fulfilling the conditions for the functional correlation of lesions are numerous and some of them were discussed here in detail. Even if the function of an area cannot be determined from lesion evidence, the clinicopathologic correlation with modern techniques can further the sophistication of functional analysis and vice versa. An integration from psychology to lesion localization may seem far away, but many strides have been undertaken. This book has recorded some of them.

References

Ades, H. W., & Raab, D. H. (1946). Recovery of motor function after two-stage extirpation of area 4 in monkeys. *Journal of Neurophysiology, 9,* 55–60.

Basser, L. S. (1962). Hemiplegia of early onset and the faculty of speech with special reference to the effects of hemispherectomy. *Brain, 85,* 427–460.

Benton, A. L. (1977). Reflections on the Gertsmann Syndrome. *Brain and Language, 4,* 45–62.

Broca, P. (1861). Remarques sur le siège de la faculté du langage articulé, suivies d'une observation d'aphémie (perte de la parole). *Bulletin et Memoires de la Societe Anatomique de Paris, 36,* 330–357.

Caplan, D. (1981). On the cerebral localization of linguistic functions. *Brain and Language, 14,* 120–137.

Fritsch, G. T., & Hitzig, E. (1870). Uber die elektrische Erregbarkeit des Grosshirns. *Archiv fuer Anatomie und Physiologie, Leipzig,* 300–332.

Geschwind, N. (1965). Disconnexion syndromes in animals and man. *Brain, 88,* 237–294, 584–644.

Geschwind, N., & Levitsky, W. (1968). Human brain: Left-right asymmetries in temporal speech regions. *Science, 161,* 186–187.

Glassman, R. B. (1978). The logic of the lesion experiment and its role in the neural sciences. In S. Finger (Ed.), *Recovery from brain damage.* New York: Plenum.

Gloning, I., Gloning, K., Haub, G., & Quatember, R. (1969). Comparison of verbal behaviour in right-handed and non-right-handed patients with anatomically verified lesions of one hemisphere. *Cortex, 5,* 43–52.

Goodglass, H., & Kaplan, E. (1972). *Assessment of Aphasia and Related Disorders.* Philadelphia: Lea & Febiger.

Head, H. (1926). *Aphasia and kindred disorders of speech.* London/New York: Cambridge University Press.

Henschen, S. E. (1920–1922). *Klinische und anatomische Beiträge zur Pathologie des Gehirns* (Vols. 5–7). Stockholm: Nordiska Bokhandel.

Hubel, D., & Wiesel, T. (1965). Receptive fields and functional architecture in two nonstriate visual areas (18 and 19) of the cat. *Journal of Neurophysiology, 28,* 229–289.

Jackson, H. J. (1878). On affections of speech from disease of the brain. *Brain, 1,* 304–330.

Kertesz, A., Lesk, D., & McCabe, P. (1977). Isotope localization of infarcts in aphasia *Archives of Neurology,* 34:590–601.

Kertesz, A. (1979). *Aphasia and associated disorders.* New York: Grune & Stratton.

Kertesz, A., & Sheppard, A. (1981). The epidemiology of aphasic and cognitive impairment in stroke—age, sex, aphasia type and laterality differences. *Brain, 104,* 117–128.

Klein, V. B. (1978). Inferring functional localization from neurological evidence. In E. Walker (Ed.), *Explorations in the biology of language.* Montgomery Bradford.

Lashley, K. S. (1938). Factors limiting recovery after central nervous lesions. *Journal of Nervous and Mental Disease, 88,* 733–755.

Mesulam, M. M. (1981). A cortical network for directed attention and unilateral neglect. *Annals of Neurology, 10* (4), 309–325.

Munk, H. (1881). *Ueber die Funktionen der Grosshirnrinde. Gesammelte Mitteilungen aus den Jahren 1877–1880.* Berlin: Hirschwald.

Schiller, F. (1947). Aphasia studied in patients with missile wounds. *Journal of Neurology, Neurosurgery and Psychiatry, 10,* 183.

von Monakow, C. (1914). *Die Lokalisation in Grosshirn und der Abbau der Funktionen durch cortikale, Herde.* Wiesbaden: Bergmann.

Zulch, K. J., Creutzfeldt, O., & Galbraith, G. C. (1975). *Cerebral localization.* New York: Springer-Verlag.

2

Neuroanatomical Aspects of Cerebral Localization*

*Albert M. Galaburda
and Marek–Marsel Mesulam*

Introduction

Localization in neurology implies that discrete brain regions subserve discrete brain functions and that circumscribed brain lesions
result in delimited brain dysfunction. One way to study localization
is through the employment of neuroanatomical means aimed at correlating results of behavioral and physiological testing and features
of neuroanatomy. Another way would be to correlate neuroanatomical features of lesions and deficits documented during life. Modern

*Some of the work reported here was supported by NIH grant NS14018, a biomedical
support grant to the Beth Israel Hospital, Boston, Massachusetts, and a grant from
the Orton Dyslexia Society, Baltimore, Maryland.

21

day contributions to localization might be achieved through better descriptions of functional deficits paired with more precise outlines of the lesion's anatomy. The anatomical approach to lesion analysis falls into three categories: (1) the topographical localization and extent of lesions with reference to features of cortical folding, lobes, lobules, gyri, fissures, and sulci; (2) the correlation of lesions with features of architectonic regional differentiation of the cortex and subcortical gray masses; and (3) the correlation of lesions with features of regional differentiation of fiber pathways. This chapter deals with these three aspects of neuroanatomical localization.

Although ideas about cerebral localization date back to antiquity, their scientific exploration had its beginnings in the nineteenth century. The introduction of hardening techniques provided the first possibility for the success of blunt dissections of human brains. These dissections were able to show that some fiber pathways appeared to be discretely organized, having a specific origin and a specific termination, and that the same bundles could be found in all brains (Arnold, 1838; Burdach, 1819–1826; Foville, 1844; Gall & Spurtzheim, 1810; Reil, 1809). Later, it was possible to refine knowledge concerning fiber connections with the aid of special stains and experimental techniques. Thus, connections could be traced in whole-brain serial sections stained for myelinated axons (Dejerine & Dejerine–Klumpke, 1895; Luys, 1865; Weigert, 1906). However, the ability to determine the exact origin and termination of these fascicles was still severely limited. Following descriptions of retrograde cellular atrophy after axonal damage (Gudden, 1870; Nissl, 1894) and a demonstration of anterograde axonal degeneration of Waller (1850) and Türck (1851) the examination of human brains with circumscribed lesions enabled the productive study of neuronal connectivity.

Although the suspicion that discrete fiber bundles arose and terminated in equally discrete cortical areas dates back to the time of the discovery of these bundles in the early nineteenth century (Remak, 1838), the actual demonstration of areas of distinctive cellular differentiation in cortex and subcortical nuclear structures had to wait until the development of adequate cell stains and improved microscopes. Early descriptions of regional cellular differentiation were made by Bevan–Lewis (1879), Betz (1881), and Meynert (1884), but the first serious attempts to map out architectonically distinct areas on the cortex came around the time of the introduction of formalin fixation (Blum, 1893), improved celloidin embedding (Weigert, 1895), and Nissl staining (Nissl, 1894). The early maps of

Hammarberg (1895) and Campbell (1905) were extended and increasingly detailed by Brodmann (1909), Economo and Koskinas (1925), later by students of the famed Vogt School of Brain Research in Berlin, and subsequently, in Neustadt (see, for example, Sanides, 1962). The study of human cerebral architectonics and connectivity gradually diminished after World War I to be replaced by studies of descriptive and experimental neuroanatomy in animals. However, recent advances have occurred in architectonics as well as in tracing fiber pathways. These advances are of potential relevance to functional localization.

Methods

TOPOGRAPHICAL ANALYSIS OF THE GROSS BRAIN

REMOVAL AND PHOTOGRAPHY

Topographical localization in the gross specimen depends on a well-preserved, undistorted brain. Therefore, great care must be taken at the time of brain removal at postmortem examination that the specimen is not lacerated or abraded by the bone saw passing deep to the inner table of the cranium, since the cortex will be immediately vulnerable at that point. In this regard, it should be noted that the commonly employed planes of sawing (see, for example, Escourolle and Poirier, 1973) overlie the fronto-opercular region anteriorly and the temporoparietal region posteriorly—both areas relevant to studies of language localization that can be rendered useless to architectonic and connectional analysis by the overzealous use of the saw. After removal of the bony calvarium, as much dura as possible should be left attached to the underlying brain for separation later in the procedure, since, after fixation, it is possible to remove the dura with less chance of avulsion of underlying cortex. Avulsion with dural removal is common in areas of disease where the dura often is adherent to the underlying brain, and in the parasagittal regions where the dura is normally attached to the brain by bridging vessels. The parasagittal regions are of special significance for language localization studies since they contain the supplementary motor regions, and special efforts should be made to leave them intact. Another source of distortion and trauma during removal is found upon attempting to free infratentorial structures.

Incision of the tentorium for this purpose may be accompanied by laceration of neighboring temporal and occipital lobes. Finally, the brain should be cut away from the spinal cord as low in the cervical canal as possible, in order to have the pyramidal decussations available for examination.

The fresh specimen should be weighed in an oval pan conforming to its shape, and its weight recorded. Yakovlev (1970) recommends that the brain then be put in an oval dish and perfused through the carotid and vertebral arteries, first with normal saline and then with formalin solution hung at a height of about 2 m until the exiting fluid is clear. This is to ensure optimal Nissl staining. After weighing and clearing the blood by perfusion, the brain is identified by a tag tied to the basilar artery. The brain is then suspended in formalin by a durable string, usually passed through the walls of both carotid arteries and then secured at both ends to a string that is tied around the container near its edges. The container should be sufficiently large to permit free flotation of the specimen (about eight liters) and firm enough to resist distortion. Ten percent buffered formalin is used for a fixative; the formalin is changed after 24 hours, then once a week for 4 weeks, and once a month for additional months. The brain is kept in fixative for 3 months before further processing. Yakovlev recommends that the fluid be changed by siphoning it out to minimize the handling of the brain.

After fixation, the brain is washed with tap water for several days to permit detailed gross anatomical analysis without the irritating effects of formalin. The brain is then photographed. The number and type of photographs depends on whether the brain is to be processed in whole-brain serial sections or blocks are to be taken of areas of interest. It is clear that the preparation of the brain in whole-brain serial sections is the best method able to guarantee the largest amount of pertinent information. However, under certain conditions, it is reasonable to process relevant blocks and avoid the expense and time required for the whole brain. When the decision is made to process the whole brain, six views of the brain are photographed: frontal view, occipital view, dorsal view, undersurface, and right and left convexities. Best results are obtained when the specimen is submerged in water at photography. Photography should be repeated after the careful stripping of the meninges; this is required because, with the meninges in place, it is often difficult to distinguish fissures from blood vessels on the photographs and therefore to correlate lesions to fissural patterns.

In the event that blocks are taken for sectioning instead of whole-brain sections, it is suggested that the hemispheres be divided in the midsagittal plane by a longitudinal section through the middle of the corpus callosum. For this purpose, the best method is to spread the interhemispheric fissure with thumb and forefinger, to pass a long, straight-bladed knife down the midline so that it touches the dorsum of the corpus callosum, and to invert the brain to allow its own weight to divide the hemispheres. If this is done, the medial surfaces of the hemispheres should be photographed as well with and without meninges. After blocks are chosen and taken, their orientation should be noted and the blocks photographed. During the preparation of blocks, and whenever possible, photographs should be taken of the superior temporal plane and its planum temporale (the portion lying posterior to Heschl's gyrus) before the removal of blocks (Figure 1). The superior temporal plane is prepared for photography after separation of the temporal lobe from the remainder of the brain. For this purpose, after the hemispheres have been divided, the Sylvian fissures are gently spread apart with the thumb and forefinger, thus allowing visualization of the insula. A knife's edge is then passed from the anterior border of the insula through the thickness of the hemisphere in the direction of the plane of the Sylvian fissure, taking care not to graze the banks of the fissure. This procedure will provide a wider separation of the Sylvian fissure; it will be possible to identify clearly the posterior edge of the fissure. The knife is then placed carefully against this edge (the posterior angle at which the temporal and parietal opercula join) and the blade is drawn backward through the substance of the brain toward the occipital pole until the temporal lobe is separated from its roof. The superior temporal plane is now available for photography.

At this time, it is also useful to take pictures of the roof of the Sylvian fissure to provide a view of the frontal and parietal opercula (Figure 1). In our laboratory, we mark the undersurface of the central region (frontoparietal operculum, subcentral region) with black india ink to facilitate the later identification of the frontal from the parietal portions of the operculated hemisphere on the photograph (Figure 1). At this point, it is pertinent to add that it is not necessary to separate the temporal lobe to evaluate the superior temporal plane and planum temporale. Any portion of the brain can be easily reconstructed from a serially sectioned whole brain. This is accomplished by projecting a section onto graph paper and mapping the structure in question at a spacing determined from knowledge of distance between sections and magnification factor of the pro-

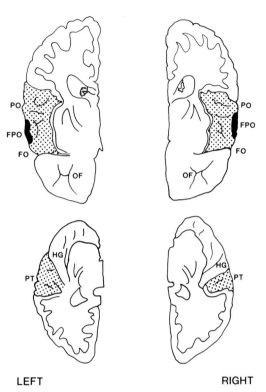

LEFT   RIGHT

Figure 1. Diagram to show the opercular portions of the frontal and parietal lobes (above) and the temporal lobes (below). The oribitofrontal surface of the frontal lobe (OF) is seen, as well as the frontal operculum (FO), the parietal operculum (PO) and the blackened area which corresponds to the frontoparietal operculum (FPO)—the region directly below the precentral and postcentral gyri. The temporal plane with Heschl's gyrus (HG) and the planum temporale (PT). Note the size correspondence between PO and PT on either side. (From Yakovlev, 1970.)

jection apparatus (Galaburda, Sanides, & Geschwind, 1978). For instance one might want to reconstruct the intraparietal sulcus. The rostralmost section containing the sulcus is projected onto graph paper. The sulcus on the section may measure, let us say, 1 cm in depth and the projected image 10 cm; that would reflect a 10× linear magnification factor. The brain's midline is marked and the edges of the sulcus are marked on the paper at the appropriate distance from the midline. A more caudal section is then selected. If the following section is 700 μm away from the first one, the sulcal edges should be marked 7 mm away on the graph paper, thus ensuring a proportional reconstruction. The marks denoting the sulcal edges are then joined and the resulting figure represents the outline of the intraparietal sulcus magnified linearly by a factor of 10.

Whenever possible, it is useful to relate lesion findings on CT scans to gross anatomical observations of the fixed brain and to mark these on the photographic templates. In other words, if a given portion of cortex is visibly affected in the CT scan, its shape and extension should be noted on the photograph of the fixed specimen. This procedure may prove difficult when sulci are not seen clearly on the CT scan or when the accurate identification of visible sulci is not possible. In a very young patient, or in a brain with significant edema and distortion, even major fissures such as the Sylvian fissure and the central sulcus are often difficult to identify on the CT scan. Under these circumstances, a CT scan can be taken of the fixed specimen with radio-opaque markers placed in a clearly identified fissure and gyri, thus allowing for a direct comparison with a living scan and more accurate gross topographical localization of a lesion.

TOPOGRAPHICAL LANDMARKS AND GROSS RIGHT–LEFT
ASYMMETRIES

A diagram of the external configuration of the lateral surface of the brain is shown in Figure 2. Although the illustration shows many standard landmarks, there is enormous variability in external topography in the normal state. The best guide to the accurate description of a gross brain is experience. The repetitive systematic survey of lobes, fissures, gyri, sulci, and fissurets provides a sense of the normal spectrum of gross configuration, and comparison with this mental standard may disclose the presence of aberration from the normal gross anatomy. Thus, for instance, one can detect abnormalities in the contour of the hemispheres because of focal swelling or cortical depression. There may be abnormalities in the shape and size of a given lobe. For instance, the occipital lobes are foreshortened and the temporal lobes are malformed in Down's syndrome (Davidoff, 1928), and early lesions may produce regional absence or curtailment of brain tissue. The ability to notice abnormalities in minor sulci is more difficult to acquire, but it is possible—with experience—to realize that, for example, the brains of

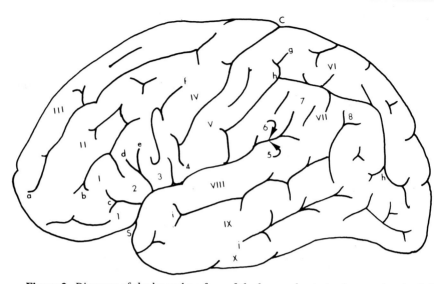

Figure 2. Diagram of the lateral surface of the human brain to show gyri and sulci relevant to current aspects of localization: (I) Inferior frontal gyrus; (II) Middle frontal gyrus; (III) Superior frontal gyrus; (IV) Precentral gyrus; (V) Postcentral gyrus; (VI) Superior parietal lobule; (VII) Inferior parietal lobule; (VIII) Superior temporal gyrus; (IX) Middle temporal gyrus; (X) Inferior temporal gyrus; (1) Pars orbitalis (frontal operculum); (2) Pars triangularis (frontal operculum); (3) Pars opercularis (frontal operculum); (4) Frontoparietal operculum (subcentral region); (5) Planum temporale; (6) Parietal operculum; (7) Supramarginal gyrus; (8) Angular gyrus; (a) Superior frontal sulcus; (b) Inferior frontal sulcus; (c) Horizontal limb of the Sylvian fissure; (d) Ascending limb of the Sylvian fissure; (e) Diagonal sulcus; (f) Precentral sulcus; (g) Postcentral sulcus; (h) Intraparietal sulcus; (i) Superior temporal sulcus; (j) Inferior temporal sulcus; (C) central sulcus; (S) Sylvian fissure.

some patients with mental retardation may exhibit only a diminution in the number of minor sulci as compared to normal brains (Yakovlev, 1959), whereas others may show a focal exaggeration in the number of small gyri (polymicrogyria) (Galaburda & Kemper, 1979).

Ever since the early days of comparative neuroanatomy, it has been noted that the brain in man is not only more convoluted than that of other primates, but also more asymmetrical. There is a variety of normal gross anatomical left–right differences which can be noted on the fixed brain. For instance, the right frontal lobe tends to be broader than the left and occasionally protrudes ahead of its contralateral homologue, therefore appearing longer. This finding has been demonstrated in computed brain tomograms (LeMay & Kido, 1978) and often the plain skull X-ray shows a bony indentation known as petalia on the side of the longer lobe. The parietal lobes are also often asymmetric in configuration. On the right side, there is commonly a bulge in the central region when the brain is viewed from above. On the other hand, the brain tends to broaden more posteriorly in the left parieto-occipital region, and the occipital lobe on that side often is broader and longer, producing left occipital petalia. This left occipital petalia may also be demonstrated on CT scans (LeMay & Kido, 1978) and in plain skull radiographs. Asymmetries in the size of the frontal and the occipital lobes should be compared, when possible, to asymmetries in the ventricular system. Ventricular asymmetries can often be demonstrated by CT scan and by pneumoencephalography (Knudson, 1958; McRae, Branch, & Milner, 1968). The left occipital horn is often longer than the right and the asymmetry has been correlated with handedness (McRae *et al.*, 1968). Obviously, left–right ventricular asymmetries can also be the result of lesions causing loss of substance. An old left posterior lesion, for instance, may be accompanied by a dilated occipital horn. However, in that case, the left occipital lobe would be atrophied and therefore smaller than the right. In an early brain lesion, the specific pattern of ventricular asymmetries can be the only clue to the diagnosis of early damage. On the other hand, some cases can be more difficult to assess. For instance, a mild enlargement of the right frontal horn with a slight reduction in the size of the frontal lobe on that side can be easily missed since the commonly occurring right frontal preponderance may simply be lessened. The discovery of CT asymmetries in life and findings of gross anatomical right–left differences in the actual brain may be useful in suggesting further studies of asymmetry (architectonic) as well as in explaining the effects of lateralized lesions on cognitive functions.

Note should be made of the brain's external fissuration pattern. This is particularly relevant to the study of left–right asymmetries. Lateral differences in the length and orientation of the Sylvian fissures have been described in normal adult and fetal brains (Chi, Dooling, & Gilles, 1977; LeMay & Culebras, 1972). The left fissure is usually longer and more horizontal than the right, which, in addition to being shorter, tends to curve upward in its posterior end. This pattern of Sylvian asymmetry is present in about two-thirds of brains of right handed individuals, whereas it is less common in lefthanders (Hochberg & LeMay, 1974). Furthermore, the more common pattern of Sylvian asymmetry is seen predominantly in subjects whose speech lateralization has been demonstrated to be in the left hemisphere by amytal testing (Ratcliff, Dila, Taylor, & Milner,

1980). The Sylvian asymmetry, therefore, represents one instance of anatomical right–left differences in the brain which can aid in the localization of language to the left hemisphere in most righthanders.

It appears that the longer fissure on the left reflects a longer lateral edge of the planum temporale and a larger parietal operculum as well (see Figure 1). Sulcal asymmetries also exist in the frontal opercular region (Eberstaller, 1884; Galaburda, 1980). Here, it is necessary to first identify the ascending limb of the Sylvian fissure (Figure 2). This deep vertical branch forms the posterior limit of the *pars triangularis* or the frontal operculum at the border with the *pars opercularis*. The ascending limb, sometimes branched, occurs more often on the left side. If a branch is present, it is called the diagonal sulcus because it runs obliquely (posteriorly and superiorly) from the ascending limb (Figure 2). The relationship of this sulcal branching to handedness and speech lateralization is not known; however, branching may suggest a greater folding (therefore greater amount of cortex) in the left pars opercularis, a structure relevant to speech localization in the left hemisphere (Galaburda, 1980). Finally, the left cingulate sulcus may be branched more often than the right (Eberstaller, 1884), a situation which may reflect left–right differences in the region of the supplementary motor area, although no systematic studies have been made to show statistical significance. Characteristics of the pattern should be recorded for each brain and additional comments may be made of any other striking asymmetries in folding as well as possible fissural abnormalities.

The shape and size of main gyri should be noted. Of particular interest in localization of higher functions is the configuration of the opercular portions of the hemispheres and of the planum temporale. The frontal operculum consists of three main divisions: the *pars triangularis* (the cap of Broca) in the middle, bordered anteriorly by the horizontal limb of the Sylvian fissure, and posteriorly by the ascending limb (Figure 2). In front of the horizontal limb lies the *pars orbitalis* of the operculum. In back of the ascending limb lies *pars opercularis* (the foot of Broca).

The foot of Broca has been thought to be important for the localization of anterior lesions causing aphasia. It usually assumes a U-shaped configuration whereby the posterior limb of the U is attached to the subcentral region (fronto-parietal operculum) and the anterior limb represents the posterior bank of the ascending limb of the Sylvian fissure (Figure 2). In some specimens, the *pars opercularis* is difficult to visualize as it is excessively cloistered within the Sylvian fossa. In such cases, it is useful to have photographs of the operculum and to reconstruct the region from the serial sections.

In some brains, the central sulcus reaches all the way to the Sylvian fissure; in most, it does not, ending instead a centimeter or two above the Sylvian fissure in a T-shaped configuration with the precentral gyrus joining with a postcentral gyrus in the so-called subcentral region or frontoparietal operculum (Figure 2). Asymmetries in this configuration should be noted and may reflect asymmetries in opercularization of the subcentral region on the two sides. The subcentral region's role in language localization is not clear, but lesions producing long-lasting Broca's aphasias appear to involve this area of the operculum as well as the *pars opercularis* (Kertesz, 1977).

Paralleling the asymmetry and the temporal operculum, the left parietal operculum is also larger than the right. This is to be expected since the longer left Sylvian fissure would have to have a larger roof (the parietal operculum) as well as a large floor (planum temporale) (see Figure 1). There may be additional examples of gyral asymmetries which have, however, tended to be less consistent and for which structural functional correlations have not been specified.

In the medulla, it should be noted which pyramid begins its decussation closer to the pons. It has been reported that the left pyramid, destined to the right side of the spinal cord, decussates higher in the brain stem (Kertesz & Geschwind, 1971). This has been interpreted to mean that the left pyramidal tract is larger because it innervates the dominant hand or is more fully decussated. However, insufficient numbers of lefthanders were examined to prove a correlation between the pattern of pyramidal decussation and handedness.

Distortions of gyri and sulci may take place in brains with lesions. These brains should be scrutinized in the usual manner, and attempts made to relate lesion location and size to cognitive deficits and the presence of asymmetries. Additional care should be taken to outline the surface extent of lesions on the appropriate photographic views of the brain or on photographs of brain sections whenever possible.

MICROSCOPIC STUDY OF THE BRAIN

In order to obtain a permanent record of a normal or lesioned brain, it is necessary to prepare the brain in whole-brain serial sections. For a detailed description of methods of embedding, cutting, and staining, the reader is referred to the Appendix of this chapter. Celloidin embedding and cutting are described in Appendix I; the staining method for myelin is described in Appendix II; cresyl violet staining for Nissl substance is described in Appendix III; the frozen section method and accompanying variations in staining are described in Appendix IV; the Braak method for pigment architectonics is described in Appendix V; and the method for silver impregnation of degenerated axons is described in Appendix VI.

ARCHITECTONIC ANALYSIS

Except for some restricted applications of technologies directed at the demonstration of fiber connections, the microscopic analysis of localization is based primarily on architectonic studies. Such studies may be applied to unlesioned brains in which specific functional characteristics were specified during life, thus allowing for structure–function relationships. They may also be applied to the analysis of lesioned brains, thus permitting structure-deficit relationships. Although an elucidation of the available data on the architectonic organization of the human brain is well beyond the scope of this chapter, we will outline some useful general principles. We will stress cytoarchitectonics, which is based on cell stains, typically of Nissl substance. Myeloarchitectonics outlines intracortical fibers and their areal differentiation. Angioarchitectonics refers to the appearance of small blood vessels in different areas. Pigment architectonics is used to refer to the differential accumulation of lipofuscin pigment. Chemoarchitectonics is based on specific histochemical staining and the distribution of given enzymes or other neurochemicals in the brain.

A major aid in architectonics is the presence of gross anatomical landmarks which correspond to architectonic differentiation. Thus, gyri often contain separate architectonic areas, while sulci, fissurets, and often even small cortical dimples commonly outline a border between two architectonic areas. For example, the precentral gyrus contains the gigantopyramidal motor area; the central sulcus delimits its posterior margin; and the precentral sulcus (at least dorsally) delimits its anterior border. Also in the frontal lobe, the opercular portions of the hemisphere contain architectonic areas of distinctive appearance which are often separated from other areas on the frontal convexity by portions of the inferior frontal sulcus. These areas, some of which appear to be relevant to the localization of language function, are themselves separated by sulci (the horizontal and vertical branches of the Sylvian fissure). In the frontal opercular region, the most striking appearance is provided by an area lying on the pars opercularis characterized by large pyramids in IIIc (the deepest third of Layer III), a well-developed granular Layer IV, and coarse pyramids in Va (the superficial half of Layer V) mingling with Layer IV cells (area 44 of Brodmann, 1909) (Figure 3). In pigment architectonic preparations, the IIIc pyramids accumulate large amounts of densely packed lipofuscin (Braak, 1979). Furthermore, this architectonic area is distinctive in the frontal opercular region in that it alone tends to be larger on the left side (Galaburda, 1980). Area 6 lies dorsal to Area 44 and is much less granular, especially near the interhemispheric fissure. In parts of Area 6, Braak (1979) has demonstrated similar (though less striking) lipofuscin-rich cells as in Area 44 which correspond in location to the physiologically determined supplementary motor area.

In the parietal lobe, the central sulcus limits the anterior extension of granular somatosensory Area 3 (Figure 4). A small area having features of both areas 4 and 3 is found at the depth of the central sulcus—the intersensory motor area (Sanides, 1962). As with other primary sensory cortices, the somatosensory Area 3 is extremely fine and sandy in appearance (koniocortex) because of its wealth of small granular elements. Layer IV is broad and dense, and Layer V is cell-poor, which produces a contrast with its neighboring dense layers, IV and VI. Adjacent to this primary area is Area 1, which is also fine and granular, although less so than Area 3, thus illustrating a general feature of those cortices which surround primary sensory fields: They contain large pyramids in IIIc (Figure 4). Most of the remainder of the parietal lobe, as well as most of the frontal convexities, contain the so-called homotypical cortices which are striking by virtue of their highly laminated appearance. In the frontal lobe, they tend to be more pyramidal, whereas in the parietal lobe, they are more granular. In both regions, however, all cell layers are sharply demarcated, thus providing the laminated appearance.

The primary auditory cortex (Area 41) is easily identified on Heschl's gyrus. When more than one transverse temporal gyrus is present, Area 41 is present only on the most anterior one. This cortex is also extremely granular and has a strikingly depopulated Layer V typical of koniocortex, and a characteristic feature is the presence of narrow columns of small pyramids and granule cells in Layer III, giving this layer the appearance of a heavy rain shower. Several areas with well-developed IIIc pyramids surround Area 41,

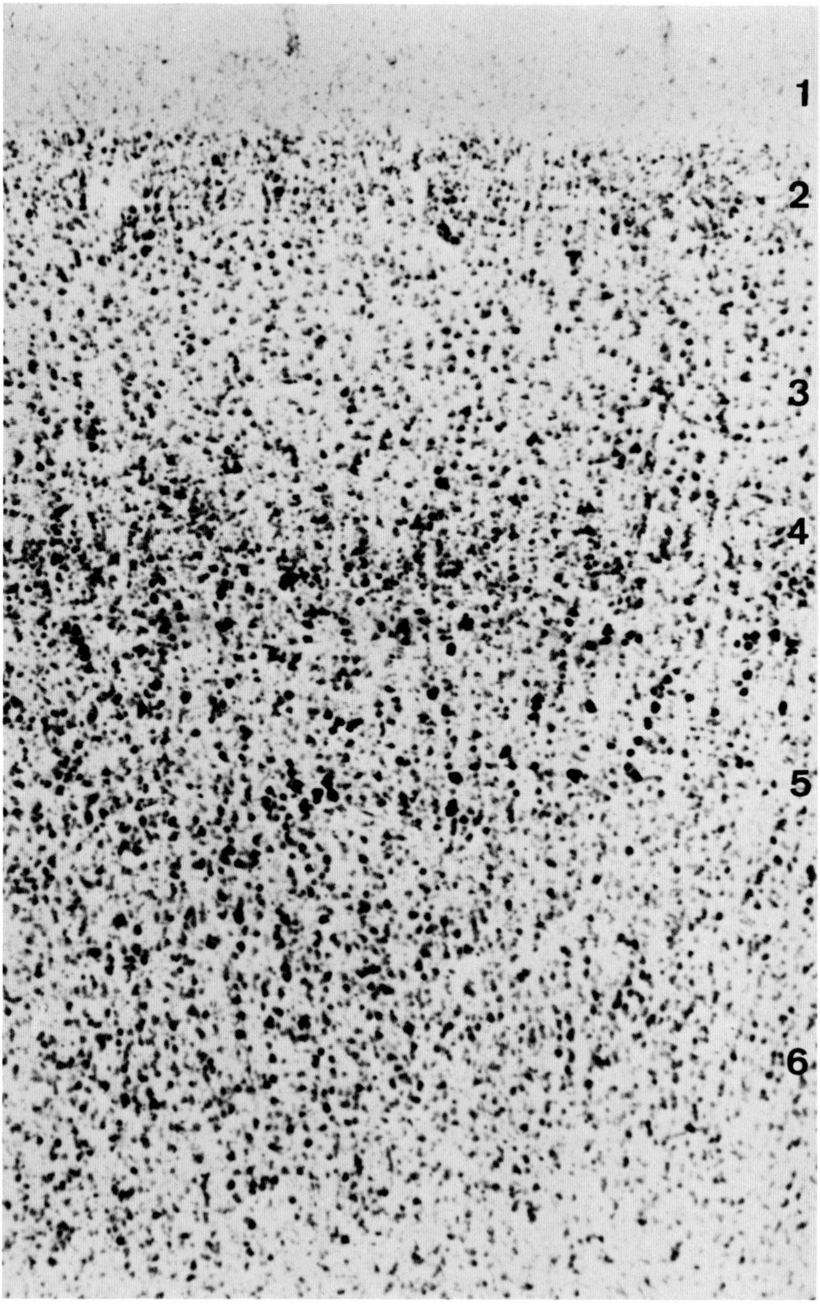
1
2
3
4
5
6

and some reach nearly to the temporal pole (Galaburda & Sanides, 1980). One of these areas is found on the lateral posterior corner of the planum temporale and has been called area "Tpt" (Galaburda & Sanides, 1980) because it has some temporal as well as parietal architectonic features (Figure 5). This area is important to localization because of its strategic location vis-à-vis lesions causing Wernicke's aphasia. Tpt is equivalent to the caudal portion of Brodmann's Area 22 and von Economo's and Koskinas' TA_1. In some ways, this area is similar in appearance to the area on pars opercularis (see preceding description). It also contains large IIIc pyramids and Va pyramids which mingle into Layer IV. However, as might be predicted for a cortex with closer sensory ties, it is more granular and it has a less populated Layer V than the frontal opercular field. In pigment architectonic preparations (Braak, 1978), the region of the planum temporale which, in Nissl preparations contains Tpt, also demonstrates dense accumulations of lipofuscin in IIIc pyramids. Area Tpt volumes in the left and right hemispheres are different and tend to match asymmetries in the planum temporale (Galaburda *et al.*, 1978). Thus area Tpt is more often larger on the left. Architectonic areas on the second and third temporal gyri, especially caudally, tend to look homotypical and are similar in appearance to the parietal homotypical areas on the inferior parietal lobule.

In the occipital lobe, the calcarine sulcus and its banks contain the primary visual Area 17. This area is easily recognized because of its laminated fourth layer of striking appearance and the presence of periodic large Layer V pyramids. Once again, the area surrounding the primary visual cortex (Area 18) has large IIIc pyramids. Area 19 is slightly more laminated and heralds the change to the homotypical fields of the parietal and temporal lobes.

Primitive cortices in the cingulate gyrus, posterior orbitofrontal regions, medial and polar temporal regions, and rostral insula differ from each other in details but share in common a lesser degree of cellularity than the previously discussed cortices, an emphasis in the cell size and packing densities of the deeper layers, a coarseness and richness in Layer II and a poor development of Layer IV.

In myelin preparations, primary fields—both motor and sensory—exhibit the highest degree of intracortical myelination.

Figure 3. Cytoarchitectonic Area 44 (after Brodmann, 1909). This area lies predominantly on the pars opercularis. It is characterized by a granular Layer IV which is obscured by the encroachment of well-developed IIIc pyramids and Layer Va pyramids (see text).

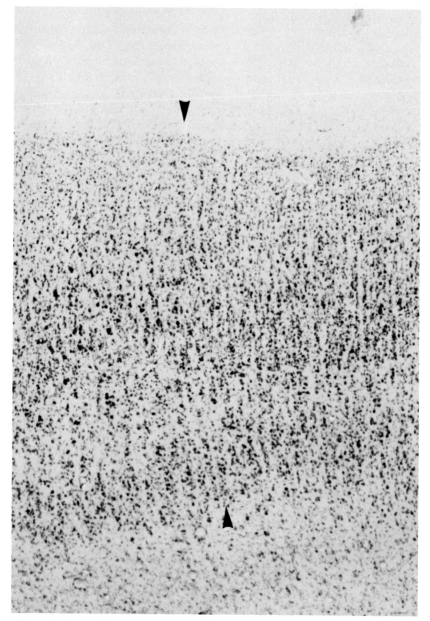

Figure 4. Cytoarchitectonic areas 3 (right) and 1 (left) (after Brodmann, 1909). Note the rich granularity of Area 3 and the prominent IIIc pyramids in Area 1. Also Layer V in 3, almost devoid of large cells acquires moderately large pyramids in Area 1.

This degree diminishes in a stepwise manner in immediately surrounding fields, and is less striking in the homotypical cortices. The more primitive cortices contain the least intracortical myelination in the neocortical formations.

The parcellation of cortical areas into architectonic subdivisions is necessary for the accurate measurements of cortical volumes in normal brains, as well as for the exact specification of lesion extent in brain damage with focal deficits. Parcellation is based on an areal impression by the use of low-power light microscopy. An "impressionistic" view, rather than the analysis of specific cellular elements, is most helpful. The ability to be developed is not unlike that of the chest radiologist who becomes skillful in the perception of shadows and in the oversight of artifacts. The average appearance of an area, rather than minute focal variations, are to be stressed. The relative strengths of layers as denoted by cell size, packing density, and depth of staining are helpful, rather than individual cellular morphology. The presence of columns of cells perpendicularly oriented with reference to the pial surface is a useful distinguishing feature. The manner in which cell layers border each other, whether sharply or indistinctly, provides a helpful clue. Occasionally, a distinctive neuronal element can be used, for example, the Betz cell in Area 4 and the Meynert pyramid in Area 17. As mentioned previously, sulci and dimples may help place architectonic borders, but often do not mark a border, and the cortex simply conforms to the folding [in a predictable manner (Bok, 1959)] and continues unchanged beyond the sulcus. Finally, it is best to begin mapping at a region where gross anatomical landmarks can ascertain proper architectonic recognition.

The same principles of parcellation must be applied whether the brain under study is a normal specimen or one with a lesion. In lesioned brains, it is pertinent to ask, if possible, what area or areas are involved, whether the lesion extends subcortically, how much of an area is involved, and whether all layers are involved. The volume of the lesion should be compared with the volume of the architectonic area(s) involved. In Figure 6, for example, it is possible to state that the lesion involves only Area 1, sparing areas 3 and 2, that all layers are involved, that the lesion extends a small distance into the subcortical white matter, and that (in this particular section) approximately one-third of Area 1 is involved.

The architectonic analysis of lesioned brains is an arduous undertaking which should be reserved to brains of patients with relatively small lesions studied carefully for deficits during life.

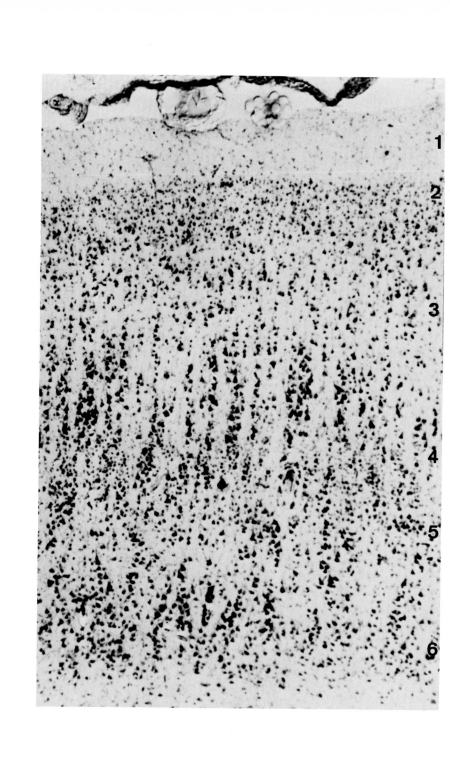

1

2

3

4

5

6

Furthermore, certain lesions are almost never suitable for statements of localization. For instance, brain tumors and other mass lesions displace nearby brain and produce clinical effects at a distance which cannot be easily explained by the analysis of the brain at postmortem, however detailed the examination. On the other hand, slowly growing masses may result in dramatic anatomical changes with relatively few functional deficits during life. This observation illustrates the claim that structure–function correlations are easiest to interpret with acute and subacute lesions. Consequently, the best lesions for architectonic localization are made up of small infarctions of vascular etiology and the occasional circumscribed wound produced by a penetrating injury or a surgical ablation. Conversely, the understanding of the anatomical localization of function and of functional deficits in chronic lesions will have to await improved knowledge of late changes and plasticity in the nervous system.

CONNECTIONAL ANALYSIS

When a substantial portion of an axon is severed from its cell body, the perikaryon undergoes a series of retrograde alterations which culminate in perikaryal lysis and reactive gliosis. Thus, following cerebral lesions, mapping the extent of this retrograde degeneration makes it possible to trace the distribution of neuronal cell bodies which give rise to afferent axonal projections into the damaged region. However, only a fraction of the axons affected by such lesions result in detectable retrograde degeneration (Powell & Cowan, 1967). Thus, this approach enables, at best, a limited mapping of afferent connections. Furthermore, damage to axons passing through the lesioned area is as likely to result in retrograde degeneration as damage to axonal endways terminating within it; this fact further impairs the ability to reach reliable conclusions concerning connectivity. With few notable exceptions, such as the investigation of corticospinal tract by Holmes and May (1909), the usefulness of retrograde degeneration has largely been confined to the delineation of thalamo-cortical connections (von Monakow, 1895; Yakovlev, Locke, & Angevine, 1966). However, recent experiments based on the

---

Figure 5. Cytoarchitectonic area Tpt (22 of Brodmann, 1909; TA$_1$ of v. Economo & Koskinas, 1925). This area lies in the posterior third of the superior temporal gyrus. Note the singular characteristics of this area illustrated by rows of Layer III pyramids waving in and out of Layer IV.

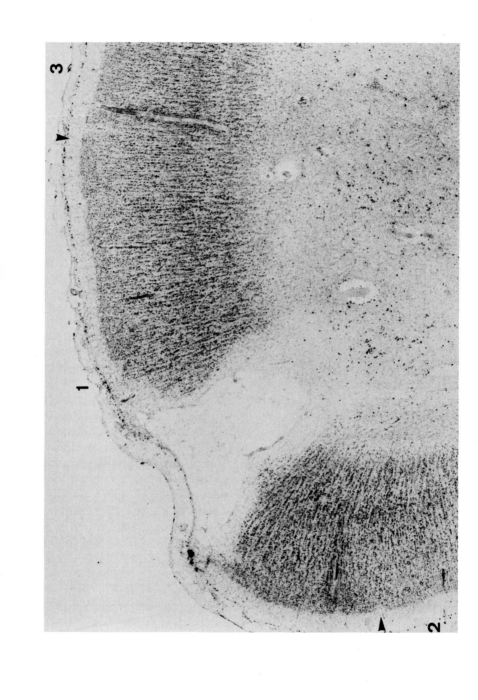

retrograde transport of horseradish peroxidase (Trojanowski & Jacobson, 1976) clearly show that observations based on retrograde degeneration have revealed an incomplete view even of thalamo-cortical connectivity.

Methods based on the principle of anterograde Wallerian degeneration have also contributed to the elucidation of neuronal connectivity. One type of observation based on Wallerian degeneration relied on the disappearance of myelin distal to the point of axonal injury. Valuable contributions were mostly limited to the delineation of spinal tracts where the organization of individual pathways into discrete bundles made the location of demyelination quite conspicuous. The application of Wallerian degeneration to the study of more diffusely organized pathways became possible with techniques introduced by Marchi and Algeri (1886) and then by Glees (1946). These methods enabled the positive visualization of the degenerated myelin and axon, respectively, rather than merely relying on their disappearance. The Marchi and Glees techniques have been successfully applied to the human brain (Meyer, 1949; Roussy, 1907; Smith, 1951, 1960). However, virtually all of these studies concentrated on the connections of cortex with subcortical structures, whereas very little information was obtained on cortico-cortical connectivity. Furthermore, although these methods constitute milestones in the history of neuroanatomy, they suffer well-recognized limitations that severely curtail their applicability.

For instance, the Glees method stains normal axons so that tracing the distribution of the beaded and swollen degenerated axons dispersed among normal fibers becomes excessively laborious. The Marchi method, on the other hand, can trace degeneration only along myelinated pathways and has a propensity for unpredictable artifact (Smith, 1956). Moreover, both methods are subject to the axon-of-passage problem. Thus, the extent of anterograde degeneration is not limited to the projection fields of the neuronal cell bodies involved by the injury, but also includes the distal portion of axons merely passing through the lesion site.

The modern era in neuroanatomy has been ushered in by the introduction of powerful techniques for the *selective* silver impregnation of degenerated axons and their terminals (Fink & Heimer, 1967; Nauta, 1957; Nauta & Gygax, 1954). These methods exploit the

---

Figure 6. Small vascular lesion entirely contained with Area 1 in the postcentral gyrus; Area 3 (right) is uninvolved, as is Area 2 (lower left). Note the sparing of the pial covering, and the extension onto the subcortical white matter.

differential argyrophilia of degenerated fibers such that the chemical manipulation of suitable brain tissue results in the deposition of black silver salts predominantly on degenerating axonal elements rather than on neuronal fibers. Although this method is also subject to the axon-of-passage problem, the distribution of anterograde degeneration resulting from a lesion may be mapped with greater ease than would have been possible with the Glees technique. However, the rather stringent requirements for specific survival and fixation parameters which are necessary for the optimal application of selective silver impregnation have emerged as significant obstacles to investigation in the human brain.

Nevertheless, in the hands of several pioneering investigators, the Nauta–Gygax methods have been applied to the human brain for the analysis of descending motor pathways (Kuypers, 1958) and of spinothalamic projections (Albrecht & Fernström, 1959; Bowsher, 1957; Mehler, 1966). Furthermore, these methods and their derivatives have also revealed the cortical distribution of the visual radiations as well as projections into the entorhinal cortex (Mesulam, 1979). Indeed, the laminar distribution of geniculocalcarine pathways was demonstrated with a resolution which had previously been obtained only in experimental animals. Thus, the silver impregnation methods offer a potentially useful tool of charting many neural connections, including cortico-cortical pathways, in the human brain (Mesulam, 1979). Naturally, the recent introduction of methods based on the axonal transport of tracer substances such as horseradish peroxidase and radiolabeled amino acids have greatly enhanced the resolution and accuracy with which neural connections can be delineated (Cowan, Gottlieb, Hendrickson, Price, & Woolsey, 1972; LaVail, 1975). However, the experimental manipulations required by these methods cannot be applied to humans so that techniques based on selective silver impregnation would appear to offer the most effective means presently available for mapping connectivity in the human brain. Therefore, it is useful to review the guidelines for applying the silver impregnation methods to the human brain.

Survival time

The interval between the occurrence of the lesion and the time of death is important in determining the quality of selective silver impregnation that can be obtained. The length of the "optimal" survival time varies with the animal species and the fiber system under study. Prior experience with the human brain indicates that survival times between 4 and 36 days are most adequate. However, it is conceivable that much longer survival times could also be compatible with successful staining of anterograde degeneration (Grafe, Schimpff, & Leonard, 1978).

Interval between death and autopsy

Following death, unfixed neural perikarya show a gradual dissolution over a period of 48 hours, while the myelin and axis cylinders appear to maintain their structural integrity (Haines and Jenkins, 1968). Thus, it would be expected that the selective staining of anterograde degeneration might not be substantially altered, even if autopsy were delayed for 24–48 hours. Naturally, prompt autopsy and fixation are desirable. However, we have obtained adequate preparations even in cases where the autopsy was delayed by 24 hours (Mesulam, 1979). We do not have experience with longer intervals.

Fixation

This is one of the most critical factors for obtaining successful staining. For experimental animals, *in situ* perfusion and subsequent fixation of the brain with unbuffered 4% formaldehyde solution for 2–6 months is generally the procedure of choice (Nauta, 1957). *In situ* perfusion is usually not possible in the human. However, whole brain immersion in unbuffered 4% formalin for 6 months is adequate. While shorter fixation times of 2 months occasionally provide acceptable specimens, consistent results are only possible with the more prolonged fixation of 6 months. We have obtained good results with specimens that had been fixed for as long as 2½ years (Mesulam, 1979).

Following this initial period in 4% formalin, it is advisable to cut out the areas of interest into tissue blocks that are approximately 7 × 4 cm on the cutting surface and no more than 8 cm thick. These blocks are then immersed in a sucrose–formaldehyde solution (300 g sucrose dissolved in 725 ml of distilled water and 100 ml of concentrated formalin) for 5 weeks and then embedded in an albumin–gelatin matrix as described by Ebbesson (1970) (also see Appendix IV). After hardening of the matrix in 2 days, the embedded block is left in concentrated formalin for 5 weeks. Excess albumin is then trimmed and one corner of the matrix cut to aid in orientation. The block is then frozen on dry ice and cut into 27 micron

(μm) sections on a freezing microtome. An adequate number of sections are collected in 4% formalin and stored for 2–20 days before staining.

Staining of degenerated axonal elements

Three distinct methods outlined in Appendix VI provide adequate selective impregnation of anterograde degeneration. Method 1 is a Nauta procedure with uranyl nitrate as the mordant (Ebbesson, 1970). Degenerated axonal elements acquire a selective argyrophilia and appear swollen, interrupted, and beaded, whereas normal fibers stain less well or not at all. Method 2 is a Nauta procedure with extensive pretreatment which greatly improves the ability to suppress normal fibers (Albrecht & Fernström, 1959) (see Figure 7). In each of these methods, degeneration is traced with greater ease if the degenerated axons are parallel to the plane of section. Method 3 is a modified Fink–Heimer (1967) procedure developed in our laboratory. In experimental animals, this procedure enables the selective demonstration of degenerated terminal boutons. We have not had the same degree of success in human specimens. However, in selected cases, and only after prolonged manipulations of the relevant parameters, it has been possible to demonstrate the "terminal fields" of certain projections within layers of cortex (Mesulam, 1979). Thus, after a lesion in the visual radiations this method has shown a concentration of degenerated elements virtually confined to Layer IVc of calcarine cortex. Initially, we obtained the most consistent results with Method 1. However, additional experience indicates that Method 2 is the most practical for human material and we employ it for most routine examinations.

Staining of normal fibers and cells

Silver impregnation methods, and especially Method 2, do not ordinarily yield adequate staining of normal fibers and cell bodies. Thus, matching sections should be processed with standard Nissl and myelin stains in order to determine the laminar and architectonic distribution of the anterograde degeneration. This can be obtained with ease when cresyl violet acetate is used as described at the end of Appendix VI.

Interpretation of the results

We plot the extent of the lesion and of the subsequent degeneration onto tracings of the sections and then transfer these to drawings of the whole brain. This process is greatly facilitated by

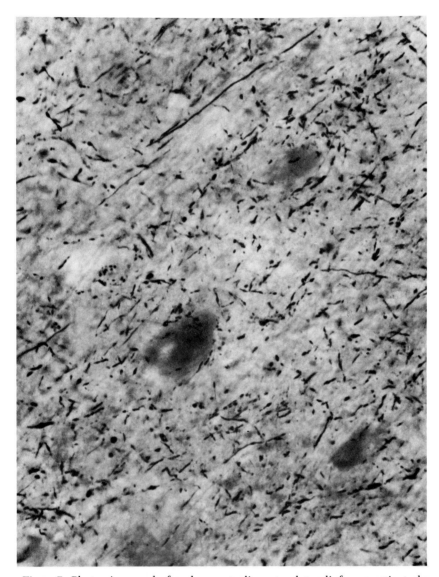

Figure 7. Photomicrograph of nucleus ventralis posterolateralis from a patient who had surgical lumbar commissurotomy 18 days before death. Fine and coarse degenerated fibers are seen, especially along magnocellular neurons. The Albrecht–Fernström method had been used as indicated in Appendix VI (from Mesulam, 1979).

obtaining photographs of the whole brain as well as of the blocks of tissue that will be used for subsequent cutting and staining.

Argyrophilia not related to anterograde degeneration may occur in glial, perivascular, perikaryal, and melanin-containing sites. Furthermore, human tissue is also excessively prone to diffuse silver precipitation in the normal neuropil and especially on myelin. It is possible to minimize this undesirable argyrophilia by several manipulations outlined in Appendix VI.

Additional difficulties arise with respect to fibers-of-passage through the lesion site. Even in experimental animals where the intended ablation is meticulously planned, the resultant lesion usually includes not only cell bodies where efferent projections are being investigated, but also passing fibers which originate in distant regions. However, useful hypotheses may still be formulated if this limitation is kept in mind and if pertinent experimental data obtained from nonhuman species are consulted as guidelines.

Moreover, in some cases, neuronal injury may spread across synapses over time. Indeed, there is evidence for retrograde as well as anterograde transneuronal degeneration in several animal species, including the human (Cowan, 1970; Torch, Hirano, & Solomon, 1977). It is not yet known how extensively such transsynaptic degeneration can be demonstrated with silver impregnation methods. However, this possibility introduces additional caution in the interpretation of neuronal connectivity, since part of the degeneration, especially in cases with long survival times, may be reflecting transsynaptic effects.

It is desirable to determine the laminar and architectonic distribution of the degeneration and to stain control areas where degeneration is not expected. A distinct laminar distribution of the degeneration and its abrupt termination at architectonic boundaries increases the level of confidence with which results may be interpreted. Similarly, if control sections from other areas, preferably from the homologous region of the contralateral hemisphere, do not show degeneration, the validity of the observations is further enhanced. Otherwise, widespread argyrophilia, even if it looks like degeneration, should be suspected of having an artifactual origin.

When all necessary blocking and staining is completed, it is advisable to examine the rest of the brain in search of additional unsuspected lesions. If present, their direct or transsynaptic contribution to the pattern of degeneration should be considered. Since it is rarely practical to stain the whole brain, it may be more practical to do a macroscopic survey on 2–3 mm sections for this purpose.

Conclusions

Before localization theory can be put to a test, it is essential that additional detailed neuroanatomical data be obtained. The data may be of the type aimed at correlating results of detailed psychological testing in normal subjects and features of the normal cerebral anatomy; or attempts may be made to carefully specify the nature, location, and extent of lesions and to correlate these with deficits demonstrated during life.

At postmortem examination, initial assessment may be made of the external topography of the brain. The size and configuration of the hemispheres, of lobes, of gyri and sulci as well as features of gross anatomical left–right asymmetry may provide the first indications that certain functions of functional deficits can be correlated with brain anatomy. Subsequently, the brain may be processed for microscopic analysis which consists primarily of an architectonic study and, if possible, analysis for features of fiber connectivity. The architectonic subdivision of the cortex reflects more closely than aspects of gross anatomy the functional organization of the brain. Thus, measurements of architectonic volumes, left–right comparisons, and correlations of lesions to architectonic areas may supply the necessary information required to make the structural–functional correlations needed for the purpose of localization. If, in addition, the exact connectivity of normal areas as well as the connectional loss occasioned by lesions can be specified, the architectonic and connectional organization of neuroanatomical substrates underlying special functions may be clarified.

Appendix I

CELLOIDIN EMBEDDING AND CUTTING

This method is particularly valuable in human material because of the excellence of the stains obtained. The thickness of cutting (35–50 μm) is ideal for cytoarchitectonics.

I. *Dehydration*
   After fixation in 10% formalin for 3 months the brain is dehydrated.
   A. 80% ethanol—3 days (the brain becomes soft and must be rested on cotton).

    B. 95% ethanol—3 days.

    C. 100% ethanol—2 days (seal edges of container with tape).

    D. 100% ethanol–ether (equal parts)—24 hours.

II. *Embedding*

    A. Transfer brain to a large rectangular glass container (a glass pet-store aquarium is useful for this purpose).

    B. Solutions of celloidin by weight are made with equal parts of 100% ethanol and ether:

        1. 3% celloidin to cover—6–8 weeks, then pour off

        2. 6% celloidin to cover—6–8 weeks, then pour off

        3. 12% celloidin to cover—several weeks

As the 12% celloidin solution thickens, it will shrink, and it is usually necessary to add more solution. The hardening process takes several weeks. When the surface is dry, add 80% ethanol to cover the surface and leave for an additional 2–3 week period until the whole block is solid and ready for cutting.

III. *Cutting*

After trimming the celloidin block to achieve a stable base (trimmings of expensive celloidin can be reused), the specimen is ready for cutting. In our laboratory, we use an especially constructed giant microtome, but there are several alternatives on the market which can accommodate a large specimen. It is important to check, however, whether the microtome intended for purchase will accept a tall feed consistent with a whole human brain standing on the occipital lobes (for coronal sections).

Our sections are cut at 35 μm thickness for cytoarchitectonics and myeloarchitectonics. Sections to be stained and spares are segregated in individual containers in 80% ethanol. Every twentieth section is stained for Nissl substance, and the adjacent section for myelin sheaths. The spares may be kept indefinitely in the ethanol containers which are properly sealed.

Appendix II

LOYEZ STAINING

The Loyez method is used to stain myelin sheaths. The steps of this staining method are illustrated on Figure 8.

The first differentiation in 4% iron alum mordant takes from 12 to 24 hours. The sections are then washed in distilled water and

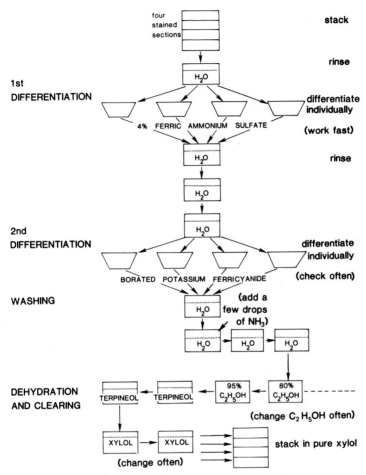

Figure 8. Diagram to show the steps of the Loyez method for staining myelinated fibers. Also see text.

placed in freshly made hematoxylin stain for 24 hours. Afterward, the sections are washed in distilled water and differentiated a second time in Weigert's borated ferricyanide. After washing again, the sections are dehydrated in graded ethanol solutions (80 and 95%), cleared with terpineol and xylol, and stored in pure xylol for mounting.

The most important aspect of mounting is the careful orientation of the sections so that front and back and left and right are consistently identifiable. Permount[R] mounting medium affords a good seal after air bubbles are pressed out. The slides dry in about 1 week, and are then ready for numbering and storage.

Appendix III

CRESYL VIOLET STAINING

Cresyl violet stains the Nissl substance. Sections are washed in distilled water and placed one at a time in 1% cresyl violet acetate solution for 10 minutes. Each section is placed in distilled water for 15 minutes and then differentiated and dehydrated in 70, 80, and 95% ethanol. A few drops of colophonium should be added to the 80 and 95% ethanol baths. If differentiation is adequate, the sections are then cleared with terpineol and passed through xylol. Sections are now ready for mounting as outlined in Appendix II.

Appendix IV

FROZEN SECTIONS

Blocks for cell and myelin stains and whole brains for the Braak method (see Appendix V) may be processed in the frozen state after embedding in albumin–gelatin.[1] After 1–3 weeks fixation in 10% formalin, the block is soaked in sucrose–formalin (300 gm of sucrose dissolved in 725 ml of distilled water and 100 ml of concentrated formalin). Soaking is complete when the block sinks to the bottom of the jar. The block is then washed in distilled water and embedded in albumin–gelatin.

A cardboard box is suitable as a container for the block and the albumin–gelatin. The box and its contents are placed in a dish with a thin layer of 40% formalin at the bottom, and the dish covered. When the albumin–gelatin block is hard, it should be placed in 40% formalin to cover and remain there for 3–4 days. For cutting, we use a hollow rectangular metal base which can be filled wtih dry ice. Water is squirted on the external cooled metal surface in order to make an icy base and the block is attached with additional water. Metal rings are then placed around the block and the spaces are

---

[1]Adapted at our laboratories through the courtesy of Professor W. J. H. Nauta, Massachusetts Institute of Technology, Cambridge, MA (see also Ebbesson, 1970).

filled with additional dry ice. When the block is frozen solid, the rings are removed and the block is cut at a thickness of 30 μm. It should be stressed that small blocks require staining of every fifth to tenth section to assure detailed analysis of lesions. Spare sections are stored in 5% formalin.

Cresyl violet staining can be accomplished in mounted frozen sections. After washing with distilled water, the sections are floated onto slides which have been tilted into the bath. The sections thus mounted are dried at room temperature (2–3 hours). The slides are then placed in 80% alcohol, washed with distilled water, and placed in a 1% aqueous solution of cresyl violet for 20 minutes. The rest of the procedure is the same as with celloidin embedding (see Appendix III).

The steps in the Loyez staining of albumin–gelatin are the same as for celloidin (see Appendix II). Differences exist in the concentration of the reactants and time of reaction. For the first mordant (iron alum), we use a 2% solution for 4–6 hours. The hematoxylin time need only be 10–12 hours. The sections are washed in water and differentiated a second time in 2% iron alum until differentiation is optimal to the naked eye. After the Weigert's potassium ferricyanide step and washing, the sections can be mounted as with cresyl violet, dried in air, passed through two changes of absolute alcohol, xylol, and coverslipped with Permount®.

Appendix V

MODIFICATION OF THE BRAAK LIPOFUSCIN METHOD

The Braak technique for the staining of lipofuscin granules in neurones has been presented elsewhere (Braak, 1978, 1979). Minor changes are introduced here because of differences in availability of certain chemicals in the United States and West Germany. The main advantages of the pigment architectonic technique is the ability to process thick sections, thus cutting down preparation and analysis times as well as costs.

After several months in formalin, fixative blocks or whole brains are embedded in albumin–gelatin and prepared for sectioning (see Appendix IV). Blocks are oriented and sectioned at thicknesses of 300–1000 μm depending on the question to be answered. Interest in small architectonic areas or small lesions would require thinner sectioning. Sections are stored in 10% formalin solution.

STAINING

1. The sections are washed and placed in performic acid solution for 30–50 minutes. For performic acid mix under the hood: 90 cc formic acid; 10 cc 30% hydrogen peroxide.
2. Rinse sections in running tap water for about 60 minutes and place in 70% ethanol for 5 minutes.
3. Place sections in a staining aldehyde-fuscin solution which has been prepared from a stock solution (see following list) and leave for 12–24 hours on a rocker platform.

   Preparation for stock solution:
   a. 0.5 gram pararosaniline
   b. 100 cc 70% ethanol
   c. 1 cc crotonaldehyde
   d. 1 cc 37% hydrochloric acid
   Let ripen for 1 week. Use only 1 week.

   Preparation of staining solution:
   The amount of stock solution to be added depends on the staining characteristics of the tissue. Initially, begin with 1 cc and run some trials. The usual amount is 2–4 cc of stock solution added to:
   a. 100 cc 95% ethanol
   b. 25 cc distilled water
   c. 12.5 cc formic acid
   d. 1.2 cc performic acid (under hood)

4. Place sections in 70% ethanol for 10 min.
5. Dehydrate in several changes of 95% ethanol (24 hours)
6. Place in absolute ethanol (24 hours)
7. Place in xylene (about 12 hours)
8. Mount with Permount® (Fisher So-P-15).

Appendix VI

SELECTIVE SILVER IMPREGNATION METHOD

EMBEDDING AND CUTTING

Fixation in 10% unbuffered formalin for at least 6 months is followed by selection of blocks in areas of interest. Blocks should be approximately 7 × 4 cm at the cutting surface, and no more than 8 cm thick. The blocks are then immersed in sucrose formalin (300 gm sucrose dissolved in 725 ml of distilled water and 100 ml of concentrated formalin solution) for 5 weeks and then embedded in an albumin–gelatin matrix as described in Appendix IV. The block hardens in 2 days and is then placed in concentrated formalin for 5 weeks. Excess albumin–gelatin is trimmed and one corner of the matrix block cut to aid with orientation. The block is then frozen on dry ice as outlined in Appendix IV and cut in 27 μm thick sections. A freezing microtome may also be used for this purpose. Sections are stored in 4% formalin and kept 2–20 days prior to staining.

STAINING

Staining is done in batches of 8–10 free floating sections except for the Laidlaw bath and steps which follow it. These sections are conveniently transferred from one solution to another by using a plexiglass cylinder that is about 1–2 cm deep and 7 cm across. This is covered at one end by a nylon mesh and fits into a Petri dish. Only distilled water is used in all sections. All procedures are performed on a rocking platform.

METHOD 1 (NAUTA PROCEDURE)

1. Rinse in three changes of water (2 min each).
2. Uranyl nitrate (1 or 5% aqueous solution). This is used as a mordant in order to improve the selectivity of the silver impregnation. Increasing the time in this solution decreases the deposition of reduced silver on normal fibers and in the neuropil. However, excessive exposure may also inhibit the staining of degeneration and should be avoided. In the human brain, the optimal times vary greatly and have ranged from 1 to 40 hours in a 5% solution.
3. Rinse in 3 changes of water (5 min each).
4. Potassium permanganate (0.05% aqueous solution). This step suppresses argyrophilia. Timing is critical since too short an exposure will result in the impregnation of many normal fibers, while too long an exposure may prevent the visualization of degenerated axons. For human material, an immersion of 40–60 minutes has yielded good results. However, different times should be tried to find the optimal time for that individual specimen. If the range of optimal times is too narrow, the 0.05% stock solution may be diluted to 80 or 60% strength in order to expand this range so that a finer adjustment of the timing becomes possible.
5. Rinse in water (2 min).

6. Bleach (10 gm oxalic acid and 10 gm hydroquinone in 2000 ml water). Place sections in this solution until they are uniformly decolorized. This usually takes 1–2 min.

7. Rinse in 3 changes of water (2 min each).

8. Silver (1.5% aqueous solution of silver nitrate). Place sections in this solution for 35 minutes.

9. Rinse in 2 changes of water (2 min each).

10. Laidlaw ([a] In a 1000 ml graduated cylinder 48 gm of silver nitrate are dissolved in 100 ml of water; [b] then, a saturated (1.33% at 9°C) lithium carbonate solution is added until the 1000 ml mark is reached; [c] shake vigorously and allow the precipitate to settle to the 300 ml mark; [d] pour off the supernatant and wash the precipitate three more times with distilled water, making sure that the precipitate settles to the 300 ml mark each time and that as much of the supernatant as possible is decanted; [e] add 10 ml of ammonium hydroxide and shake; [f] add additional drops of ammonium hydroxide (shake after each drop) until the solution turns light grey but is still slightly turbid. This should require about 44 ml of ammonium hydroxide. If the resultant solution is completely limpid or if it has a distinct ammoniacal smell, there is an excess of ammonia and more lithium carbonate should be added until the solution is slightly turbid; [g] dilute with water to the 480 ml mark; [h] filter and store in a chemically clean bottle; [i] expose to daylight for 3–4 weeks until an even mirrorlike deposit forms on the walls of the bottle; [j] filter before use).

The Laidlaw step is best carried out in a crucible containing about 10 ml of solution. Individual sections are transferred to this crucible (from the water rinse in Step 9) with the help of an L-shaped glass rod. The sections are then agitated gently in the Laidlaw solution for 30–60 seconds. Adding a couple of drops of 2.5% sodium hydroxide solution to the Laidlaw solution will impart a darker color to the section, whereas the addition of a few drops of ammonia will do the opposite. Such manipulations may become necessary for obtaining optimal results. In order to avoid "exhaustion" of the Laidlaw solution, the 10 ml in the crucible is discarded after 2–3 sections have been stained.

11. Reducer (to 1800 ml water, add 150 ml 95% ethanol, 35 ml of 10% formalin, and 40 ml of 1% citric acid). The section is immersed in this solution for 1 min until a yellowish brown color appears. If the sections are too dark, diluting the reducer to 80% of its strength may help.

12. Reducer—repeat Step 11.

13. Rinse in three changes of water (2 min each).

14. Fixation (0.5% sodium thiosulphate in aqueous solution). The tissue is placed in this solution for 10–60 sec.

15. Rinse in three changes of water (2 min each).

16. Mounting (add 5 gm gelatin to 500 ml of water and heat gently until dissolved. Then add 500 ml of 80% ethanol). Sections are transferred to this solution which facilitates mounting onto glass slides. The glass slides are then air-dried, dehydrated in graded alcohols, cleared in xylene, and cover-slipped with Permount®.

METHOD 2 (ALBRECHT & FERNSTRÖM, 1959)

1. Rinse in two changes of water (2 min each).

2. Enhancement (add 5 ml of 10% hydroquinone and 2 ml of 10% calcium chloride to 93 ml of 10% formalin). If the specimen has been overfixed (6 months or longer) and if the tissue shows a generalized lack of argyrophilia, then leaving the sections in this solution for 24–48 hours may enable successful silver impregnation. Otherwise, this step may be omitted.

3. Rinse in two changes of water (2 min each).

4. Bleach (prepared as in Method 1). Sections are placed in this solution for 30 minutes.

5. Rinse in one change of water (2 minutes).

6. Chromic acid (0.05% of aqueous solution). Sections are washed in this solution for 10 min.

7. Rinse in water (2 min).

8. Hydrobromic acid (4% aqueous solution). Sections are washed in this solution for 5 min.

9. Rinse in water (2 min).

10. Phosphotungstic acid (1% aqueous solution). Sections are washed in this solution for 15 minutes.

11. Rinse in three changes of water (2 min each).

12. Potassium permanganate (0.05% aqueous solution). Good results have been obtained with times ranging from 7 to 9 minutes in this solution. However, the considerations raised for the same solution in Method 1 also apply here and the optimal times must be determined individually for each specimen.

13. Rinse in water (2 min).

14. Bleach (prepared as in Method 1). Leave tissue until it is uniformly decolorized. This takes 1–2 min.

15. Rinse in water (2 min).

16. Silver (1.5% aqueous solution of silver nitrate). Sections are placed in this solution for 30 min.

17. Rinse in water (2 min).

18. Laidlaw (prepared as in Method 1). Place the sections in the Laidlaw solution for 3 min. The considerations concerning the parameters of this step are identical to the ones stated for Method 1.

19. Reducer (to 800 ml water, add 90 ml of absolute ethanol, 27 ml of 1% citric acid, and 27 ml of 10% formalin). Place tissue in this solution until it is uniformly dark. This takes about 1 min. If the sections become too dark, the reducer fluid may be diluted to 80% strength.

20. Reducer—repeat Step 19.

21. Rinse in water (2 min).

22. Fixation (0.5% sodium thiosulphate.) Place sections in this solution for 10 sec.

23. Rinse in water (2 min).

24. Mount and coverslip as in Method 1.

METHOD 3 (A MODIFIED FINK AND HEIMER (1967) METHOD)

1. Rinse in water (2 min).

2. Potassium permanganate (0.05% aqueous solution). The considerations stated for this step in Method 1 also apply here. The optimal times in this solution for this method have ranged from 1 to 5 min. Again, optimal times must be determined individually for each specimen.

3. Rinse twice in water (2 min).

4. Bleach as in Method 1.

5. Rinse twice in water (2 min each).

6. Solution A (mix 2 gm of uranyl nitrate and 10 gm silver nitrate in 2000 ml water). Place sections in this solution for 0–10 min.

7. Rinse in water (2 min).

8. Solution B (mix 3.5 gm uranyl nitrate and 32.5 gm silver nitrate in 2000 ml water). Place sections in this solution for 0–10 min. *Note:* Various combinations of timing must be tried between solutions A and B in order to optimize argyrophilia in degenerating terminals although minimizing the deposition of reduced silver elsewhere. Such optimal combinations may range from a full 10 min in both solutions A and B to a schedule which completely eliminates either A or B.

9. Rinse in water (2 min).

10. Solution C ([a] first prepare a 2.0% solution of silver nitrate; [b] then prepare a base mixture [always freshly prepared] of 2.5%

sodium hydroxide with concentrated ammonium hydroxide in a ratio of 9 vol of the sodium hydroxide to 6 vol of the ammonia; [c] then to each 100 ml of the silver nitrate solution, add 10 ml of the base mixture and stir until clear). Sections are placed in this solution for 0.5–2 minutes. In this procedure, this step is analogous to the Laidlaw step of methods 1 and 2.

> *Note:* This is a very crucial step. For optimal staining, it may be necessary to make slight alterations in the 9:6 ratio. Changing the base ratio, even by 0.1 ml, in favor of ammonia may decrease artifactual argyrophilia, but it may also prevent the staining of degeneration. Increasing the ratio in favor of sodium hydroxide may do the opposite. The optimal ratio is crucial for good staining and seems to be very precariously balanced in human tissue.

11. Reducer (prepared as in Method 1). Leave in this solution until sections have uniformly changed color. This takes about 45–60 sec. If the sections become too dark, the reducer may be diluted to 80% strength. A few drops of citric acid may help to eliminate nonspecific precipitation of silver.

12. Reducer—repeat Step 11.

13. Rinse in water (2 min).

14. Fixation (solution prepared as in Method 1).

15. Rinse twice in water (2 min each).

16. Mount and coverslip as in Method 1.

METHOD 4 FOR NORMAL CELLS AND FIBERS

1. Rinse in water (5 min).

2. Cresyl violet acetate (0.2% aqueous solution). Place sections in this solution for 10 min.

3. Acid–alcohol (1 part of 10% acetic acid to 2 parts absolute ethanol). Differentiate sections here until the gray matter is pale blue and the white matter is light violet.

4. Rinse in water until all dye is removed.

5. Mount and coverslip as in Method 1.

References

Albrecht, M. H., & Fernström, R. C. (1959). A modified Nauta-Gyax method for human brain and spinal cord. *Stain Technology, 34,* 91–94.

Arnold, F. (1838). *Bemerkungen über den Baue des Hirns und Rückenmarks nebst Beiträgen zur Physiologie des zehuten und elften Hirnnerven, mehren kritischen*

Mitteilungen sowie verschiedenen pathologischen und anatomischen Beobach-tungen. Zurich: S. Höhr.

Betz, W. (1881). Uber die feinere Struktur der Grosshirnrinde des Menschen. *Zentralblatt fuer die Medizinischen Wissenschaften, 19,* 193–195, 209–213, 231, 234.

Bevan-Lewis, W. (1879). On the comparative structure of the cortex cerebri. *Brain, 1,* 79–96.

Blum, F. (1893). Der Formaldehyd als Härtungsmittel. *Zeitschrift fuer Wissenschaftliche Mikroskopie, 10,* 314–315.

Bok, S. T. (1959). *Histonomy of the cerebral cortex.* Amsterdam: Elsevier.

Bowsher, D. (1957). Termination of the central pain pathway in man: The conscious appreciation of pain. *Brain, 80,* 606–622.

Braak, H. (1978). On magnopyramidal temporal fields in the human brain probable morphological counterparts of Wernicke's sensory speech region. *Anatomy and Embryology, 152,* 141–169.

Braak, H. (1979). The pigmentarchitecture of the human frontal lobe. I. Precentral, subcentral and frontal region. *Anatomy and Embryology, 157,* 35–68.

Brodmann, K. (1909). *Vergleichende Lokalisationslehre der Grosshirnrinde.* Leipzig: Barth.

Burdach, K. F. (1819–1826). *Vom Baure und Leben des Gehirns.* Leipzig: Dyk'schen Buchhandlung.

Campbell, A. (1905). *Histological studies on the localization of cerebral function.* London & New York: Cambridge University Press.

Chi, J. G., Dooling, E. C., & Gilles, F. H. (1977). Gyral development of the human brain. *Annals of Neurology, 1,* 86–93.

Cowan, W. M. (1970). Anterograde and retrograde transneuronal degeneration in the central and peripheral nervous system. In W. J. H. Nauta & S. O. E. Ebbesson (Eds.), *Contemporary research methods in neuroanatomy.* New York: Springer-Verlag, pp. 217–251.

Cowan, W. M., Gottlieb, D. I., Hendrickson, A. E., Price, J. L., & Woolsey, A. (1972). The autoradiographic demonstration of axonal connections in the central nervous system. *Brain Research, 37,* 21–51.

Davidoff, L. M. (1928). The brain in monogolian idiocy. *Archives of Neurology and Psychiatry, 20,* 1229–1257.

Déjérine, J. J., & Déjérine-Klumpke, A. (1895). *Anatomie des centres nerveux.* Paris: Ruef et Cie.

Ebbesson, S. O. E. (1970). The selective silver impregnation of degenerating axons and their synaptic endings in nonmammalian species. In W. J. H. Nauta & S. O. E. Ebbesson (Eds.), *Contemporary research methods in neuroanatomy.* New York: Springer-Verlag, pp. 132–161.

Eberstaller, O. (1884). Zur oberflächen Anatomie der Grosshirn Hemisphären. *Wiener Medizinische Blaetter, 7,* 479, 642, 644.

Economo, C., & Koskinas, G. N. (1925). *Die Cytoarchitektonik der Hirnrinde des erwachsenen Menschen.* Berlin: Springer-Verlag.

Escourolle, R., & Poirier, J. (1973). *Manual of basic neuropathology.* Philadelphia: Saunders.

Fink, R. P., & Heimer, L. (1967). Two methods for selective silver impregnation of degenerating axons and their synaptic endings in the central nervous system. *Brain Research, 4,* 369–374.

Foville, A. L. F. (1844). *Traité complet de l'anatomie, de la physiologie et de la pathologie du système nerveux cérébrospinal.* Paris: Fortin, Masson et Cie.

Galaburda, A. M. (1980). La région de Broca: Observations anatomiques faites un siècie après la mort de son découvreur. *Revue Neurologique, 136,* 609–616.

Galaburda, A. M., & Kemper, T. L. (1979). Cytoarchitectonic abnormalities in developmental dyslexia: A case study. *Annals of Neurology, 6,* 94–100.

Galaburda, A. M., & Sanides, F. (1980). Cytoarchitectonic organization of the human auditory cortex. *Journal of Comparative Neurology, 190,* 597–610.

Galaburda, A. M., Sanides, F., & Geschwind, N. (1978). Human brain: Cytoarchitectonic left–right asymmetries in the temporal speech region. *Archives of Neurology (Chicago), 35,* 812–817.

Gall, F. J., & Spurtzheim, G. (1810). *Anatomie et physiologie du système nerveux en général et du cerveau en particulier* (Vol. 1). Paris: F. Schoell.

Glees, P. (1946). Terminal degeneration within the central nervous system as studied by a new silver method. *Journal of Neuropathology and Experimental Neurology, 5,* 54–59.

Grafe, M. R., Schimpff, R. D., & Leonard, C. M. (1978). Degeneration argyrophilia following long-standing damage to the human brain. *Neuroscience Abstracts, 4,* 75.

Gudden, B. A. (1870). Experimentaluntersuchungen über das peripherische und centrale Nervensystem. *Archiv fuer Psychiatrie und Nervenkrankheiten, 2,* 693–723.

Haines, D. E., & Jenkins, T. W. (1968). Studies on the epithalamus. *Journal of Comparative Neurology, 132,* 405–417.

Hammarberg, C. (1895). *Studien über Klinik und Pathologie der Idiotie.* Upsala: Edv. Berling.

Hochberg, F. H., & LeMay, M. (1974). Arteriographic correlates of handedness. *Neurology, 25,* 218–222.

Holmes, G., & May, W. P. (1909). On the exact origin of the pyramidal tracts in man and other mammals. *Brain, 32,* 1–43.

Kertesz, A. (1977). Isotope localization of infarcts in aphasia. *Archives of Neurology (Chicago), 34,* 590–601.

Kertesz, A., & Geschwind, N. (1971). Patterns of pyramidal decussation and their relationship to handedness. *Archives of Neurology (Chicago), 24,* 326–332.

Knudson, P. A. (1958). *Ventriklernes Storrelses—forhold i' Anatomisk Normale Hjerner fra voksne.* Copenhagen theses, Odense, Andelsbogtrykkeriet.

Kuypers, H. G. J. M. (1958). Corticobulbar connections to the pons and lower brainstem in man: An anatomical study. *Brain, 81,* 364–388.

LaVail, J. H. (1975). Retrograde cell degeneration and retrograde transport techniques. In W. M. Cowan & M. Cuénod (Eds.), *The use of axonal transport for studies of neuronal connectivity.* Amsterdam: Elsevier, pp. 217–248.

LeMay, M., & Culebras, A. (1972). Human brain: Morphologic differences in the hemispheres demonstrable by carotid arteriography. *New England Journal of Medicine, 287,* 168–170.

LeMay, M., & Kido, D. K. (1978). Asymmetries of the cerebral hemispheres on computed tomograms. *Journal of Computer Assisted Tomography, 2,* 471.

Luys, J. B. (1865). *Recherches sur le système nerveux cérébrospinal; sa structure, ses functions et ses maladies.* Paris: J. B. Baillière.

Marchi, V., & Algeri, G. (1886). Sulle degenerazioni discendenti consecutive a lesioni sperimentali in diverse zone della corteccia cerebrale. *Rivista Sperimentale di Freniatria e Medicina Legale delle Alienazioni Mentali, 12,* 208–252.

McRae, D., Branch, D., & Milner, B. (1968). The occipital horns and cerebral dominance. *Neurology, 18,* 95–98.

Mehler, W. R. (1966). The posterior thalamic region in man. *Confinia Neurologica, 27,* 18–29.

Mesulam, M. M. (1979). Tracing neural connections of human brain with selective silver impregnation. *Archives of Neurology (Chicago), 36,* 814–818.

Meyer, M. A. (1949). A study of efferent connections of the frontal lobe in the human brain after leucotomy. *Brain, 72,* 265–296.

Meynert, T. (1884). *Psychiatrie: Klinik der Erkrankungen des Vorderhirns.* Vienna: Braumuller.

Nauta, W. J. H. (1957). Silver impregnation of degenerating axons. In W. F. Windle (Ed.), *New research techniques in neuroanatomy.* Springfield, Ill.: Thomas, pp. 17–26.

Nauta, W. J. H., & Gygax, P. A. (1954). Silver impregnation of degenerating axons in the central nervous system: A modified technic. *Stain Technology, 29,* 91–93.

Nissl, F. (1894). Über eine neue Untersuchungsmethode des Centralorgans speciell zur Feststellung der Localisation der Nervenzellen. *Neurologisches Zentralblatt, 13,* 507–508.

Powell, T. P. S., & Cowan, W. M. (1967). The interpretation of the degenerative changes in the intralaminar nuclei of the thalamus. *Journal of Neurology, Neurosurgery and Psychiatry, 30,* 140–153.

Ratcliff, G., Dila, C., Taylor, L., & Milner, B. (1980). The morphological asymmetry of the hemispheres and cerebral dominance for speech: A possible relationship. *Brain and Language, 11,* 87–98.

Reil, J. C. (1809). Untersuchungen über den Bau des grossen Gehirns im Menschen. *Archiv fuer Anatomie und Physiologie, 9,* 136–524.

Remak, R. (1838). *Observationes Anatomicae et Microscopicae de Systematis Nervosi Structura.* Berlin: Reimerianis.

Roussy, G. (1907). *La couche optique (étude anatomique, physiologique et clinique)— Le syndrome thalamique.* Paris: G. Steinheil.

Sanides, F. (1962). *Die architektonik des Menschlichen Stirnhirns.* Berlin: Springer-Verlag.

Smith, M. C. (1951). The use of Marchi staining in the later stages of human tract degeneration. *Journal of Neurology, Neurosurgery and Psychiatry, 14,* 222–225.

Smith, M. C. (1956). The recognition and prevention of artifacts of the Marchi method. *Journal of Neurology, Neurosurgery and Psychiatry, 19,* 74–83.

Smith, M. C. (1960). Nerve fiber degeneration in the brain in amyotrophic lateral sclerosis. *Journal of Neurology, Neurosurgery and Psychiatry, 23,* 269–282.

Torch, W. C., Hirano, A., & Solomon, S. (1977). Anterograde transneuronal degeneration in the limbic system: Clinical-anatomic correlation. *Neurology, 27,* 1157–1163.

Trojanowski, J. Q., & Jacobson, S. (1976). Areal and laminar distribution of some pulvinar cortical efferents in rhesus monkey. *Journal of Comparative Neurology, 169,* 371–392.

Türck, L. (1851). Über sekundäre Erkrankung einzelner Rückenmarksstränge und ihrer Fortsetzungen zum Gehirn, in Gesammelte neurologische Schriften. *Jahrbuch für Psychiatrie und Neurologie, 31,* 64–85.

von Monakow, C. (1895). Experimentelle und pathologisch-anatomische Untersuchungen über die Beziehungen der sogenannten Sehsphäre zu den infracorticalen Opticus Centren und zum Nervus Opticus. *Archiv fuer Psychiatrie und Nervenkrankheien, 20,* 714–781.

Waller, A. V. (1850). Experiments on the section of the glossopharyngeal and hypoglossal nerves of the frog, and observations of the alterations produced thereby in the structure of their primitive fibers. *Philosophical Transactions of the Royal Society of London, 140,* 423–429.

Weigert, C. (1895). Beiträge zur Kenntnis der normalen menschlichen Glia. *Abhandlungen der Senkenbergischen Naturforschenden Gesellschaft, 19,* 65–216.

Weigert, C. (1906). Über eine neue Untersuschungsmethode des Zentralnervensystems. *Gesammelte Abhandlungen, 2,* 533–538.

Yakovlev, P. I. (1959). *The development and functional organization of the brain as revealed by the study of malformations.* Presented at a conference on research and training in the field of mental retardation, Lynchburg Training School and Hospital, Colony, Virginia.

Yakovlev, P. I. (1970). Whole-brain serial sections. In C. G. Tedeschi (Ed.), *Neuropathology: Methods and diagnosis.* Boston: Little, Brown. pp. 371–378.

Yakovlev, P. I., Locke, S., & Angevine, J. B. (1966). The limbus of the cerebral hemisphere, limbic nuclei of the thalamus and the cingulum bundle. In D. P. Purpura & M. D. Yahr (Eds.), *The thalamus.* New York: Columbia University Press, pp. 77–97.

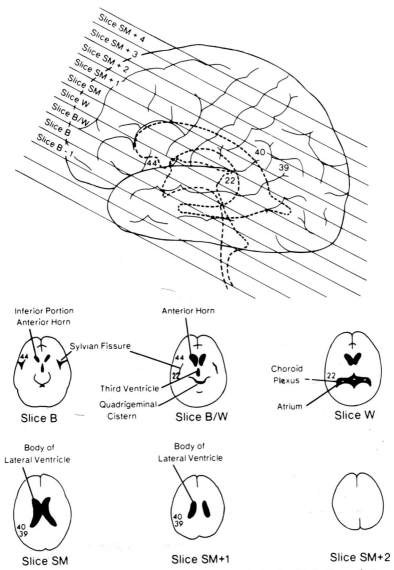

Figure 1. Lateral and cross-sectional views of the brain which show relationship of cortical language areas to shape of ventricles on CT scan slices. Broca's area is 44; Wernicke's area, 22; the supramarginal gyrus, 40; and angular gyrus, 39. (Reprinted with permission, *Neurology*, Naeser and Hayward, 1978).

cipital horns. This slice is just at the roof of the third ventricle. The calcified choroid plexus is readily observed in the left atrium at slice W. Wernicke's area is anterior and lateral to the left atrium on slice W. Slice SM (supramarginal gyrus slice) is marked by the bow-shaped bodies of the lateral ventricles. The bodies are close together at this slice, but separated one slice higher (SM + 1). The supramarginal gyrus (40) is lateral to the posterior half of the body of the lateral ventricle. The angular gyrus (39) is posterior to the supramarginal gyrus. Slice SM + 1 (one cm above slice SM) is similar to slice SM.

Most CT scans used in our research were done at 15–20 degrees above the canthomeatal line. Occasionally, scans were done at near zero (horizontal), or 25–35 degrees above the canthomeatal line. In the latter two instances, the complete shape of the ventricles obviously did not coincide with the complete shape of the ventricles observed on scans done at 15–20 degrees (Figure 1). In such unusual instances, each slice was labeled (B, B/W, W, SM, SM + 1) according to the specific region of interest—that is, if the patient's lesion was an *anterior* one, then the shape of the *frontal horns, only* was used to label the slice, not the shape of the third ventricle, temporal horns or occipital horns; if the patient's lesion was a *posterior* one, then the shape of the *third ventricle, atrium,* or *bodies of the lateral ventricles, only* were used to label the slice not the shape of the frontal horns. Because the cortical language areas are immediately lateral to the ventricular landmarks used, the angulation at which the scan was performed did not alter this fixed relationship of an immediately adjacent cortical language area to a given ventricular shape (Hanaway, Scott, & Strother, 1977; Matsui & Hirano, 1978). Equivalent lesion localization information and slice labeling ultimately was obtained for all scans, whether done at 0, 20, or 35 degrees above the canthomeatal line.

CT scans used were done either on the Syntex System 60 CT Scanner at the Palo Alto, California V. A. Medical Center or on the Ohio Nuclear Delta 50 or 2010 CT Scanners at the Boston V. A. Medical Center. Each scanner had a pixel (picture element) size of 1 mm × 1 mm. The pixels for any given CT slice were represented on a 256 × 256 X–Y coordinate matrix which could be accessed with a floating cursor on a cathode ray tube viewer (CRT). (For more information regarding CT scan terminology, see McCullough, 1977.) Each CT slice for each patient was labeled (B, B/W, W, SM, SM + 1) as described, before any detailed computer analysis was done.

SEMIAUTOMATED COMPUTER PROGRAMS USED IN ANALYZING CT SCAN LESION SIZE

Quantification of lesion size on CT scans has taken two forms in our research: absolute infarct size (number of 1 mm × 1 mm pixels contained within the lesion), and percentage of left hemisphere (LH) tissue damage. Lesion size was computed in absolute number of 1 mm × 1 mm pixels so that the CT scan data later could be compared to previously published pathology reports where lesion size was reported in cm². Lesion size was also computed in percentage LH tissue damage to adjust for variation in hemisphere (head) size. Work with our programs has shown that the left hemisphere can range in size from 6000 to 11,000 pixels, depending on the patient's head size and the slice level observed (Naeser, Hayward, Laughlin, Becker, Jernigan, & Zatz, 1981).

The two semiautomated computer programs that have been used are Automated Framing Program (AFP) (Naeser, Hayward, Laughlin, & Zatz, 1981) and Automated Hemisphere Program (AHP) (Naeser, Hayward, Laughlin, Becker, Jernigan, & Zatz, 1981). The AFP was designed to quantify the number of pixels in a lesion and the mean CT number (tissue density number) of those lesion pixels (i.e., how close was the mean lesion CT number to normal tissue or how close to lower CT numbers of cerebrospinal fluid and water levels, 0). A sample AFP lesion printout is shown in Figure 2. The AFP required the user to input the X–Y coordinates which "framed" the lesion in the left hemisphere. A 169-pixel Healthy Tissue Sample (HTS) was taken opposite the lesion from an analogous position in the right hemisphere. The mean CT number of the HTS was then compared to the framed lesion area with a t-test. Each four-pixel sample within the framed area that was significantly lower in CT number (closer to cerebrospinal fluid [CSF] or water level) was represented by a probability value marker ($-$, =, or *, referring to the p < .05, < .01, or < .001 levels, respectively) and printed out in matrix form. Note, the number of pixels in a lesion can be obtained in less than 1 minute on most CT scanners available today, without the AFP program. The investigator merely calls up the "irregular region of interest" or "map" function program at the CRT viewer screen, and traces over the lesion with the joy-stick controlled marker. The pixels are automatically counted and the total instantly appears on the CRT. These and other pixel-counting programs are standard software provided by most CT scan manufacturers today.

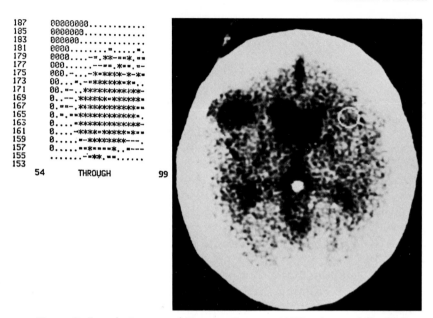

```
187    00000000............
185    0000000.............
183    000000..............
181    0000........".....".
179    0000....-=.*0K-==*.==
177    000......--==.*==.=-
175    000.-..-*=*0K0K-*-*=
173    00...=.-=*0K0K0K=*=..
171    00.=-..*0K0K0K0K0K.0K-
169    0..--.*0K0K0K=*0K0K0K=
167    0.==-.*0:0K0K0K0K0K0K==
165    0.=.==*0K0K0K0K0K0K=.
163    0....=*0K0K0K0K0K0K0K-
161    0....-*0K0K=*0K0K=*==
159    0.....=-*0K0K0K---.
157    0.....==*=====*.=---
155    .......-=*0K.==......
153
       54        THROUGH         99
```

Figure 2. Sample Automated Framing Program (AFP) printout (left) of left frontal lobe lesion on slice W (right). The lesion contained 684 pixels (2.6 cm × 2.6 cm). The white circle represents the approximate location of the 13 mm^2 (169 pixel) Healthy Tissue Sample (HTS) taken opposite the lesion in the right hemisphere. The patient, 44 years old, had a transcortical motor aphasia; the CT scan was done 1 year post-stroke. (Reprinted with permission, from *Brain and Language*, Naeser, Hayward, Laughlin, and Zatz, 1981).

The AHP (also labeled ASI–I, Automated Slice Information—I program, Jernigan, Zatz, Naeser, 1979) was designed to quantify the relative amount of LH tissue loss in percentage (Figure 3). This program requires the user to input the X–Y coordinates of the midline

Figure 3. Sample Automated Hemisphere Program (AHP) printout (right) of CT scan with left temporal lobe lesion in Wernicke's area on slice W (left). The percentage of significantly low CT number pixels in the right hemisphere representing ventricles, fissures, and sulci was 12.7% ($\frac{1301}{10,232}$ = 12.7%). The percentage significantly low CT number pixels in the left hemisphere representing ventricles, fissures, sulci, and lesion was 29.4% ($\frac{2820}{9580}$ = 29.4%). The LH %LoPix minus RH %LoPix was 16.7%. Hence, the relative percentage LH tissue damage at this slice W was 16.7%. The white circle represents the approximate location of the right hemisphere, Healthy Tissue Sample (R, HTS) which was always taken lateral to the third ventricle (or comparable midline structure) regardless of lesion locus for the AHP analysis. The patient, 60 years old, had a Wernicke's aphasia; the CT scan was done 9 months post-stroke (reprinted with permission from *Brain and Language*, Naeser, Hayward, Laughlin, Becker, Jernigan, and Zatz, 1981.)

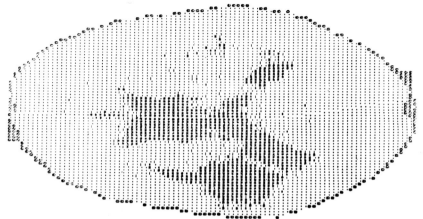

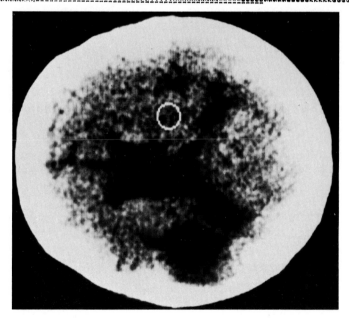

structures of the brain (interhemispheric fissure, septum pelluci-
dum, etc.) so that the right hemisphere (RH) and left hemisphere
(LH) can be compared. A 169-pixel R–HTS is taken just lateral to the
midline structures (usually mixed white and gray matter) on each
slice. The mean CT number of this R–HTS is then compared to 4-
pixel samples in the entire LH, then RH, with a t-test in a similar
manner to the AFP. The significantly low CT number areas in the
RH represented ventricle and fissures (RH % LoPix). (*LoPix* is the ab-
breviation for significantly low 4-pixel samples.) The significantly
low CT number areas in the LH represented ventricle and fissures
as well as lesion (LH % LoPix). The LH % LoPix minus RH % LoPix
represented the relative amount of LH tissue loss in percent, for
example, approximate LH lesion size.

The AFP and AHP results for six cortical aphasia groups (transcortical motor, Broca's, mixed, global, conduction, Wernicke's) and
four subcortical aphasia groups (three capsular/putaminal groups
and one thalamic case) are presented in this chapter. All aphasia
patients discussed had been examined with the Boston Diagnostic
Aphasia Exam (BDAE) (Goodglass & Kaplan, 1972), the Token Test
(TT) (Spreen & Benton, 1969), and an experimental syntactic comprehension test—the Palo Alto Syntax Test (PAST) (Naeser, Mazurski, Goodglass, Laughlin, Peraino, Pieniadz, & Leaper, 1983). These
patients had all met the criteria of righthandedness and single-ep-
isode, unilateral left hemisphere stroke (without neurosurgical intervention). Etiology was occlusive/vascular in all but three cases
where hemorrhage was present. The aphasia patients with cortical
lesions included 28 males and 4 females from 31 to 84 years of age
who were studied 2 months to 24 years post-stroke. The aphasia patients with subcortical lesions included 11 males and 1 female from
43 to 68 years of age who were studied acutely to 5 years post-stroke.

CORTICAL APHASIA GROUPS—SAMPLE CASES

CASE 1: TRANSCORTICAL MOTOR APHASIA

L. B. is a 70-year-old male former vice-president of an international bank who was studied with the BDAE at 5 months post-stroke
(MPS) (Table 1) and had a CT scan done at 6 MPS (Figure 4, top). A
mild right-sided hemiparesis had cleared within the first week.

Spontaneous speech was near normal, although sparse and
marked by obvious word-finding problems and occasional para-

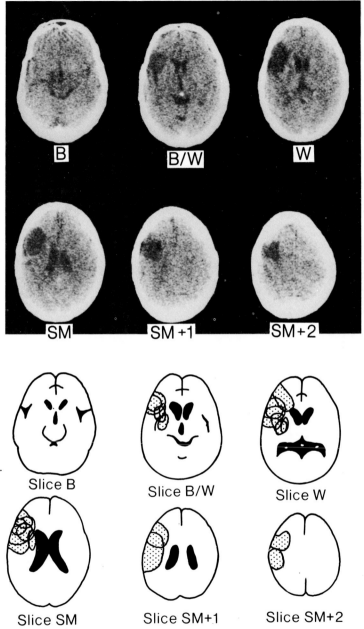

Figure 4. Transcortical Motor Aphasia CT scan for Case 1. L. B., age 70, 6 months post-stroke (above), and composite CT scan lesion sites for seven cases (below). Small lesions were primarily superior or deep to Broca's area on slices B/W and W the peak amount of tissue damage was at slice W (Figure 5). (Reprinted with permission, *Neurology*, Naeser and Hayward, 1978).

TABLE 1

Test Scores for Six Cortical and Four Subcortical Sample Aphasia Cases

	Transcortical Motor	Broca's	Mixed	Global	Conduction	Wernicke's	Caps/ Putamin. Ant–Sup.	Caps/ Putamin. Post.	Caps/ Putamin. Ant–Sup. & Post.	Thalamic
Age at Onset	70	51	69	61	53	55	53	43	64	69
Testing—Months Post Stroke	5	54	6	1/12	2/13	1/12	2/13	1	15	1/3
Fluency of Spontaneous Speech	Sparse, Gd. Artic. & Syntax	Nonfluent	Stereo-typed Phr.	None, only Monosyl.	Fluent, Literal Paraph.	Fluent, verbal Paraph.	Grammatical, Slow Dys-arthria	Fluent, Verbal Paraph.	None, only Monosyl.	Fluent Hypo-phonic
Number of Words per Phrase Length (7)	7	3	—	—	7/7	7/7	4/7	7	1	5/6
Articulatory Agility (7)	7	2	—	—	6/6	7/7	2.5/2	6	1	5/6
Grammatical Form (7)	7	2	—	—	7/7	7/7	5/7	7	1	5/6
Timed Verbal Oral Agility (14)	14	5	7	4/2	13/14	3/8	–/8	14	—	7/–
Timed Nonverbal Oral Agility (12)	12	9	7	4/2	5/6	4/4	11/10	6	—	5/–
Comprehension BDAE Z–Score (+1)	+.2	+.66	–.2	–1.5/–1.7	+.5/+.9	–.7/–.2	+.5/+1.0	–.6	–1.05	–.5/+.5
Body Parts (20)	17	18	7	2/0	14.5/18	6/12	18/20	13.5	11	12/16
Complex Ideat. Material (12)	7	9	9	0/0	10/11	5/4	6/10	1	0	8/–

Test	70%	90%	55%	–/27%	89%/84%	48%/67%	90%/91%	—	61%	–/80%
Token Test (100%)	70%	90%	55%	–/27%	89%/84%	48%/67%	90%/91%	—	61%	–/80%
Repetition—Words (10)	8	7	6	2/4	8/9	4/7	4/9	9	0	10/10
Repetition—High Probability Phrases (8)	8	2	0	1/0	2/7	0/0	7/8	4	0	7/8
Repetition—Low Probability Phrases (8)	6	0	0	0/0	0/7	0/0	2/3	4	0	4/5
Naming Pictures (105)	94	98	0	0/12	76/105	44/66	–/102	61	0	62/99
Objects (18)	18	18	0	0/4	9/18	0/4	–/18	9	0	12/18
Letters (18)	16	13	0	0/0	18/18	15/15	–/18	15	0	18/18
Category Recall Animal Names (19)	6	10	—	–/–	5/11	3/7	–/6	2	—	3/–
Word-Fluency Letters F, A, S (41)	3	10	—	–/–	12/12	–/11	–/6	—	—	–/–
Silent Reading Sentence Comp. (10)	7	8	8	0/0	7/10	4/8	–/3	3	0	1/8?
Bucco-Facial Apraxia	None	Mod.	None	Sev.	Mild	None	Mild	None	Sev.	Mild
Left Limb Apraxia	Mild	Mod.	Sev.	Sev.	Mild	Mild	None	Mild	Sev.	Mild

73

phasias. When asked to describe his profession, he said, "Well, International Bank, I was vice chairman of the International Bank. . . . I 'prognose' the work that was done . . . uh . . . uh . . . that's all."

Comprehension was only mildly impaired at 5 MPS and improved to near normal at 18 MPS (+.75). Sentence repetition was good. Although picture naming was good, category word recall was extremely poor. He named only six animals in 1 minute at 5 MPS, and seven at 18 MPS. He could name only one word per letter (F, A, or S) in the Spreen Benton word fluency test. A score of three words placed him in the eighth percentile for aphasics on this test (18 MPS). This problem with word recall had also been obvious in his spontaneous speech, which was sparse, and marked with many word-finding pauses. This patient did not return to work. He was able to golf and made several trips. At 2 years post-stroke, he died from a massive second stroke.

CT SCAN FINDINGS IN TRANSCORTICAL MOTOR APHASIA

The CT scan of patient L. B. in Figure 4 (top) revealed a small lesion in Broca's area lateral to the left frontal horn, on slice B/W. There was no lesion in Broca's area on slice B. The remainder of the lesion extended into the higher left frontal lobe. The number of lesion pixels at slice B/W was only 400 (approximately 2 cm × 2 cm); the largest portion of the lesion was present above Broca's area at slice W 1108 lesion pixels (3.3 cm × 3.3 cm). At slice SM, there were only 724 lesion pixels (2.7 cm × 2.7 cm). The percentage LH tissue damage at slice B/W was 7.9%; at slice W, 11.6%; and at slice SM, 11.1%.

Previous studies have shown that transcortical motor aphasia (TCM) is often observed with small frontal lobe lesions which are, primarily, either superior or deep to Broca's area (Benson & Geschwind, 1971). These are often labeled "watershed lesions," because they are located between the distribution of the left middle and left anterior cerebral arteries. In addition, TCM has been observed in cases where branches of the anterior cerebral artery have been occluded (Alexander & Schmitt, 1980; Kertesz, Lesk, & McCabe, 1977; Rubens, 1975).

The results of the AFP and AHP lesion-size analyses on the CT scan slices of seven TCM aphasics are shown in Tables 2 and 3. The mean number of lesion pixels per CT scan slice where lesion was present was 483 or only 2.2 cm × 2.2 cm. Figure 5 shows in bar

TABLE 2

Number of Lesion Pixels at Each CT Slice for Six Cortical Aphasia Groups
(Total per Patient and Mean per Lesion Slice, below)

	Tcm	Broca's	Mixed	Global	Conduction	Wernicke's
Slice B						
No. Pts.:	2	2	3	4	0	1
x̄:	308	834	1026	2260	—	336
S.D.:	22	659	834	696	—	—
Slice B/W						
No. Pts.	6	3	5	4	1	1
x̄:	326	994	1396	2446	716	816
S.D.:	97	648	617	532	—	—
Slice W						
No. Pts.:	6	3	6	5	4	4
x̄:	536	1026	1477	2370	347	737
S.D.:	356	273	711	662	271	406
Slice SM						
No. Pts.:	5	3	6	5	5	4
x̄:	517	945	1221	2100	518	675
S.D.:	304	91	711	398	576	615
Slice SM + 1						
No. Pts.:	2	3	3	5	3	3
x̄:	866	1072	1585	1896	813	962
S.D.	42	128	946	890	354	285
Slice SM + 2						
No. Pts.:	2	3	2	4	3	2
x̄:	500	956	2754	1674	492	618
S.D.:	237	590	2005	1032	114	223
Total lesion pixels per patient						
No. Pts.:	7	3	6	5	5	4
x̄:	1588	5723	6852	12,477	1816	2731
S.D.:	1341	2314	4575	5580	1956	1538
Mean number lesion pixels per lesion slice						
No. Slices:	23	18	27	32	18	15
x̄:	483	953	1522	1949	504	728
S.D.:	272	379	873	790	382	397

graph form the relative percentage LH tissue damage (LH % LoPix − RH % LoPix) at each CT scan language slice for six cortical aphasia groups. The peak amount of tissue damage for these TCM aphasics was 7.6% at slice W. Patient L. B. fits well into this lesion-size profile because the peak lesion size for this case was also at

TABLE 3

Percentage LH Tissue Damage[a] (LH %LoPix Minus RH %LoPix) at Each CT Slice for Six Cortical Aphasia Groups and One Negative Control Group

	Tcm		Broca's		Mixed		Global		Conduction		Wernicke's		Aphasics		Controls	
	x̄	S.D.	x̄	S.D.	x̄	S.D.	x̄	S.D.	x̄	S.D.	x̄	S.D.	x̄	S.D.	x̄	S.D.
Slice B																
RH %	14.3	4.4	15.7	5.5	17.0	2.8	18.5	11.4	11.3	4.4	15.3	4.4	15.3	6.0	10.1	7.6
LH %	18.3	4.7	21.4	2.6	29.7	9.8	40.4	14.1	13.6	3.8	16.9	4.1	23.1	11.5	10.6	7.8
L–R %	4.0	4.4	5.7	7.2	12.7	9.6	21.9	11.2	2.3	2.9	1.7	2.4	7.9	9.6	.5	1.9
Slice B/W																
RH %	14.0	5.2	10.6	4.8	15.2	3.6	14.2	5.4	11.5	2.7	11.4	3.8	13.0	4.4	10.1	6.3
LH %	18.9	5.6	20.4	9.4	27.8	9.4	42.7	14.8	13.7	3.6	17.7	5.8	23.4	12.4	9.4	6.7
L–R %	4.8	3.3	9.8	9.1	12.5	6.8	28.5	12.0	2.2	2.2	6.3	3.4	10.4	10.6	-.7	1.7
Slice W																
RH %	13.5	6.8	16.9	5.0	15.9	4.7	20.0	6.7	11.3	2.7	15.5	8.4	15.4	6.5	8.2	5.2
LH %	21.2	6.9	31.9	4.8	32.6	8.2	50.7	12.6	13.8	2.9	25.8	10.8	28.9	13.8	8.5	4.7
L–R %	7.6	3.4	15.0	5.9	16.8	8.6	30.7	7.4	2.5	1.3	10.4	4.1	13.5	10.3	.3	1.4
Slice SM																
RH %	14.4	5.0	20.5	3.8	19.6	4.7	21.7	5.9	12.5	3.7	17.9	7.2	17.5	5.8	12.6	4.1
LH %	21.2	6.4	36.4	4.3	37.6	6.1	52.7	15.3	18.4	4.9	28.8	8.5	31.9	13.9	13.3	4.6
L–R %	6.9	6.1	15.9	5.2	18.1	6.8	31.1	11.0	5.9	2.7	10.9	4.9	14.4	10.5	.8	1.6
Slice SM + 1																
RH %	5.3	3.4	12.3	3.1	13.4	9.9	15.4	5.3	6.9	3.7	11.8	13.1	10.5	7.6	10.4	4.6
LH %	10.4	8.6	33.0	3.7	28.4	13.1	43.8	18.5	12.2	6.7	19.0	18.5	23.6	16.7	9.2	3.9
L–R %[a]	5.1	6.4	20.7	4.2	15.1	9.7	28.4	15.6	5.2	5.4	7.2	5.9	13.1	12.0	-1.2	2.5
Overall slices																
RH %	12.3	2.1	15.2	3.1	16.1	3.3	18.0	6.6	10.7	2.3	14.4	5.7	14.3	4.4	10.3	3.3
LH %	18.0	4.1	28.6	3.7	31.3	6.0	46.1	14.7	14.3	3.4	21.9	7.7	26.2	12.5	10.3	3.4
L–R %	5.7	3.3	13.4	5.5	15.2	5.8	28.1	11.2	3.6	2.4	7.5	2.9	11.9	9.8	.02	.9

[a] LH tissue damage is defined here as the LH %LoPix minus the RH %LoPix. LoPix refers to CSF. See text for further description of %LoPix.

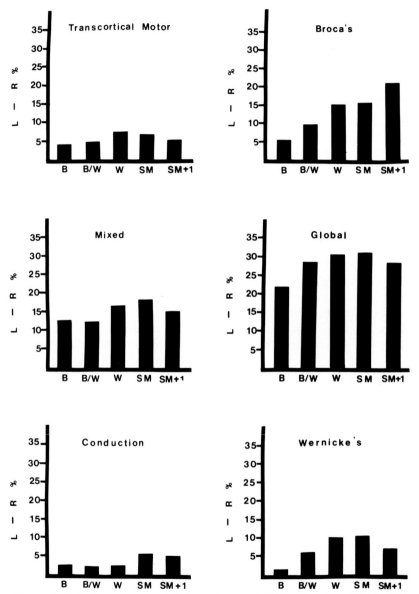

Figure 5. Relative percentage LH tissue damage (LH %LoPix minus RH %LoPix) at each CT scan slice for six cortical aphasia groups. (Reprinted with permission from *Brain and Language*, Naeser, Hayward, Laughlin, Becker, Jernigan, and Zatz, 1981.)

slice W—that is, 3.3 cm × 3.3 cm, or 11.6% LH tissue damage at that slice.

In summary, TCM aphasia was defined in our study as a milder form of aphasia with good comprehension (BDAE z – score, +.8 to +1.0; Token Test, 88–97%) and good sentence repetition. Speech was sparse but well articulated and syntactically correct, although marked with obvious word-finding problems and occasional paraphasias. The CT scan lesion sites were, primarily, superior or deep to Broca's area (Figure 4, bottom). The mean lesion size was approximately 500 pixels per slice (2.2 cm × 2.2 cm) and the peak amount of tissue damage was at slice W.

CASE 2: BROCA'S APHASIA

O. F. is a 51-year-old male who was studied with the Boston Diagnostic Aphasia Examination at 4½ years post-stroke (Table 1) and had a CT scan done at 7 years post-stroke (Figure 6, top). He had a lasting right hemiplegia.

Speech was nonfluent, with reduced number of words, slow rate of speech, telegraphic syntax, more nouns than verbs, and absence of functor words (Goodglass & Berko–Gleason, 1960). When asked to describe the "Cookie Theft Picture" from the BDAE, the patient said the following: "Well . . . mess . . . uh 'sggaa . . . dder' cookie, uh-oh, fall down . . . wife spill water . . . and uh 'dis . . . ez' . . . and, uh 'tsups' and saucer and plate . . . I, uh . . . no . . . done!" The description was spoken in a monotone and with great motoric effort in articulation.

Comprehension was good. Sentence repetition was poor, with nonfluent responses. "Down to earth" was repeated "Down to erts" (distorted articulation) and "Go ahead and do it if possible" was repeated "Go . . . to . . . do . . . it" (word omissions, telegraphic syntax). At 10 years post-stroke, this patient's hemiplegia and aphasia remained essentially unchanged.

CT SCAN FINDINGS IN BROCA'S APHASIA

The CT scan of patient O. F. in Figure 6 (top) revealed a large lesion in Broca's area lateral to the left frontal horn on both slices B and B/W. The lesion extended medially from Broca's area to reach the frontal horn, and included the caudate, internal capsule, and

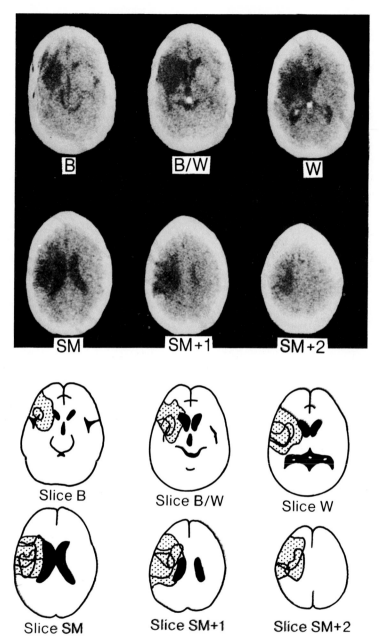

Figure 6. Broca's Aphasia. CT scan for Case 2. O. F., age 51, 7 years post-stroke (above), and composite CT scan lesion sites for four cases (below). Large lesions were located in Broca's area on slices B and/or B/W and the peak amount of tissue damage was high in the frontoparietal areas at slices SM and SM + 1 (Figure 5) (reprinted with permission, *Neurology*, Naeser and Hayward, 1978).

basal ganglia. In addition, the large lesion extended superiorly to include the pre- and post-Rolandic areas in the frontal and parietal lobes at slices W, SM and SM + 1. The temporal lobe was spared. The number of lesion pixels at slice B was 1300 (3.6 cm × 3.6 cm) and at B/W, 1740 (4.2 cm × 4.2 cm). The lesion size at each remaining slice was large, 1000–1300 pixels. The percentage LH tissue damage at slice B was 15.8%, at B/W, 23.4%, and 21–23% on the remaining slices (W, SM, SM + 1).

Long-lasting Broca's aphasia is associated with large lesions which often extend from Broca's area to the anterior portions of the parietal lobe (Kertesz *et al.*, 1979; Mazzocchi & Vignolo, 1980; Mohr, Pessin, Finkelstein, Funkenstein, Duncan, & Davis, 1978; Naeser & Hayward, 1978). Occlusive-vascular type lesions producing Broca's aphasia have been associated with occlusion of the superior division, left middle cerebral artery (Altemus, Roberson, Miller Fisher, & Pessin, 1976).

The results of the AFP and AHP lesion-size analyses on the CT scan slices of four Broca's aphasics are shown in Tables 2 and 3. The average number of lesion pixels per CT scan slice where lesion was present was 953 or 3.1 cm × 3.1 cm. Figure 5 shows, in bar graph form, the relative percentage LH tissue damage at each CT scan language slice for the Broca's aphasia group. The lesion-size profile for this group has a stair-step shape, with the largest amount of tissue damage at the higher slices. Patient O. F. fits well into this lesion-size profile as the lesion was large at slice B (15.8%) and even larger at the higher slices, SM and SM + 1 (21–23%).

In summary, Broca's aphasia was defined in our study as a moderate form of aphasia with good comprehension (BDAE *z*-score, +.5 to +.9; Token Test, 65–91%) but poor sentence repetition. Speech was nonfluent. The CT scan lesion sites extended from Broca's area to the anterior parietal lobe, frequently including deep structures such as the caudate, internal capsule and/or basal ganglia (Figure 6, bottom). The lesion size was approximately 1000 pixels (3.2 cm × 3.2 cm) per slice and the tissue damage profile was stair-step in shape with large lesions at each slice, especially the higher slices.

Melodic Intonation Therapy (MIT) (Albert, Sparks, & Helm, 1973; Sparks, Helm, & Albert, 1974) has been shown to be effective in reducing the impaired articulation and increasing number of words per phrase length in Broca's aphasics treated with this singing, rhythm-tapping program. A recent study has shown that Broca's aphasics with CT scan lesion sites similar to those described in Figure 6 are particularly amenable to treatment with the MIT approach (Helm-Estabrooks, Naeser, & Kleefield, 1980).

CASE 3: MIXED APHASIA

S. E. is a 69-year-old male business executive who was studied with the Boston Diagnostic Aphasia Examination at six MPS (Table 1), and also had a CT scan done at six MPS (Figure 7, top). The patient had a lasting right hemiplegia, right sensory deficit, and right homonymous hemianopia.

Speech was very limited, yet marked with paraphasias. His description of the Cookie Theft Picture was as follows: "Well, the, uh, 'shesus Christ.' Well, what do you want? Oh, the 'bi passage is going strong.' Kitchen run." At 13 MPS, there was no improvement in information content, although paraphasias were reduced. "That's fine 'n' dandy . . . uh (uda) How's the . . . god damn, god damn . . . I don't see the point, but . . . that's fine and dandy . . . you see, I don't know what the hell."

Comprehension was only moderately impaired at six MPS. Although he could repeat single words such as "what," "chair," "hammock," and "fifteen," polysyllabic words and sentences were very difficult. Neologisms and paraphasic errors were common: "You know how" was repeated "Ho hay tsu" and "Down to earth," "Earth deduct one, no," and "Limes are sour," "Sour milk," and "I got home from work," "I work to work . . . I want to work."

The ability to name pictures was extremely impaired; most errors were "no response" although he did say "ring" for "key." He scored 8/8 in Word Picture Matching and there was remarkable sparing for silent reading comprehension. Writing with his left hand was almost nonexistent. He could sign his name or copy words but did not write letters or words.

The patient was classified as a "mixed" aphasic because, although speech output was severely impaired (limited to stereotyped phrases), his comprehension was moderately impaired and his reading mildly impaired. The "mixed" group of aphasics in this study generally were considered to be more severely involved in speech output and comprehension than the Broca's, but not as severely involved as the globals. The Token Test scores ranged from 52% to 67% for these "mixed" cases, 65% to 91% for the Broca's, and 33% to 47% for the globals. This was a group of aphasics whose aphasia

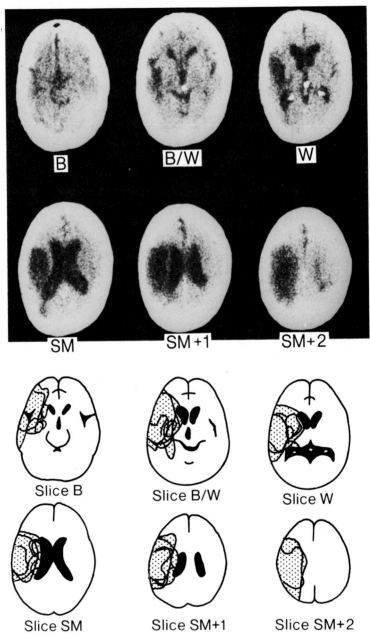

Figure 7. Mixed Aphasia. CT scan for Case 3. S. E., age 61, 6 months post-stroke (above) and composite CT scan lesion sites for seven cases (below). Lesions were more heterogeneous and some spared Broca's or Wernicke's areas.

was generally considered moderate-to-severe. Future studies may reveal that the subjects within this group actually comprise many subgroups.

CT SCAN FINDINGS IN MIXED APHASIA

The CT scan for patient S. E. in Figure 7 (top) revealed no cortical lesion in Broca's or Wernicke's areas, but did show a large temporal lobe lesion deep to Wernicke's area on slice B/W and W, including auditory radiations in the temporal isthmus area (see Figure 12, within Subcortical Aphasia section). There was also some involvement of the insula, extreme capsule, claustrum, and external capsule at slices B/W and W. The major portion of the lesion was in the frontal and parietal lobes (including pre- and post-Rolandic and supramarginal gyrus areas) at slices SM, SM + 1, and SM + 2.

The lesion sizes were as follows: slice B, no isolated lesion; slice B/W, 876 pixels; slice W, 1672 pixels; slice SM, 2028 pixels; slice SM + 1, 2596 pixels; and SM + 2, 4170 pixels (6.5 cm × 6.5 cm). The percent LH tissue damage was as follows: slice B/W, 11%; W, 13.6%; SM, 18.5%; SM + 1, 22.2%.

It is important to note that although this "mixed" aphasia case had a stair-step lesion-size profile similar to the Broca's group, the size of the lesion (no lesion at slice B and 11% at slice B/W) and location of the lesion (deep in left temporal lobe at slice B/W) were not compatible with the lesion sizes or sites of Broca's aphasics.

The results of the AFP and AHP lesion-size analyses for six mixed aphasics are shown in Tables 2 and 3. The average number of lesion pixels present per CT scan slice where lesion was present, was 1522 or 3.9 cm × 3.9 cm.

In summary, the mixed aphasics were defined in our study as a moderate-to-severe form of aphasia where, although the patients had severe speech and repetition problems, their comprehension was moderately impaired (BDAE z-score, -1.0 to $+.1$; Token Test, 52–67%). The CT scan lesion sites were rather heterogeneous and, in some cases, did not even include Broca's or Wernicke's cortical language areas, although other cortical and subcortical lesion areas were obvious (Figure 7, bottom). The lesion size was approximately 1500 pixels (3.9 cm × 3.9 cm) per slice and the mean percentage LH tissue damage ranged 12–18% per slice.

CASE 4: GLOBAL APHASIA

L. P. is a 61-year-old male painting contractor who was studied with the BDAE at one and 12 MPS (Table 1) and had a CT scan done at seven MPS (Figure 8, top). The patient had a dense right hemiplegia, right sensory deficit, and right homonymous hemianopia.

Speech was nonexistent or limited to short, perseverated, stereotyped syllables or phrases spoken with motoric effort and distorted articulation. This patient's Cookie Theft Picture description was limited to "Go place . . . pl . . . place."

The patient had severe language comprehension problems. Repetition of single words was severely impaired. He was able to repeat only "purple" and "brown" in single-word repetition. He was not able to repeat any sentences and tended to echo back only the last word—that is, "Down to earth" was repeated "Nearth, birth, no," and "Limes are sour," "bour," and "I got home from work," "work." Severe deficits were also observed in naming, reading, and writing.

CT SCAN FINDINGS IN GLOBAL APHASIA

The CT scan of L. P. in Figure 8 (top) showed a large left frontal, temporal, and parietal lobe lesion on all CT scan slices, including complete involvement of Broca's, Wernicke's, and supramarginal gyrus areas, surface, and deep. The deep extension of the lesion included internal capsule and basal ganglia (slice B/W as well as white matter and the arcuate fasciculus (Slice SM). The number of lesion pixels at slice B was 2688 (5.2 cm × 5.2 cm); B/W, 3316 (5.8 cm × 5.8 cm); W, 3436; SM, 2720; and SM + 1, 1904. The percentage LH tissue damage at slice B was 17.2%; B/W, 33.1%; W, 40.8%; SM, 31.1%; and SM + 1, 27.0%.

The lesion locus and extent is compatible with other published CT scan research papers that have dealt with cortical global aphasics (Kertesz et al., 1979; Mazzocchi & Vignolo, 1980). These large lesions are compatible with complete occlusion of the left middle cerebral artery and/or the left internal carotid, with varying amounts of collateral blood flow (Kertesz et al., 1977; Yarnell et al., 1976).

The results of the AFP and AHP lesion-size analyses on the CT scan slices of five global aphasics are shown in Tables 2 and 3. The average number of lesion pixels per CT scan slice where lesion was present was 1942 (4.4 cm × 4.4 cm). Figure 5 shows the bar graph profile of relative percentage LH tissue damage for the global group.

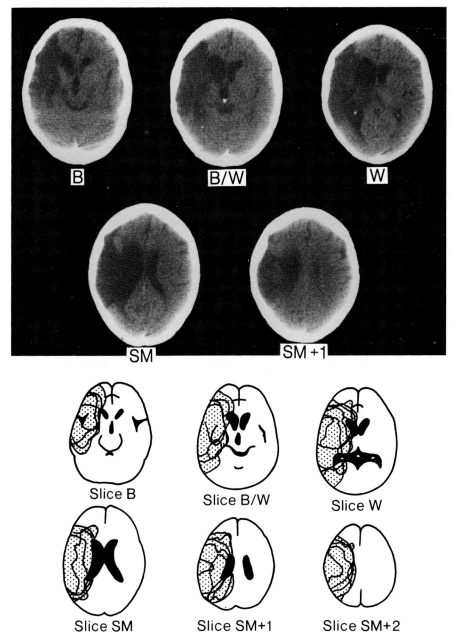

Figure 8. Global Aphasia. CT scan for Case 4. L. P., age 61, 7 months post-stroke (above) and composite CT scan lesion sites for five cases (below). Large lesions were present in every language area, Broca's, slices B and B/W; Wernicke's, slices B/W and W; supramarginal gyrus and arcuate fasciculus, slices SM and SM+1.

Each slice has a mean percentage LH tissue damage which ranged from 21.9% (slice B) to 31.1% (slice SM). The lesion size for patient L. P. extended beyond the mean lesion-size profile for globals. He had a range of 17.2–40.8% LH tissue damage at each slice.

In summary, global aphasia was defined in our study as a severe form of aphasia. The CT scan lesion sites included both Broca's and Wernicke's cortical language areas as well as structures deep to them. The large lesion always involved at least three lobes: frontal, parietal and temporal (Figure 8, bottom). The lesion size was approximately 2000 lesion pixels (4.5 cm × 4.5 cm) per slice and the tissue damage profile revealed 21–31% LH tissue damage at each slice.

The prognosis was extremely limited in all cases; we have only one patient who returned to gainful employment. Our records show one younger case, age 24, who was able to return to work in a quarry 5 years following bilateral head trauma and stroke. The patient was right-handed and had reversed CT scan hemispheric (skull) asymmetries—that is, the right occipital width and length were greater than the left. Increased left occipital width and length is the most common CT-scan hemispheric asymmetry observed in right handers (LeMay, 1977). Studies are currently investigating the relationship between CT scan hemispheric (skull) asymmetries and exceptional recovery patterns in aphasia (Pieniadz, Naeser, Koff, & Levine, 1979). Previous publications have suggested that some left handers have better recovery from aphasia than right handers (Gloning, Gloning, Haub & Quatember, 1969; Luria, 1970). A recent study by Pieniadz & Naeser (1981) has shown that in 15 cases where CT-scan measurements and planum temporale length measurements were possible at postmortem, the correlation between CT scan occipital length at slice SM and planum temporale length was .674 ($p < .01$). These authors hypothesize that the aphasics with reversed CT-scan hemispheric (skull) asymmetries may have better recovery, possibly due to anomalous (reversed or bilateral) cerebral dominance (Galaburda, LeMay, Kemper, & Geschwind, 1978).

CASE 5: CONDUCTION APHASIA

F. J. is a 53-year-old male house painter who was studied with the BDAE at 2 and 13 MPS (Table 1) and had a CT scan done at 4 MPS (Figure 9, top). The patient had a mild right hemiparesis which cleared within the first few weeks.

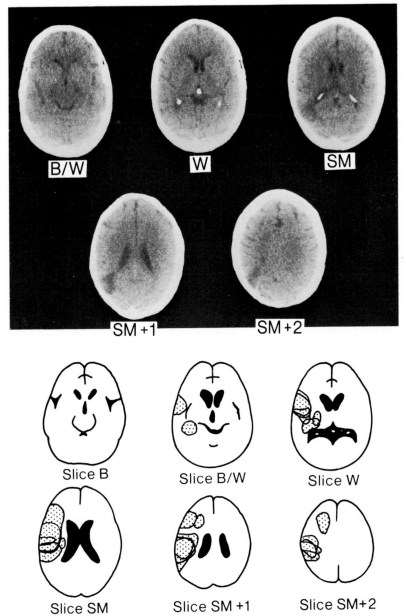

Figure 9. Conduction Aphasia. CT scan for Case 5. F. J., age 53, 4 months post-stroke (above), and composite CT scan lesion sites for six cases (below). Small lesions were primarily deep to Wernicke's area (slice W or in supramarginal gyrus at slices SM and SM + 1. The peak amount of LH tissue damage was at slice SM (Figure 5).

Speech was predominately fluent with literal paraphasias and word-finding problems. When asked to describe the Cookie Theft Picture, he said: "Well, the girl is want'in uh . . . a c'c'cookie, and, her brother is up on the stool to the cood-cookie . . . jar. Uh, he's fall'n, uh fall'n off the stool, and uh the mother is . . . uh . . . cleaning uh . . . dishes, and uh . . . a sink is . . . uh . . . over . . . flowing. There's a plate . . . and two . . . over there . . . and ch'cabinet in back."

The literal paraphasias included the "ch" in "cabinet" and "cood" in "cood-cookie jar." The sentences were spoken with normal intonation and ease of articulation. The patient was aware of his errors.

Comprehension was good at two MPS and near normal at nine MPS (+.9). Sentence repetition was poor, and fluent paraphasic responses were present. More literal than verbal paraphasias were present. The patient was aware of his errors, but was unable to correct them. "The vat leaks" was repeated "The vat kleaks"; "Near the table in the dining room" was repeated as "Near the table in the din . . . dan . . . dining land"; "No ifs, ands, or buts" was repeated as "Nos, ifs, buts, or nuts." Numbers were particularly difficult to repeat and were most often repeated as other numbers (verbal paraphasias). This patient repeated "forty-eight divided by sixteen" as "forty-nine divided by sixteen."

This patient received speech therapy for 1 year but was unable to return to work. One of the mild conduction aphasia cases was able to return to work as a travel clerk dispatcher approximately 1 year following stroke onset.

CT SCAN FINDINGS IN CONDUCTION APHASIA

The CT scan of patient F. J. in Figure 9 (top) revealed a small left parietal lobe infarct in the area of the supramarginal and angular gyri at slices SM and SM + 1 with further extension into the parietal lobe on slice SM + 2. Because the lesion extended deep from the supramarginal gyrus to the body of the lateral ventricle, the white matter arcuate fasciculus was also involved. This small, primarily parietal lobe lesion is compatible with occlusion of the posterior parietal or angular branches of the left middle cerebral artery.

The number of lesion pixels at slice SM was only 568 (2.4 cm × 2.4 cm) and at slice SM + 1, 656 (2.6 cm × 2.6 cm) and at slice SM + 2, 524 (2.3 cm × 2.3 cm). The percentage LH tissue damage at each slice was also small: at slice SM, 4.6%; at slice SM + 1, 4.7%.

Previous studies have shown conduction aphasia to be observed with lesions in the supramarginal gyrus area as well as posterior temporal lobe area (Benson, Sheremata, Bouchard, Segarra, Price, & Geschwind, 1973; Geschwind, 1965; Green & Howes, 1977; Kertesz *et al.*, 1979; Naeser & Hayward, 1978). In addition Damasio and Damasio (1980) recently have reported cases of conduction aphasia associated with small lesions in the insular area and extreme capsule area where a temporofrontal portion of the arcuate fasciculus is located.

Results of the AFP and AHP lesion-size analyses on the CT scan slices of five conduction aphasics are shown in Tables 2 and 3. The average number of lesion pixels per CT scan slice where lesion was present was only 504 (2.2 cm × 2.2 cm). Figure 5 shows the relative percentage LH tissue damage at each CT scan language slice for the conduction aphasics. The peak amount of tissue damage for the conduction aphasics occurred at slice SM (5.9%) and SM + 1 (5.2%). Patient F. J. fits well into this lesion-size profile because the peak lesion sizes for this case were also at slice SM (4.6%) and SM + 1 (4.7%).

In summary, conduction aphasia was characterized in our study as a milder form of fluent aphasia with good comprehension (BDAE z-scores ranged from +.5 to +1.0; Token Test scores, 82 to 100%), but poor repetition with fluent paraphasic responses. Speech was better than repetition and was predominantly fluent with literal paraphasias and word-finding problems. The patient was aware of his errors but could not correct them. The CT scan lesion sites were primarily superior to Wernicke's area on slices SM and SM + 1 in the supramarginal gyrus and arcuate fasciculus area and/or deep to Wernicke's area, on slice W, in the arcuate fasciculus (Figure 9, bottom). The mean lesion size was approximately only 500 pixels per slice (2.2 cm × 2.2 cm). The peak amount of tissue damage was at slices SM and SM + 1.

CASE 6: WERNICKE'S APHASIA

M. L. is a 55-year-old male undertaker who was studied with the BDAE at 1 and 12 MPS (Table 1) and had a CT scan done at 4 MPS (Figure 10, top). A mild right hemiparesis (arm greater than leg) and right visual field deficit were present.

Speech was fluent, with multiple verbal and literal paraphasias. Variety of grammatical form was present and speech was produced rapidly with clear articulation and good intonation. The patient was

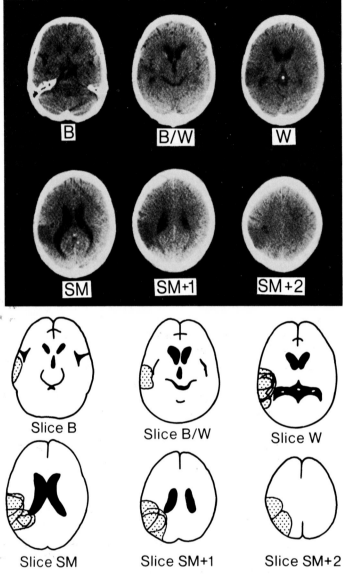

Figure 10. Wernicke's Aphasia. CT scan for Case 6. M. L., age 55, 4 months post-stroke (above) and composite CT scan lesion sites for four cases (below). Lesions were located in Wernicke's area at Slice W and in the supramarginal gyrus area at slice SM. The peak amount of LH tissue damage was at slices W and SM (Figure 5).

not aware of most errors. A sample from the picture description is as follows: "The mother's washing with some besses . . . dishes . . . plus the sink is 'falling down,' on the ground . . ."

Comprehension was poor at one MPS and still moderately impaired 1 year later. He had particular problems with body part and sentence comprehension (Table 1). Sentence repetition was extremely poor and responses contained multiple verbal paraphasias and extended English jargon. "Down to earth" was repeated "Off down to birth . . . on to earth," and "The spy fled to Greece," "The spy . . . spoke to Greece"; and "I stopped at his front door and rang the bell," "I stopped at the door to help the bell."

CT SCAN FINDINGS IN WERNICKE'S APHASIA

The CT scan of patient M. L. in Figure 10 (top) showed a left temporal lobe infarct in Wernicke's area on slices B/W and W. The temporal lobe lesion extended into the parietal lobe in the area of the supramarginal gyrus on slice SM. There was supramarginal and angular gyrus involvement on slice SM + 1 with additional extension into the inferior parietal lobule on higher slices. The deep extension of this lesion on slice W from the superior temporal gyrus to the left atrium included involvement of the optic radiations.

The number of lesion pixels at slice B/W was 640 (2.5 cm × 2.5 cm); at W, 944 (3.1 cm × 3.1 cm); SM, 936 (3.1 cm × 3.1 cm); and at SM + 1, 1068 (3.3 cm × 3.3 cm). The percentage LH tissue damage at each slice was as follows: slice B, 6.3%; B/W, 7.9%; W, 12.6%; SM, 14.9%; and SM + 1, 18.7%.

Previous studies have shown Wernicke's aphasia to be primarily associated with large left temporoparietal lesions (Benson & Geschwind, 1971; Benson & Patten, 1967; Kertesz et al., 1977, 1979; Mazzocchi & Vignolo, 1980; Naeser & Hayward, 1978). In stroke patients, these lesion sites are compatible with occlusion of the inferior division of the left middle cerebral artery (Altemus et al., 1976).

Results of the AFP and AHP lesion-size analyses on the CT scan slices of five Wernicke's aphasics are shown in Tables 2 and 3. The average number of lesion pixels per CT scan slice where lesion was present was 728 (2.7 cm × 2.7 cm). Figure 5 shows, in bar graph form, the relative percentage LH tissue damage at each CT scan language slice. The peak amount of tissue damage for the Wernicke's aphasics occurred at slices W (10.4%) and SM (10.9%). Patient M. L. fits well into this lesion-size profile because greater than 10% LH tissue damage was present at slice W (12.6%) as well as slice SM (14.9%).

In summary, Wernicke's aphasia was characterized in our study as a moderate–severe fluent aphasia with poor comprehension (BDAE z-score, -1.0 to $+.7$; Token Test, 47–77%) and poor repetition. Spontaneous speech was characterized by verbal paraphasias and extended English jargon. The patients were unaware of their errors. The CT scan lesion sites were located in Wernicke's area on slices B/W and W, and in the supramarginal gyrus area on slices SM and SM+1 (Figure 10, bottom). The mean lesion size per slice was approximately 750 pixels (2.7 cm $\times$ 2.7 cm). The peak amount of tissue damage was both infra-Sylvian on slice W and supra-Sylvian on slice SM.

Statistical Comparison of Lesion-Size Data between Aphasia Groups: Transcortical Motor versus Broca's Aphasics

The TCM aphasia group had significantly smaller mean number lesion pixels per slice (483) than did the Broca's aphasics (953) ($p <$ .001). T-tests applied to the L–R %LoPix differences for these two groups revealed significantly smaller lesions for the TCM group both at slice SM ($p < .05$) and slice SM+1 ($p < .001$) than for the Broca's. Thus, the CT scan data supported the behavioral data (smaller frontal lobe lesions, mild TCM aphasia versus larger frontal lobe lesions, Broca's aphasia).

A discriminant analysis was done with the AHP data, utilizing mean L–R %LoPix differences at each of the five language slices for seven TCM and four Broca's aphasics. In this analysis, 6/7 TCM aphasics and 4/4 Broca's aphasics were correctly classified (91% correct). To make the classifications, the discriminant analysis utilized the L–R %LoPix differences at slice SM+1 only.

BROCA'S VERSUS MIXED APHASICS

There was no significant difference in lesion size at any single CT scan slice between the mixed and the Broca's aphasics. There was, however, a significant difference between the mixed and the Broca's in mean number lesion pixels per slice ($p < .01$): mixed, 1522; Broca's 953.

A discriminant analysis was done with the AHP data, utilizing mean L–R %LoPix differences at each of the five language slices for five mixed and four Broca's aphasics. In this analysis, 4/5 mixed and 4/4 Broca's were correctly classified (89%). The discriminant analysis utilized L–R %LoPix differences first at slice B, then slices SM + 1, SM, and slice B/W to make the classifications.

MIXED VERSUS GLOBAL APHASICS

The global aphasics' mean number of lesion pixels was significantly larger than that for the mixed aphasics at slices B/W ($p < .01$), W ($p < .01$), and SM ($p < .05$). T-tests applied to the L–R %LoPix differences for these two groups revealed significantly larger lesions for the globals at slice B/W ($p < .05$) and slice W ($p < .05$).

A discriminant analysis was done with the AHP data, utilizing mean L–R %LoPix differences at each of the five language slices for five mixed and five global aphasics. In this analysis, 5/5 mixed and 4/5 globals were correctly classified (90% correct). The discriminant analysis utilized the L–R %LoPix differences, first at slice W, then slice B, then slice SM to make the classifications. Thus, the quantitative CT scan data supported the behavioral data in terms of severity of aphasia—that is, the larger lesions (21–31% LH tissue damage per slice) were associated with the more severe global aphasia, and the smaller lesions (12–18% LH tissue damage per slice) with the more moderate-to-severe mixed aphasia.

CONDUCTION VERSUS WERNICKE'S APHASICS

There was no significant difference in mean number lesion pixels per lesion slice between the conduction and Wernicke's aphasics (504 versus 728) although the Wernicke's aphasics did have significantly larger mean percentage LH tissue damage than the conductions at slice W ($p < .01$) (10.4 versus 7.6%). Thus, at slice W, the more severe aphasia was associated with the larger temporal lobe lesion.

A discriminant analysis was done with the AHP data, utilizing the mean percentage LH tissue damage at each of the five language slices for five conduction aphasics and four Wernicke's aphasics. In this analysis 5/5 conduction aphasics and 4/4 Wernicke's aphasics were correctly classified (100%). The percentage LH tissue damage only at slice W was used to make the classification.

TRANSCORTICAL MOTOR VERSUS CONDUCTION
APHASICS

The mild TCM aphasics were similar to the other mild aphasia
group, the conduction aphasics, in that they also had two peak lesion slices which were above a primary language area. The TCMs
had their *peak* amount of tissue damage anteriorly at slices W and
SM (frontal lobe lesions above Broca's area), and the conductions
had their peak amount of tissue damage posteriorly at slices SM and
SM + 1 (supramarginal gyrus, parietal lobe lesions above Wernicke's
area). There was no significant difference between the mild TCM
and mild conduction aphasia groups in mean number lesion pixels
per lesion slice (each was approximately 500 pixels). The TCM
aphasics had significantly (p < .01) greater percentage LH tissue
damage at slice W than the conduction aphasics (7.6 versus 2.5%)
and this was much more anteriorly located.

Correlations between lesion size (AFP and AHP data) and severity
of aphasia (BDAE, Token Test, and PAST data) are listed in Table 4.
Note, the highest correlations with the AFP lesion-size data were
−.86 with Token Test at slice B/W, and −.85 with syntactic comprehension at slice W. The highest correlation with the AHP lesion-
size data was −.74 with syntactic comprehension at slice W.

TABLE 4

CT Scan Lesion Size/Aphasia Severity Correlations: Summary of Results of
Two Methods
(Cortical Aphasia Cases Only)

	BDAE z-score	n	Token Test	n	PAST	n
Percentage LH tissue damage (AHP data)						
Slice B/W—L–R% Difference	−.63/**	32	−.64/**	32	−.71/**	29
Slice W—L–R% Difference	−.65/**	32	−.68/**	32	−.74/**	29
Slice SM—L–R% Difference	−.60/**	32	−.68/**	32	−.70/**	29
All Slices—Mean L–R% Difference	−.61/**	32	−.67/**	32	−.75/**	29
Number lesion pixels (AFP Data)						
Slice B/W—Number Lesion Pixels	−.81/**	20	−.86/**	20	−.78/**	19
Slice W—Number Lesion Pixels	−.71/**	28	−.76/**	28	−.85/**	25
Slice SM—Number Lesion Pixels	−.57/*	28	−.68/**	28	−.71/**	25
All Slices—Total Lesion Pixels	−.63/**	30	−.70/**	30	−.81/**	27
All Slices—Mean Number Lesion Pixels	−.66/**	30	−.72/**	30	−.82/**	27

*p<.01.
**p<.001.

10% mean left hemisphere (LH) tissue damage at slices SM and SM + 1.

The term C/P with *posterior* extension is used in this chapter to describe C/P lesion areas that extended posteriorly across the auditory radiations in the temporal isthmus as described by Nielsen (1936) (Figure 12). The auditory radiations are present on CT scan slice B/W; inferior to the Sylvian fissure and superior to the temporal horn. At this level, they are ascending from the medial geniculate body to Heschl's gyrus and Wernicke's area (DeArmond, Fusco, & Dewey, 1976).

Small differences in subcortical lesion extension on the CT scan (a few millimeters in one direction or another) were associated with large differences in language behavior; hence, the complete CT scan for each case is presented and described in detail here. Slices B/W,

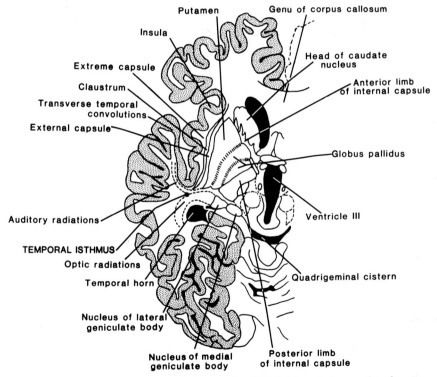

Figure 12. Schematic drawing of CT scan slice B/W (left hemisphere only), showing location of deep structures (putamen, internal capsule) and auditory radiations within the temporal isthmus. (Reprinted with permission from *Archives of Neurology*, Naeser *et al.*, 1982, 39, p. 5. Copyright 1982, American Medical Association.)

SM, and SM + 1 are the most important slices in these subcortical aphasia cases.

SAMPLE SUBCORTICAL APHASIA CASES

CASE 7: CAPSULAR/PUTAMINAL WITH ANTERIOR– SUPERIOR LESION EXTENSION

R. N. is a 53-year-old male lawyer who was studied with the BDAE at 2 and 13 MPS (Table 1), and had a CT scan done acutely and at 13 MPS (Figure 13, top half). The patient had a lasting right hemiparesis (arm greater than leg).

Speech was grammatical, but a slow, severe dysarthria was present. At 2 MPS, his picture description was as follows: "Well, here the wind coming 'du' the curtains. . . . Here the boy going in 'coodie' jar, getting 'coodie' out." At 13 MPS, the grammatical, slow dysarthric speech was still present and occasional verbal paraphasias were noted, that is, "The stool is 'kilking'—tilting, and he's going into the cookie 'department.' The two cups and a platter are to the end, having been dried." The impaired articulatory agility rating of only 2/7 in spontaneous speech was compatible with a poor Verbal Oral Agility score of only 8/14 in the timed Verbal Oral Agility task on the BDAE (how many times can the patient repeat the same word in 5 seconds, e.g., caterpillar, caterpillar, and so on.)

Comprehension was good. Repetition of low probability sentences was impaired at both 2 and 13 MPS. Most errors were due to poor articulation, "I 'shopped' (stopped) at his front door and rang the bell" and "The Chinese fan had a rare 'enwald' (emerald)." Eventually, the right upper extremity paresis resolved enough so that he was able to drive a specially adapted car. The patient was unable to return to work. He died 3 years later following a left pontine infarction.

CT SCAN FINDINGS IN SUBCORTICAL APHASIA CASES WITH CAPSULAR/PUTAMINAL LESIONS WITH ANTERIOR–SUPERIOR LESION EXTENSION

The acute CT scan of patient R. N. in Figure 13 (top row) revealed a large low-density area consistent with occlusive–vascular etiology in the region of the left internal capsule and basal ganglia (see slice B/W). CT scan at 13 MPS (Figure 13, bottom row) revealed a much

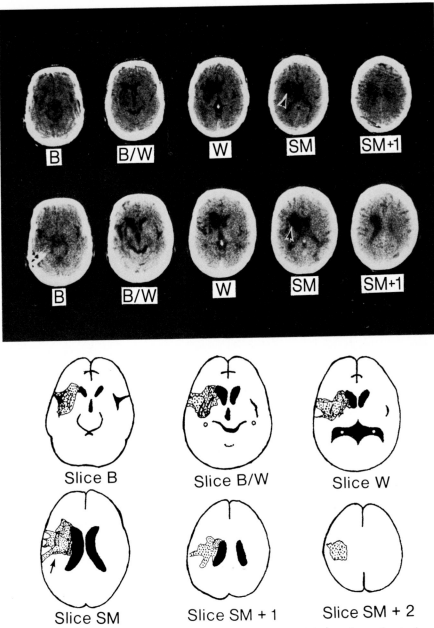

Figure 13. Subcortical aphasia with capsular/putaminal lesion site and anterior–superior lesion extension. CT scan for Case 7, R. N., age 53; acute, (top row) and at 13 months post-stroke (bottom row). The composite CT scan lesion sites for three cases are shown in the lower portion. The lesions were located primarily in the putamen with anterior lesion extension into periventricular white matter deep to Broca's area

smaller low-density focal area on slice B/W limited to the left putamen and part of the anterior limb, internal capsule, and PVWM
deep to Broca's area. Additional superior lesion extension was present in PVWM at slices SM and SM + 1 (arrows in Figure 13). No cortical lesion sites were visualized on either set of CT scans. The left
frontal horn was enlarged at 13 MPS.

At 13 MPS, the number of lesion pixels on slice B/W was only 284
(1.7 cm × 1.7 cm). The largest portion of the lesion was present at
slice SM + 1 (874 pixels, 3.0 cm × 3.0 cm). The percentage LH tissue
damage at each slice was as follows: slice B, no lesion; B/W, 11.2%;
W, 8.6%; SM, 7.2%; and SM + 1, 13.1%. Although no angiography
was done in this case, one of the C/P aphasia cases with anterior–
superior lesion extension was found to have occlusion of the left
internal carotid artery at its origin.

The results of the AFP and AHP lesion-size analyses for four C/P
aphasia cases with anterior–superior lesion extension are shown in
Tables 5 and 6. The mean number of lesion pixels per CT scan slice
where lesion was present was 944 (3.1 cm × 3.1 cm). Figure 14
shows, in bar graph form, the relative percentage LH tissue damage
at each CT scan language slice for four subcortical aphasia types.
This figure shows a flat lesion-size profile for this C/P aphasia group
with anterior–superior lesion extension with 15% LH tissue damage
at slice B/W and 14.4% at slices SM and SM + 1. Patient R. N. fits
well into this lesion-size profile because the lesion size for this case
was 11.2% at slice B/W and 13.1% at slice SM + 1.

In summary, the predominant aphasia pattern for subcortical
aphasia cases with C/P lesions with anterior–superior lesion extension was that of good comprehension and grammatical, but slow,
dysarthric speech output. See Figure 15. The impaired articulatory
agility scores of only 2 to 4/7 in spontaneous speech were compatible
with the poor timed Verbal Oral Agility Scores of only 4 to 8/14. Repetition was impaired primarily on low probability sentences; errors
were severe articulatory distortions and word omissions with occasional verbal paraphasias.

The composite CT scan lesion sites for three cases of this type of
subcortical aphasia are shown in Figure 13 (bottom). At slice B/W,

---

at slice B/W and large, superior lesion extension into periventricular white matter–corona radiata at slice SM (arrow). The amount of LH tissue damage was about
the same at each slice; the lesion-size profile was flat (Figure 14). (Reprinted with permission from *Archives of Neurology*, Naeser *et al.*, 1982, 39, p. 5. Copyright 1982,
American Medical Association.)

TABLE 5

Number Lesion Pixels at Each CT Slice for Four Subcortical Aphasia Groups
(Total per patient and mean per lesion slice, below)

	Capsular/ putaminal with anterior– superior lesion extension	Capsular/ putaminal with posterior lesion extension	Capsular/ putaminal with both anterior– superior and posterior lesion extension	Thalamic aphasia
Slice B				
No. Pts.:	3	1	1	—
$\bar{x}$:	721	1136	280	—
S.D.:	378	—	—	—
Slice B/W				
No. Pts.:	4	3	3	1
$\bar{x}$:	930	1057	674	120
S.D.:	555	660	282	—
Slice W				
No. Pts.:	4	3	3	1
$\bar{x}$:	1190	1025	906	360
S.D.:	380	640	131	—
Slice SM				
No. Pts.:	4	3	3	1
$\bar{x}$:	969	517	633	148
S.D.:	182	323	160	—
Slice SM + 1				
No. Pts.:	3	1	2	—
$\bar{x}$:	828	261	1078	—
S.D.:	249	—	330	—
Total lesion pixels per patient				
No. Pts.:	4	3	3	1
$\bar{x}$:	4252	3065	3027	628
S.D.:	1122	2247	496	—
Mean number lesion pixels per lesion slice				
No. Slices:	18	11	12	3
$\bar{x}$:	944	836	756	209
S.D.:	368	536	289	131

each case had a lesion in the putamen and part of the anterior limb, internal capsule with anterior lesion extension into PVWM deep to Broca's area. At slice SM, each case had large superior lesion extension (greater than 10% LH tissue damage) into PVWM–corona radiata deep to the precentral gyrus facial area. This lesion at slice

TABLE 6

Percent LH Tissue Damage* (LH %LoPix minus RH %LoPix) at Each CT Slice for Four Subcortical Aphasia Groups

	Capsular/ Putaminal with Anterior– Superior Lesion Extension	Capsular/ Putaminal with Posterior Lesion Extension	Capsular/ Putaminal with both Anterior– Superior and Posterior Lesion Extension	Thalamic Aphasia
Slice B				
No. Pts.:	2	1	1	1
$\bar{x}$*:	14.7	14.0	11.7	2.7
S.D.:	1.4	—	—	—
Slice B/W				
No. Pts.:	4	3	2	1
$\bar{x}$*:	15.0	12.2	15.1	3.5
S.D.:	4.7	6.8	2.3	—
Slice W				
No. Pts.:	4	3	3	1
$\bar{x}$*:	16.4	12.5	14.5	7.6
S.D.:	5.9	5.8	1.4	—
Slice SM				
No. Pts.:	4	3	3	1
$\bar{x}$*:	14.1	7.8	13.4	4.2
S.D.:	4.9	1.8	1.9	—
Slice SM + 1				
No. Pts.:	3	2	3	—
$\bar{x}$*:	14.4	2.8	12.7	—
S.D.:	2.1	.4	6.2	—
Overall slices				
Number slices:	17	12	12	4
$\bar{x}$:	15.1	9.8	13.6	4.5
S.D.:	4.2	5.5	3.1	2.2

SM extended from the body of the lateral ventricle at least halfway toward the cortex. The mean lesion size was approximately 944 pixels per slice (3.1 cm × 3.1 cm) and the mean percentage LH tissue damage was 14–16% at each CT slice. There was a flat lesion-size profile.

These cases did not resemble Broca's or Wernicke's aphasics in neurological findings, CT scan lesion sites, or language behavior. They were similar to Broca's in that they had a right hemiparesis (plegia), impaired articulatory agility, and good comprehension.

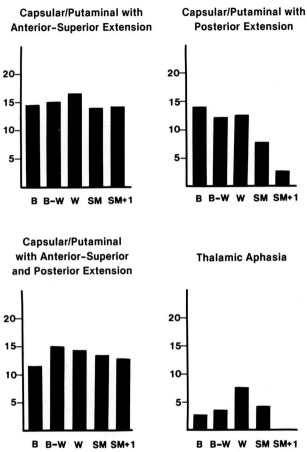

Figure 14. Relative percentage LH tissue damage (LH %LoPix minus RH %LoPix) at each CT scan slice for four subcortical aphasia types.

They were similar to Wernicke's in that they had more grammatical speech with four to six words per phrase length, and some paraphasias. Their preserved ability to name objects better than letters was more compatible with Broca's aphasics (Goodglass, Klein, Carey, & Jones, 1966). These C/P aphasia cases with anterior–superior lesion extension were also similar to Broca's aphasics in that Melodic Intonation Therapy has been found to be effective in reducing the impaired articulation and increasing the number of words per phrase length in their speech (Helm-Estabrooks, Naeser & Kleefield, 1980).

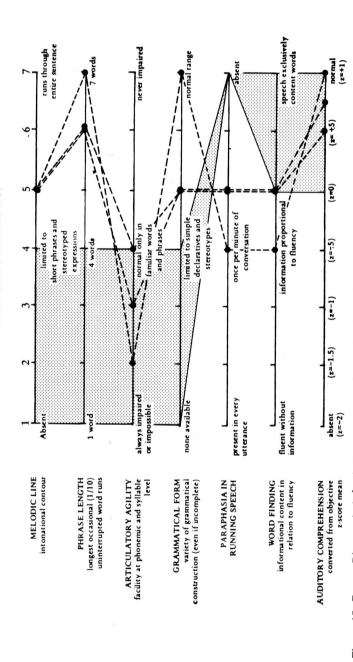

Figure 15. Boston Diagnostic Aphasia Exam rating-scale profile of speech characteristics. Characteristics typical of Broca's aphasia are shown in the shaded area. Characteristics for three subcortical aphasia cases with capsular/putaminal lesion sites and anterior–superior lesion extension are shown with the dotted lines. Note, impaired articulatory agility and good comprehension are the only two areas of overlap in scores.

CASE 8: CAPSULAR/PUTAMINAL WITH POSTERIOR
LESION EXTENSION

B. E. is a 43-year-old male high school teacher who suffered an intracerebral hemorrhage confirmed by acute CT scan. He was studied with the BDAE at one MPS (Table 1) and had a CT scan done at four MPS (Figure 16, top half). The patient had a lasting right hemiparesis (arm greater than leg), mild right sensory loss, and right visual field deficit.

Speech output was fluent with multiple verbal paraphasias and neologisms. There was no dysarthria or impairment of articulatory agility. Picture description was as follows: "It's a girl . . . a short girl with long hair . . . has a 'tenti service.' The boy is 'scooting' the jar of cookies. He's 'losting' the bowl. The faucet is 'off'...the faucet is on." The good articulatory agility rating of 6/7 in spontaneous speech was compatible with the perfect score of 14/14 in the Timed Verbal Oral Agility task. However, this same patient had a poor score of only 6/12 in the timed Nonverbal Oral Agility task (how many times the patient can open and close the mouth, move his tongue in and out, etc., in 5 seconds). This disparity in good timed Verbal Oral Agility versus poor timed Nonverbal Oral Agility appears to be unique and is a combination not often observed with Wernicke's aphasics. In addition, this case differed from Wernicke's aphasics in neurological findings in that a dense right hemiparesis was present.

Comprehension was poor. Sentence repetition was impaired; most response errors were paraphasic, with extended English jargon—for example *They heard him speak on the radio last night.* "They heard him speak on the radio 'with voices they learned from.'" *The lawyer's closing argument convinced him.* "The lawyer's closing argument 'consisted of his words.'" The patient was unable to return to teaching and died 1 year and 8 months later, following a second stroke.

CT SCAN FINDINGS IN SUBCORTICAL APHASIA CASES
WITH CAPSULAR/PUTAMINAL LESIONS WITH POSTERIOR
LESION EXTENSION

The CT scan of patient B. E., done at four MPS, is shown in Figure 16 (top half). The scan in the top row (without contrast enhancement) shows at slices B/W and W a lesion in the area of the left putamen, part of the anterior limb, internal capsule, and PVWM in

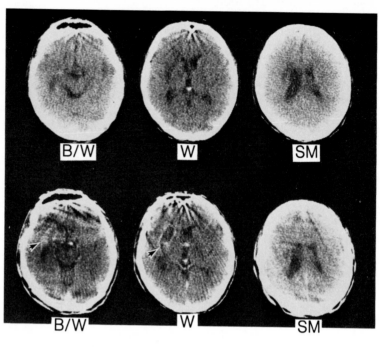

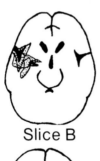

Slice B

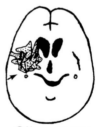

Slice B/W

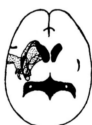

Slice W

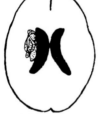

Slice SM

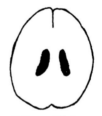

Slice SM + 1

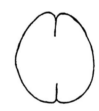

Slice SM + 2

the frontal lobe. The scan in the bottom row (with contrast enhancement) shows enhancement of the lesion site—previously mentioned—at slices B/W and W as well as extension across the auditory radiations in the temporal isthmus superior to the left temporal horn and atrium (arrows in Figure 16).

The number of lesion pixels on slice B/W was only 307 (1.8 cm × 1.8 cm). The lesion was approximately the same size at slices W and SM, that is, 419 and 396 pixels, respectively. The percentage LH tissue damage at slice B/W was 4.5%, at slice W, 5.8%, and at slice SM, 5.8%.

The results of the AFP and AHP lesion-size analyses for three C/P aphasia cases with posterior lesion extension are shown in Tables 5 and 6. The mean number of lesion pixels per CT scan slice was 836 (2.9 cm × 2.9 cm). Figure 14 shows, in bar graph form, the relative percentage LH tissue damage at each CT scan slice for this C/P aphasia group with posterior lesion extension and reveals a flat lesion-size profile for this group at slices B, B/W and W with a sharp reduction in lesion size at slices SM and SM + 1 (2.8–7.8%). Patient B. E. fits well into this lesion-size profile for the C/P cases with posterior lesion extension only, because the lesion size for this case was 5–6% at slices B/W and W and only 6% at slice SM. When this lesion-size profile is compared to the previous group (C/P with anterior–superior extension), the difference at slices SM and SM + 1 is particularly striking.

In summary, the predominant aphasia pattern for the cases with C/P lesions with posterior lesion extension was that of poor comprehension and rapid fluent speech with paraphasias and extended English jargon (see Figure 17). The good articulatory agility scores of 4.5 to 6/7 in spontaneous speech were compatible with the good timed Verbal Oral Agility scores of 9 to 14/14. Performance was poor, however, in the timed Nonverbal Oral Agility task. Repetition was impaired on both low and high probability sentences. Errors on repetition consisted primarily of paraphasias and extended English jargon.

Figure 16. Subcortical aphasia with capsular/putaminal lesion site and posterior lesion extension. CT scan for Case 8. B. E., age 43, at 4 months post-stroke (top row, without contrast, bottom row, with contrast). The composite CT scan lesion sites for three cases are shown in the lower portion. The lesions were located primarily in the putamen at slice B/W with posterior extension across the auditory radiations in the temporal isthmus (arrows). The amount of LH tissue damage was about the same at slices B, B/W and W, but there was a dramatic reduction at slices SM and SM + 1 (Figure 14). (Reprinted with permission from *Archives of Neurology*, Naeser *et al.*, 1982, 39, p. 7. Copyright 1982, American Medical Association.)

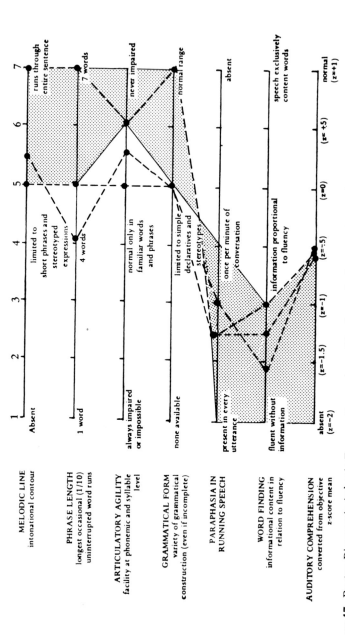

Figure 17. Boston Diagnostic Aphasia Exam rating-scale profile of speech characteristics. Characteristics typical of Wernicke's aphasia are shown in the shaded area. Characteristics for three subcortical aphasia cases with capsular/putaminal lesion sites and posterior lesion extension are shown with the dotted lines. Note, all characteristics including poor comprehension overlap in scores.

The composite CT scan lesion sites for three cases (two occlu-sive–vascular, one hemorrhage) of this type of subcortical aphasia are shown in Figure 16 (bottom). At slice B/W, each case had a le-sion in the left putamen, anterior limb, and part of the posterior limb, internal capsule, with posterior extension across the auditory radiations in the temporal isthmus (see arrows, Figure 16). There was only minimal superior extension (less than 10% LH tissue dam-age) on slice SM and none on slice SM + 1. The lesion area in PVWM at slice SM extended less than halfway, laterally, toward the cortex. The mean lesion size was approximately 836 pixels (2.9 cm × 2.9 cm) and the mean percentage LH tissue damage as 12–14% at slices B, B/W, or W and only 3–8% at slices SM or SM + 1. There was a flat lesion-size profile at slices B, B/W and W, with a sharp drop-off in le-sion size as slices SM and SM + 1.

These cases did not completely resemble Broca's or Wernicke's aphasics in neurological findings, CT scan lesion sites, or language behavior. They were similar to Broca's only in that they had a right hemiplegia (or paresis). They were similar to Wernicke's in that they had a comprehension deficit and fluent paraphasic speech; their preserved ability to name letters better than objects was also more compatible with Wernicke's aphasics (Goodglass, Klein, Carey, & Jones 1966). However, the presence of a right hemiplegia and the obvious disparity in the timed Verbal and Nonverbal Oral Agility scores made these cases different from most Wernicke's aphasics.

CASE 9: CAPSULAR/PUTAMINAL WITH BOTH
ANTERIOR–SUPERIOR AND POSTERIOR LESION
EXTENSION

A. G. is a 64-year-old male senior research report analyst who was studied with the BDAE at 15 MPS (Table 1) and had a CT scan done at 15 MPS (Figure 18, top). The patient had a lasting dense right hemiplegia, mild right sensory deficit, and right homonymous hemi-anopia.

Speech output was severely limited and consisted of only stereo-typed monosyllables, "guh . . . dee, guh . . . dee." There was a se-verely impaired articulatory agility rating of only 1/7 for spontane-ous speech; the patient was unable to be tested in the timed Verbal and Nonverbal Oral Agility tasks. A severe comprehension deficit was present and he was unable to repeat even single words or to count. In singing "Happy Birthday," the melody was adequate but

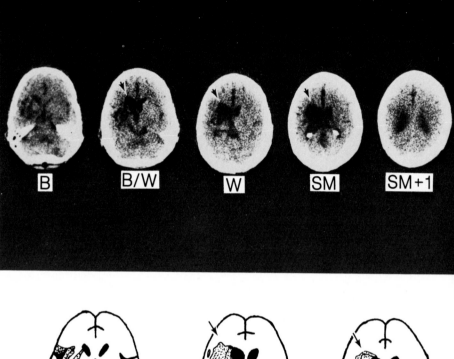

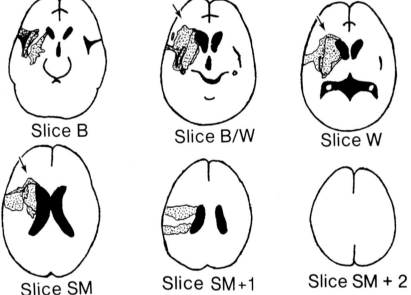

Figure 18. Subcortical global aphasia with capsular/putaminal lesion site and both anterior–superior and posterior lesion extension. CT scan for Case 9. A. G., age 64, 15 months post-stroke (above) and composite CT scan lesion sites for two cases (below). The lesions were located primarily in the putamen at slice B/W with anterior lesion extension in periventricular white matter deep to Broca's area including fibers to the genu of the corpus callosum beyond the frontal horn (arrows). The lesions also

the words were mostly unintelligible. He was classified as a global aphasic. He was able to live at home, although he spent most of his time in a wheelchair. He died 3 years later (without any improvement) following a second stroke.

CT SCAN FINDINGS IN SUBCORTICAL APHASIA CASES
WITH CAPSULAR/PUTAMINAL LESION SITES WITH BOTH
ANTERIOR–SUPERIOR AND POSTERIOR LESION
EXTENSION

The CT scan of patient A. G., done at 15 MPS, is shown in Figure 18 (top). The infarct on slice B/W is located in the area of the left putamen, globus pallidus, and anterior and posterior limbs, internal capsule with posterior extension across the temporal isthmus all the way to the left temporal horn. At the same slice, there was further anterior extension to PVWM deep to Broca's area. This anterior extension of PVWM continued beyond the anterior border of the left frontal horn (arrows in Figure 18) and included fibers to the genu of the corpus callosum (Figure 12).

The number of lesion pixels on slice B/W was 732 (2.7 cm × 2.7 cm); on slice W, 1024 (3.2 cm × 3.2 cm); and on slice SM, 464 (2.2 cm × 2.2 cm). The percentage LH tissue damage at slice B/W was 9.2%; at slice W, 13.4%; at slice SM, 14.4%; and at slice SM + 1, 6.8%.

The results of the AFP and AHP lesion-size analyses for three C/P aphasia cases with both anterior–superior and posterior lesion extension are shown in Tables 5 and 6. The mean number of lesion pixels per CT scan slice was 756 (2.7 cm × 2.7 cm). Figure 14 shows, in bar graph form, the relative percentage LH tissue damage at each CT scan slice for this C/P aphasia group with both anterior–superior and posterior lesion extension. This figure reveals a flat lesion-size profile for this group at all slices including 15% LH tissue damage at slice B/W and 13% at slices SM and SM + 1.

Patient A. G. fits well into this lesion-size profile because the lesion size for this case was 14% at slice B/W and 12.2% at slice SM.

---

extended posteriorly completely across the temporal isthmus. Each case also had large superior lesion extension at slice SM. The percentage LH tissue damage was about the same at each slice; there was a flat lesion-size profile (Figure 14). (Reprinted with permission from *Archives of Neurology*, Naeser *et al.*, 1982, 39, p. 10. Copyright 1982, American Medical Association.)

The scan also fits well with the lesion-site information, because there is anterior white matter lesion extension beyond the frontal horn to fibers of the genu of the corpus callosum as well as complete posterior extension across the temporal isthmus. Visual comparison of the bar graph lesion-size profile for this group versus the first group (C/P with anterior–superior lesion extension) does not reveal obvious differences. Therefore, in these two subcortical groups, it was lesion site, NOT lesion size, which determined the severity of aphasia. The milder subcortical aphasia group (C/P with anterior–superior lesion extension) had 15% mean LH tissue damage at slice B/W; the global subcortical aphasia group (C/P with both anterior–superior and posterior lesion extension) also had 15% mean LH tissue damage at slice B/W. The latter group, however, had anterior extension which extended beyond the frontal horns to the fibers in the genu of the corpus callosum and posterior extension across the temporal isthmus; the former group did not.

In summary, the predominant aphasia pattern for subcortical aphasia cases with C/P lesions with both anterior–superior and posterior lesion extension was that of lasting global aphasia (one case was observed "unchanged," 3 years later).

The composite CT scan lesion sites for two of these subcortical global aphasia cases are shown in Figure 18 (bottom). At slice B/W, each case had a lesion centered in the putamen, globus pallidus, and anterior and posterior limb, internal capsule. The lesions extended anteriorly in PVWM deep to Broca's area, including fibers to the genu of the corpus callosum beyond the frontal horn (see arrows, Figure 18, bottom). The lesions extended posteriorly, completely across the temporal isthmus. Each case also had large superior lesion extension (greater than 10% LH tissue damage) to the PVWM–corona radiata at slice SM. The mean lesion size was approximately 756 pixels per slice (2.7 cm × 2.7 cm) and the mean percentage LH tissue damage was 12–15% at each CT slice. There was a flat lesion-size profile.

Visual comparison of the bar graph lesion-size profile for the subcortical global group (C/P with both anterior–superior and posterior lesion extension) (Figure 14) versus the cortical global group (Figure 5) reveals an obvious difference in lesion size at each CT slice. At slice B/W, the mean percentage LH tissue damage for the subcortical global group was 15%; for the cortical global group 28.5%. This further suggests that it was lesion SITE, not lesion SIZE, which determined the type and severity of aphasia.

The severely limited speech output in these subcortical global aphasics probably was related to isolation of Broca's area both in afferent pathways (via temporal isthmus, extreme capsule, and arcuate fasciculus) and in efferent pathways (via anterior limb, internal capsule, and genu of corpus callosum). Thus, although Broca's cortical area as well as the surrounding U-fibers were still intact, there was no efferent pathway available for left hemisphere speech output. This isolation of the intact Broca's area is similar to the severe aphasia case of Bonhoeffer (1914) discussed by Geschwind (1965) and a global putaminal hemorrhage case reported by Hier, Davis, Richardson & Mohr (1977).

CASE 10: THALAMIC APHASIA

S. V. is a 69-year-old male department store worker who was studied with the BDAE at one and three MPS (Table 1), and had a CT scan done acutely (hemorrhage) and at four MPS (Figure 19). The patient had a lasting dense right hemiparesis (arm greater than leg) and a right sensory deficit. Although there was no visual field deficit, abnormalities were noted in eye movements, especially on the left.

Speech output initially was hypophonic and fluent with paraphasias, for example, "Taking the . . . the jar out of the thing those . . . that's what he's doing . . . this guy . . . He can't do it . . . on account of operation . . . She's getting off the base . . . I'm a going away from . . . oh . . . a woman . . . she's washing the dishes." The patient spoke in a low volume, appeared very tired, and was occasionally inattentive. At three MPS, the picture description was complete and accurate without word-finding difficulties or paraphasias.

Although comprehension was poor at one MPS, it was much improved at three MPS. Repetition was good for words and high-probability phrases at one and three MPS, but was poor on low-probability phrases at both times. Errors consisted primarily of paraphasias, e.g., *The phantom soared across the foggy heath* was repeated, "The phantom crossed the soggy heath," and *The barn swallow captured a plump worm*, became, "The barn swallow captured a plump 'bird'". The patient had made very good progress toward recovery from the aphasia by three MPS.

CT SCAN FINDINGS IN THALAMIC APHASIA

The acute CT scan of patient S. V. in Figure 19 (top row) shows hemorrhage in the area of the thalamus and roof of the third ventricle at slice W. The CT scan done at four MPS (Figure 19, bottom

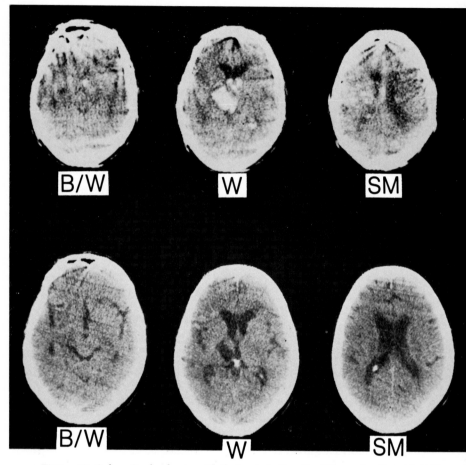

Figure 19. Subcortical aphasia with thalamic lesion site. CT scan for Case 10. S. V., age 69; acute, (hemorrhage, top row), and at 4 months, post-stroke (bottom row). The small lesion was located primarily in the pulvinar and posterior limb, internal capsule slice W, bottom row). The percentage LH tissue damage was very small compared to the other subcortical, capsular/putaminal cases (Figure 14); there was no anterior, superior, or posterior lesion extension.

row) shows resorption of the hematoma and a large, low-density area in the left thalamus (primarily pulvinar) and left posterior limb, internal capsule. There was no cortical lesion nor was a lesion observed in the anterior limb, internal capsule, putamen, or temporal isthmus. There was no superior PVWM–corona radiata lesion extension. Except for overlap onto the posterior limb, internal capsule, the lesion site did not coincide with any of the lesion sites observed in the three C/P aphasia patterns discussed above.

The peak lesion size (slice W) was only 360 pixels (1.9 cm × 1.9 cm) and 7.6% LH tissue damage. The mean number lesion pixels at each CT slice and percentage LH tissue damage for this case are listed in Tables 5 and 6. This is the only case of thalamic aphasia we have been able to study quantitatively. The mean number lesion pixels per slice was only 209 (1.4 cm × 1.4 cm). The percentage LH tissue damage at each CT scan slice (in bar graph form in Figure 14) shows a lesion-size profile with a peak amount of tissue damage at slice W (7.6%). When this profile is compared to the previous three C/P subcortical aphasia groups, an obviously smaller lesion-size is noted in this case.

In summary, the predominant aphasia pattern for this thalamic aphasia case due to hemorrhage was one of fluent, hypophonic speech, mild comprehension deficit, and mild repetition deficit only for low-probability phrases. The hypophonic fluent speech plus comprehension deficit have been mentioned in previous thalamic aphasia cases, but the impairment in low-probability phrase repetition has not been mentioned before in the literature. Indeed, the most recent thalamic aphasia study (Cappa & Vignolo, 1979) stressed the preserved repetition ability and "transcortical features" of thalamic aphasia. Further studies with controlled sentence repetition tasks need to be done to establish the cases (and presumably, lesion sites) that have preserved sentence repetition.

The lesion was located primarily in the pulvinar of the thalamus and the posterior limb, internal capsule. The mean lesion size per CT slice was only 209 pixels (1.4 cm × 1.4 cm) and the percentage LH tissue damage only 3–7.6% at each CT slice. The peak amount of tissue damage was only 7.6% at slice W.

The lesion size for this subcortical thalamic case is much smaller than that observed with the subcortical C/P aphasia cases at every CT scan slice. The peak amount of tissue damage, 7.6% (slice W), was more compatible with that observed with the mild cortical aphasia cases—that is, transcortical motor, 7.6% (slice W), and conduction, 5.9% (slice SM). This thalamic aphasia case did have good recovery from most of the language deficits (see Table 3.1).

Further studies with additional thalamic aphasia cases will be necessary to confirm the frequency of small lesion sizes associated with thalamic aphasia. It may be that only those with relatively small hemorrhages survive to be studied and do well, the large hemorrhages do not.

Discussion

This chapter has presented six sample cortical aphasia cases and four sample subcortical aphasia cases representing 10 aphasia types. Brief BDAE language descriptions and detailed CT scan lesion-site and lesion-size information have been provided. The purpose has been to show how quantitative CT scan information on a single aphasia case can help to classify that case within a given group of cases in the presence of similarity in language behavior, lesion size, and lesion site.

Highly significant correlations were observed between lesion size (slices B/W and W and severity of aphasia in cases representing six groups of cortical aphasia. In the cortical aphasia cases, an increased number of lesion pixels was generally associated with an increased severity of aphasia, that is, mild TCM and conduction aphasics had approximately only 500 lesion pixels per slice, whereas the Broca's had 1000; the Wernicke's, 750; the mixed, 1500; and the globals, 2000. Lesion site was, of course, also very important in establishing the "fluency" of the speech output and the aphasia type.

Correlations between lesion size and severity of aphasia have not yet been done on the C/P subcortical aphasia cases. Revew of lesion-size data presented here for three C/P aphasia groups (10 cases) would suggest that for these subcortical cases, the lesion-size aphasia severity correlations will probably not be as high as they were for the cortical aphasia cases. The C/P aphasia cases with the *largest* mean number lesion pixels per slice (944) also had the *best* comprehension scores (C/P aphasia cases with anterior–superior lesion extension). The C/P aphasia cases with both anterior–superior and posterior lesion extension with a *smaller* mean number of lesion pixels per slice (756) had the *worst* comprehension test scores. This information suggests that with the C/P subcortical aphasia cases, lesion *site* is more important than lesion *size*. It was observed, for example, that a lesion extending just a few mm in the posterior direction across the temporal isthmus was always associated with a comprehension deficit. Among all subcortical aphasics, however, the single thalamic aphasia case had the smallest lesion (only 209 lesion pixels per slice) and the best recovery. Future studies with many more subcortical aphasia cases (both C/P and thalamic) will be necessary to establish the relationship between lesion size and severity in the subcortical aphasias.

The information provided within this chapter is intended to help the clinician decide which aphasics can be classified into one of the 10 aphasia types presented here. The atypical cortical lesion cases, the subcortical lesion cases, the two- and three-lesion cases, and the bilateral lesion cases are certainly among the most difficult and challenging at the present time. Continued detailed study of language behavior and CT scan lesion-size and lesion-site information is likely to improve our understanding of these more complex cases.

Acknowledgements

The Radiology Services at the Boston V.A. Medical Center and the Palo Alto V.A. Medical Center provided valuable assistance with the CT scans. The author is also grateful to Gale Haas, Carole Palumbo, Jean Pieniadz, and Alison York for their assistance in preparation of the manuscript.

References

Albert, M., Sparks, W., & Helm, N. (1973). Melodic intonation therapy for aphasia. *Archives of Neurology (Chicago)*, *29*, 130–131.

Alexander, M. P., & LoVerme, S. R. (1980). Aphasia following left hemispheric intracerebral hemorrhage. *Neurology*, *30*, 1193–1202.

Alexander, M. P., & Schmitt, M. A. (1980). The aphasia syndrome of stroke in the left anterior cerebral artery territory. *Archives of Neurology (Chicago)*, *37*, 97–100.

Altemus, L. R., Roberson, G. H., Miller Fisher, C., & Pessin, M. (1976). Embolic occlusion of the superior and inferior divisions of the middle cerebral artery with angiographic-clinical correlation. *AJR, American Journal of Roentgenology*, *126*, 576–581.

Barat, M., Constant, P. H., Mazaux, J. M., Caille, J. M., & Arné, L. (1978). Correlations anatomo-cliniques dans l'aphasie. Apport de la tomo densitometrie. *Revue Neurologique*, *134*, 611–617.

Benson, D. F. (1979). *Aphasia, Alexia, Agraphia*. London & New York: Churchill-Livingstone, pp. 93–100.

Benson, D. F., & Geschwind, N. (1971). The aphasias and related disturbances. In A. B. Baker & L. H. Baker (Eds.), *Clinical Neurology* (Vol. 1). Hagerstown, Md.: Harper & Row.

Benson, D. F., & Patten, D. H. (1967). The use of radioactive isotopes in the localization of aphasia-producing lesions. *Cortex*, *3*, 258–271.

Benson, D. F., Sheremata, W. A., Bouchard, R., Segarra, J. M., Price, D. L., & Geschwind, N. (1973). Conduction aphasia: A clinico-pathological study. *Archives of Neurology (Chicago)*, *28*, 339–346.

Bonhoeffer, K. (1914). Klinischer und Anatomischer Befund zür Lehre von der Apraxie und der 'motorischen Sprachbahn. *Monatsschrift für Psychiatrie und Neurologie*, *35*, 113.

Cappa, S. F., & Vignolo, L. A. (1979). "Transcortical" features of aphasia following left thalamic hemorrhage. *Cortex*, *15*, 121–130.

Ciemins, V. A. (1970). Localized thalamic hemorrhage: A cause of aphasia. *Neurology,* *20,* 776–782.

Damasio, H., & Damasio, A. (1980). The anatomical basis of conduction aphasia. *Brain,* *103,* 337–350.

DeArmond, S. J., Fusco, M. M., Dewey, M. M. (1976). *Structure of the human brain.* London & New York: Oxford University Press.

Galaburda, A. M., LeMay, M., Kemper, T. L., & Geschwind, N. (1978). Right-left asymmetries in the brain. *Science, 199,* 852–856.

Geschwind, N. (1965). Disconnexion syndromes in animals and man. Part II. *Brain,* *88,* 585–644.

Gloning, I., Gloning, K., Haub, G., & Quatember, R. (1969). Comparison of verbal behavior in right-handed and non-right-handed patients with anatomically verified lesions of one hemisphere. *Cortex, 5,* 43–52.

Goodglass, H., & Berko-Gleason, J. (1960). Agrammatism and inflectional morphology in English. *Journal of Speech and Hearing Research, 3,* 257–267.

Goodglass, H., & Kaplan, E. (1972). *The assessment of aphasia and related disorders.* Philadelphia: Lea & Febiger.

Goodglass, H., Klein, B., Carey, P., & Jones, K. J. (1966). Specific semantic word categories in aphasia. *Cortex, 2,* 74–89.

Green, E., & Howes, D. H. (1977). The nature of aphasia: A study of anatomic and clinical features and of underlying mechanisms. In H. Whitaker & H. A. Whitaker (Eds.), *Studies in neurolinguistics* (Vol. 3). New York: Academic Press, pp. 125–156.

Hanaway, J., Scott, W. R., & Strother, C. M. (1977). *Atlas of the human brain and the orbit for computed tomography.* St. Louis, Mo.: Warren H. Green, Inc.

Hayward, R. W., Naeser, M. A., & Zatz, L. M. (1977). Cranial computed tomography in aphasia. *Radiology, 123,* 653–660.

Helm-Estabrooks, N. A., Naeser, M. A., & Kleefield, J. (1980). CT scan lesion localization and response to melodic intonation therapy. Paper presented at Academy of Aphasia meetings, Cape Cod, Massachusetts, October.

Hier, D. B., Davis, K. R., Richardson, E., & Mohr, J. P. (1977). Hypertensive putaminal hemorrhage. *Annals of Neurology, 1,* 152–159.

Hounsfield, G. N. (1973). Computerized transverse axial scanning (tomography): Description of system. *British Journal of Radiology, 46,* 1016–1025.

Jernigan, T. L., Zatz, L. M., & Naeser, M. A. (1979). Semiautomated methods for quantitating CSF volume on cranial computed tomography. *Radiology, 132,* 463–466.

Kertesz, A., Harlock, W., & Coates, R. (1979). Computer tomographic localization, lesion size and prognosis in aphasia and nonverbal impairment. *Brain and Language, 8,* 34–50.

Kertesz, A., Lesk, D., & McCabe, P. (1977). Isotope localization of infarcts in aphasia. *Archives of Neurology (Chicago), 34,* 590–601.

LeMay, M. (1977). Asymmetries of the skull and handedness: Phrenology revisited. *Journal of the Neurological Sciences, 32,* 243–253.

Luria, A. R. (1970). *Traumatic aphasia.* The Hague: Mouton.

Matsui, T., & Hirano, A. (1978). *An atlas of the human brain for computerized tomography.* Tokyo: Igaku-Shoin.

Mazzocchi, F., & Vignolo, L. A. (1980). Localization of lesions in aphasia: Clinical-CT scan correlation in stroke patients. *Cortex, 15,* 627–654.

McCullough, E. C. (1977). Factors affecting the use of quantitative information from a CT scanner. *Radiology, 124,* 99–107.

Miller Fisher, C. (1959). The pathologic and clinical aspects of thalamic hemorrhage. *Transactions of the American Neurological Association, 84*, 56–59.

Mohr, J. P., Pessin, M. S., Finkelstein, S., Funkenstein, H. H., Duncan, G. W., & Davis, K. R. (1978). Broca's aphasia: Pathologic and clinical. *Neurology, 28*, 311–324.

Mohr, J. P., Walters, W. C., & Duncan, G. W. (1975). Thalamic hemorrhage and aphasia. *Brain and Language, 2*, 3–17.

Naeser, M. A., & Hayward, R. W. (1978). Correlation between CT scan findings and the Boston Diagnostic Aphasia Exam. *Neurology, 28*, 545–551.

Naeser, M. A., & Hayward, R. W. (1979). The resolving stroke and aphasia: A case study with computed tomography. *Archives of Neurology (Chicago), 36*, 233–235.

Naeser, M. A., Hayward, R. W., Laughlin, S., & Zatz, L. M. (1981). Quantitative CT scan studies in aphasia. Part I. Infarct size and CT numbers. *Brain and Language, 12*, 140–164.

Naeser, M. A., Hayward, R. W., Laughlin, S., Becker, J. M. T., Jernigan, T., & Zatz, L. M. (1981). Quantitative CT scan studies in aphasia. Part II. Comparison of the right and left hemispheres. *Brain and Language, 12*, 165–189.

Naeser, M. A., Alexander, M. P., Helm-Estabrooks, N., Levine, H. L., Laughlin, S. A., & Geschwind, N. (1982). Aphasia with predominantly subcortical lesion sites: Description of three capsular/putaminal aphasia syndromes. *Archives of Neurology (Chicago), 39*, 2–14.

Naeser, M. A., Mazurski, P., Goodglass, H., Laughlin, S. A., Peraino, M., Pieniadz, J. M., & Leaper, C. (1983). Palo Alto Syntax Test: A sentence level comprehension test for aphasics. (Manuscript submitted)

Nielsen, J. M. (1936). *Agnosia, apraxia, and aphasia: Their value in cerebral localization.* New York: Hafner, pp. 119–120.

Noel, G., Collard, M., Dupont, H., & Huvelle, R. (1977). Nouvelles possibilités de corrélations anatomo-cliniques en aphasiologie grace à la tomodensitometrie cérébrale. *Acta Neurologica Belgica, 77*, 351–362.

Penfield, W., & Roberts, L. (1959). *Speech and brain mechanisms.* Princeton, N.J.: Princeton University Press.

Pieniadz, J. M., Naeser, M. A., Koff, E., & Levine, H. L. (1979). CT scan cerebral hemispheric asymmetry measurements in stroke cases with global aphasia: Atypical asymmetries associated with improved recovery. Paper read at the 17th annual Academy of Aphasia meeting, San Diego, California, October. (In Press, *Cortex.*)

Pieniadz, J. M., Naeser, M. A. (1981). Correlation between CT Scan Cerebral Hemispheric Asymmetries and Morphological Brain Asymmetries of the Same Cases at Postmortem. Paper read at the 19th Annual Academy of Aphasia Meeting, London, Ontario, Canada, October 12, 1981. Manuscript submitted.

Ross, E. D. (1980). Localization of the pyramidal tract in the internal capsule by whole brain dissection. *Neurology, 30*, 59–64.

Rubens, A. B. (1975). Aphasia with infarction in the territory of the anterior cerebral artery. *Cortex, 11*, 239–250.

Sparks, R., Helm, N., & Albert, M. (1974). Aphasia rehabilitation resulting from melodic intonation therapy. *Cortex, 10*, 303–318.

Spreen, O., & Benton, A. L. (1969). *Neurosensory center comprehensive examination for aphasia.* Victoria, Can.: Department of Psychology, University of Victoria.

Walshe, T. M., Davis, K. R., & Miller Fisher, C. (1977). Thalamic hemorrhage: A computer tomographic-clinical correlation. *Neurology, 27*, 217–222.

Yarnell, P. R., Monroe, M. A., & Sobel, L. (1976). Aphasia outcome in stroke: A clinical and neuroradiological correlation. *Stroke, 7*, 516–522.

4

Positron-Computed Tomography in Neurobehavioral Problems

D. Frank Benson,
E. Jeffrey Metter,
David E. Kuhl,
and Michael E. Phelps

Introduction

As discussed in Chapter 1, different techniques have been used in the attempt to localize the brain abnormality underlying neuropsychological disorder. That no single technique is ideal for neuropsychological localization is evidenced by the many different means that *have* been tried and the immediate trial of any new neurodiagnostic tool for this purpose. This chapter presents both preliminary experience and discussion of the future potential of a new technique, Positron Emission-computed Tomography (positron CT) in neuropsychological research.

Presented here are most of the major localization techniques, subdivided to emphasize the approach they make to localization.

The most meaningful and accurate techniques are clinical with the remainder best used to confirm the localization deduced from the clinical techniques. The most commonly used localizing techniques are a second group whose characteristics are apparent— they produce a neuroanatomical localization of a static lesion. Postmortem neuropathological studies, neurosurgical case material, and implications from the localization of skull defects in serious head trauma all imply a stable, static lesion as the source of the neuropsychological disturbance. Most radiologic techniques also provide static information. The angiogram, pertechnetate isotope scan and X-ray-computed tomogram all provide an outline of the structural area that is abnormal at the moment of the evaluation. Even the neurologic examination, the most powerful of localizing tools, relies on a basically stable central nervous system (CNS) function.

Neuropsychologic defects exist within a dynamic nervous system, one that alters over time and probably changes on a periodic basis. A technique capable of gauging dynamic alterations occurring within the damaged central nervous system would be a valuable tool for correlations with neuropsychologic studies. A technique that could demonstrate nonfunctioning but structurally intact neural tissues would provide valuable information. Only two currently used localizing tools probe this dynamic quality. One is the *electroencephalogram* (EEG), an instrument that accurately samples the electrical activity over the cortical surface from a distance but, to date, has proved inadequate for most neuropsychologic correlations. The other is the study of *regional cerebral blood flow* (rCBF) (see Chapter 5) with ^{133}Xe gas, a procedure that has given new insights into regional brain response to functional activation (Ingvar & Schwartz, 1974; Larsen, Skinhøj, & Lassen, 1978). Both the EEG and the rCBF studies concentrate on cortical activity with considerably less information available on subcortical activity. Against this background, we can present our early experience, using positron CT in neuropsychological research at UCLA.

Positron-Emission Computed Tomography

Emission Computed Tomography (ECT) (Kuhl & Edwards, 1963; Kuhl, Edwards, Ricci, & Reivich, 1973; Phelps, 1977) is a noninvasive scanning method that produces a cross-sectional image of brain radioactivity following intravenous injection of a radioactive indicator. The process resembles X-ray CT which shows anatomic structure or cerebrovascular membrane permeability, but ECT has the potential for measuring blood flow, metabolism, and other cerebral functions, dependent upon the labeled compound chosen as a tracer. A positron-emitting isotope was used in these studies. For positron CT (Phelps, Hoffman, Mullani, & Ter-Pogossian, 1975), a cyclotron is used to prepare compounds labeled with short-lived isotopes of carbon, oxygen, nitrogen, or fluorine immediately before scanning. With radioactive decay, the emitted positrons annihilate

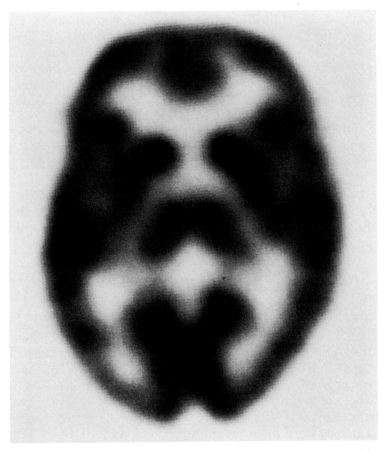

Figure 1. Normal FDG scan showing a slice of cerebrum outlined by metabolic activity. The dark image portrays glucose uptake whereas the light image indicates little or no uptake.

with electrons, producing two photons arising 180° apart; these can be detected by electronic coincidence counting. At UCLA, we have had experience in positron CT, using the ECAT® positron tomograph (Phelps, Hoffman, Huang & Kuhl, 1978) and [^{18}F]-fluorodeoxyglucose (^{18}FDG) (Huang, Phelps, Hoffman, Sideris, Selin, & Kuhl, 1980; Kuhl, Hoffman, Phelps, & Ricci, 1977; Phelps, Huang, Hoffman, Selin, Sokoloff & Kuhl, 1979; Reivich, Kuhl, Wolf, Greenberg, Phelps, Idom, Casella, Fowler, Hoffman, Alvai, & Sokoloff, 1979; Sokoloff, Reivich, Kennedy, Des Rosiers, Patlak, Pettigrew, Sakurada, & Shinohara, 1977) for mapping local cerebral glucose utilization (LCMRglc) but other compounds and other scanning devices have been used by ourselves and others.

Determination of LCMRglc by the ^{18}FDG scan requires an intravenous injection of the tracer, continuous sampling of arteriolized venous blood, and a brain scan beginning 40 minutes after injection. FDG enters the brain like glucose, is phosphorylated by brain hexokinase, but the resulting metabolic product remains primarily fixed. The 40-minute delay allows this metabolic action to reach a steady state. Calculations of LCMRglc depend on local cerebral activity concentration as measured by the positron CT technique, the time course of measured blood specific activity, and predetermined constants (Phelps *et al.*, 1979; Huang, *et al.*, 1980). Images are made at multiple levels throughout the brain in the manner of an X-ray tomogram. Figure 1, an FDG scan of a healthy normal subject, shows the normal appearance of gray-and-white matter structures, displayed according to their relative metabolic rates.

Examples of Positron CT in Neurobehavioral Research

Positron CT is a complex technique demanding considerable effort to assure replicable results. Only in the past few years has there been opportunity to use positron CT in the evaluation of patients with neurobehavioral problems. Most of this chapter presents early experiences in the use of positron CT with selected neurobehavioral problems at the UCLA School of Medicine, supplemented by reports of experience from other laboratories and initial studies dealing with normal subjects, depicting cerebral metabolism in chosen environmental situations.

Among the early clinical studies was the demonstration of metabolic alteration during the course of cerebral infarction secondary to cerebral vascular accident (CVA). Positron CT scans in the first few days showed decreased blood flow in the area of the cerebral infarct but almost normal cortical glucose utilization (LCMRglc). Later, even though blood flow returned to normal, the metabolism of some cortical and subcortical areas progressively decreased (Kuhl, Phelps, Kowell, Metter, Selin, & Winter, 1980). Permanent zones of hypometabolism remained in cortical and subcortical tissue even though they appeared structurally normal on X-ray CT.

In a similar manner, in cases of epilepsy, cortical zones considered responsible for seizures were hypometabolic in positron CT scans, although no abnormality was seen on X-ray CT (Kuhl, Engel, Phelps, & Selin, 1980). Results in these two disorders give promise that altered cerebral function may be assessed sensitively by positron CT in other disorders. The use of positron CT in the study of neurobehavioral problems has just commenced. The following represents a preliminary report of some early observations.

APHASIA

Localization of the pathology underlying aphasia has been a major concern of neurology for over 100 years. Most studies have relied on methods that determine static, structural changes within the brain and assume that the damaged tissue is directly responsible for the observed language disturbance. From such studies, nothing can be said about functional alterations occurring throughout the nondestroyed brain. On this basis, a study evaluating LCMRglc in aphasia offers promise.

Figure 2 presents data tabulated from 14 individuals with aphasia in which both X-ray CT and FDG tomograms were obtained. A number of these patients have been reported previously (Kuhl, Phelps, Kowell, Metter, Selin, & Winter, 1980; Metter, Wasterlain, Kuhl, Hanson, & Phelps, 1981). A check in any column represents metabolic or structural involvement to a given territory. All determinations were made visually from tomograms and no attempt was made to grade the severity of the structural damage on X-ray CT or of the depression of LCMRglc. It is readily apparent that metabolic abnormalities were considerably more widespread than structural changes. For instance, although structural changes were not always present on the X-ray CT, depression of LCMRglc was constantly

COMPARISON OF FDG PCT & X-RAY CT IN 14 CASES OF APHASIA

PATIENT	TYPE OF APHASIA	FRONTAL		BROCA		TEMPORAL		WERNICKE		PARIETAL		OCCIPITAL		BASAL GANGLIA		THALAMUS	
SA	ANOMIA	—	—	—	—	—	+	—	+	—	—	—	—	+	+	—	+
MP	WERNICKE	+	+	+	+	+	+	+	+	+	+	—	+	—	+	—	+
WJ	BROCA	+	+	+	+	+	+	+	+	+	+	—	—	+	+	—	+
RH	MIXED	+	+	—	—	—	+	—	—	+	+	—	—	+	+	—	+
MP	WERNICKE	—	+	—	—	+	+	+	+	+	+	—	+	—	+	—	+
AA	MIXED	+	+	+	+	+	+	+	+	+	+	—	+	—	+	—	+
JR	MIXED	—	+	—	—	—	—	—	—	—	—	—	—	+	—	—	+
GL	MIXED	+	+	+	+	+	+	+	+	+	+	—	+	+	+	—	+
JV	ANOMIA	—	+	—	—	—	—	—	—	—	—	—	—	—	+	—	+
JH	MIXED	—	+	—	+	—	+	—	+	—	+	—	+	+	+	—	+
GW	MIXED	—	+	+	+	+	+	.+	+	+	NT	—	—	—	+	—	+
MR	MIXED	+	+	—	+	—	+	—	—	—	NT	—	+	+	+	—	+
CG	MIXED	—	+	+	+	+	—	—	—	NT	NT	—	—	—	+	—	+
PH	MIXED	+	+	+	+	—	+	+	+	NT	NT	—	+	+	+	—	+
TOTAL		7	13	7	9	7	11	7	9	7/12	7/10	0	7	8	13	0	14

Figure 2. Chart showing a comparison of the abnormalities present in x-ray CT and in FDG PCT scans in 14 individuals with aphasia. A negative sign indicates no abnormality, a plus sign indicates abnormality. NT indicates not testable. Under each anatomic area there are two columns, the left hand column indicating x-ray CT, the right hand column FDG PCT results.

noted in the thalamus. To demonstrate the value of positron CT in aphasia, three cases are presented.

1. A 48-year-old male had a sudden onset of a mild right hemiparesis and aphasia. Language evaluation 6 weeks post-onset demonstrated good comprehension of conversational speech and single words, but some difficulty in understanding more complex language. Repetition of words and phrases was good. Comprehension of written sentences was good, with better understanding of nouns and adjectives than prepositions. When reading aloud, however, he often omitted words or substituted a semantically related word. He spoke in sentences of adequate length and complexity but word-finding difficulties were evident. Articulation was imprecise and the endings of words were omitted frequently. A Boston Diagnostic Aphasia Examination (BDAE) demonstrated a moderately severe aphasia of nonspecific pattern. X-ray CT demonstrated punctate areas of decreased density in the left and right caudate nuclei and in left internal capsule, with no involvement of the cortex (Figure 3). On the other hand, FDG positron CT showed a 24% decrease in LCMRglc in the left thalamus as compared to right, and a 15% decrease in metabolism of the left middle and inferior temporal gyri.

2. A 57-year-old male suddenly became aphasic. The clinical pic-

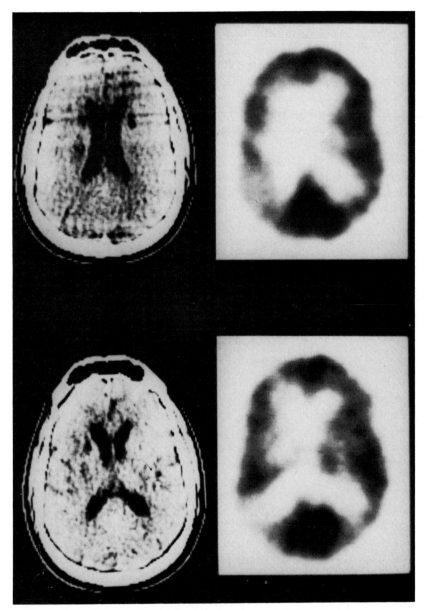

Figure 3. Case 1. Composite illustration of X-ray CT and FDG scan illustrating the marked hypometabolism of the left subcortical nuclear areas and the lesser degree of left cortical hypometabolism. Note that the X-ray CT of the cortex appears normal.

ture and the **BDAE** findings were consistent with a moderately severe Wernicke's aphasia. X-ray CT showed an area of decreased density involving the left superior and middle temporal, the angular and the supramarginal gyri. [18]FDG positron CT (Figure 4) demonstrated a 67% reduction of LCMRglc in the area of structural damage. In addition, lesser degrees of metabolic depression were noted throughout the temporal, parietal, and posterior frontal lobe above Broca's area, as well as the thalamus and basal ganglia.

3. A 68-year-old male had a sudden onset of a mild right hemiparesis along with a severely reduced verbal output. There was a history of right parietal–occipital meningioma removed 10 years before. Cerebral angiography showed occlusion of the right internal carotid artery with good collateral circulation and 98% occlusion of the left internal carotid with a large ulcer. One—possibly two—candelabra branches of the left middle cerebral artery were occluded. Left carotid endarterectomy was performed; postoperatively, there was a right hemiplegia and severe aphasia. With time, the paresis improved significantly, leaving only a mild paresis of the arm; language also improved, particularly comprehension, leaving a residual picture of a severe Broca type of aphasia.

FDG positron CT (Figure 5) demonstrated a severe metabolic disturbance in the left frontal cortex including Broca's and the precentral areas. In addition, depression of LCMRglc was present in the left basal ganglia and thalamus. Lesser metabolic depression was also present in the right parietal, temporal, and occipital areas (the site of earlier neurosurgery). The left posterior temporal area may also show some metabolic depression but an accurate judgment cannot be made because of the right hemisphere changes secondary to the previous craniotomy.

These three cases suggest that reliance on structurally oriented localizing procedures for correlation with aphasia phenomenology may be misleading. In the first case, the metabolic abnormality explains the clinical picture much more convincingly than the findings from the X-ray CT. In cases 2 and 3, some degree of metabolic depression occurred in many language areas, but the area of major depression of LCMRglc was posterior in Case 2 and anterior in Case 3, in agreement with the clinical aphasiologic designations as Wernicke and Broca aphasia, respectively. In each case, metabolic depression was present in the dominant hemisphere thalamus and basal ganglia. In Case 1 the depression of LCMRglc was greatest in the thalamus and basal ganglia, suggesting that these areas were the sites of primary pathology.

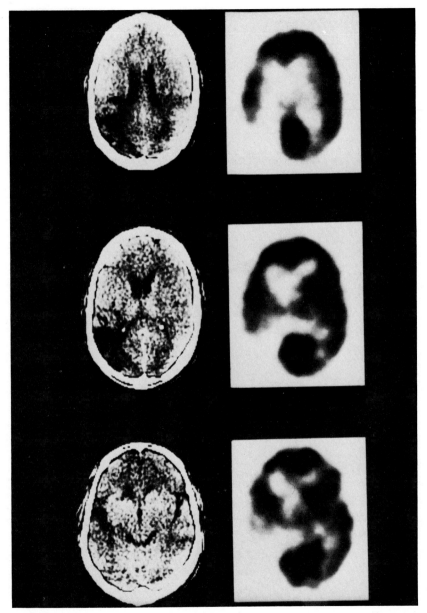

Figure 4. Case 2. Composite illustration of X-ray CT and FDG scan illustrating marked left posterior cortical hypometabolism and lesser left subcortical hypometabolism. Note that the X-ray CT of the subcortical structures appears normal.

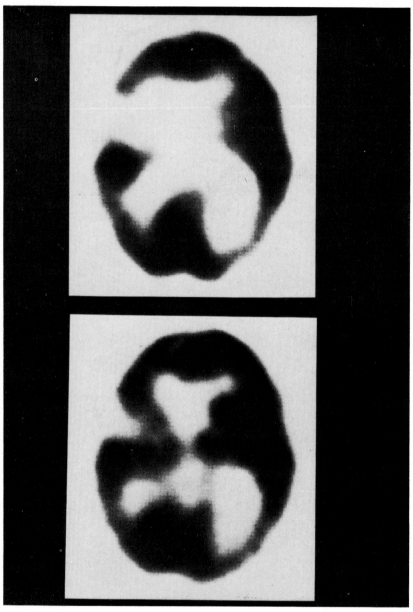

Figure 5. Case 3. FDG scan illustrating anterior cortical hypometabolism. There is also some hypometabolism in the subcortical nuclei on the left.

The results from the 14 cases listed in Figure 2 suggest several conclusions:

1. FDG imaging demonstrates a wider area of metabolic abnormality than indicated by the structural abnormality demonstrated with X-ray CT. In a number of cases, the depression of LCMRglc involved much of the left hemisphere. The area of maximal depression seemed to correlate with the area of structural damage.

2. In all aphasic patients, metabolic depression was noted in the ipsilateral thalamus and caudate. Metabolic depression in the thalamus cannot be easily explained on the basis of ischemia or hypoxia as this area receives much of its blood supply from the posterior cerebral circulation. Thalamic suppression is not specific to aphasia as it is noted in most stroke patients (Kuhl, Phelps, Kowell, Metter, Selin, & Winter, 1980). In individuals with primarily cortical pathology, the degree of depression of thalamic LCMRglc has been less than the depression in the cortically involved areas, whereas with subcortical pathology, thalamic depression has been greater than cortical depression. These findings are consistent with the suggestion of Ojemann (1975) that the role of the thalamus in language is not that of a "primary language center" but operates either as an activation resource or through involvement with short-term memory.

3. With subcortical lesions, LCMRglc depression is not confined to subcortical areas but also is noted in various cortical areas. This finding appears consistent with the extensive interconnections and interactions between subcortical and cortical structures. One implication is that following subcortical damage, cortical activation is decreased, leading to a lower metabolic demand.

4. Finally, in several cases, the LCMRglc as determined by FDG positron CT explained the clinical syndrome in a more consistent manner than X-ray CT, suggesting that reliance on areas of structural abnormality for the correlation of neuroanatomic localization and the aphasia syndromes may be misleading; it fails to consider functional abnormalities within the structurally intact tissues.

DEMENTIA

The past few years have witnessed a massive increase of both interest in, and study of, the dementias. Numerous neurobehavioral studies have featured clinical evaluations (neurologic and psychiatric evaluations) and extensive neuropsychologic batteries; some have been correlated with X-ray CT, EEG, or neuropathologic studies. Results to date have been limited by several factors, however. For example, most studies treat dementia as a unitary entity, ignoring the considerable variation in clinical presentation among the different causes of dementia. Another limiting factor concerns the widespread (nonfocal) nature of the pathology producing many varieties of dementia. X-ray CT and other static localizing techniques demonstrate only a diffuse decrease in cerebral mass, usually reported as central and/or cortical atrophy. Because of the dynamic qualities outlined above, metabolic techniques such as FDG positron CT offer considerable promise as tools to correlate abnormal cerebral function with the various progressive dementias. To date, however, only preliminary studies have been completed; these will be illustrated by several case reports.

4. A 51-year-old male had a 1½ year history of slowly progressive intellectual deterioration without accompanying elementary neurologic disorder. Examination showed severe memory loss (both recent and remote), loss of cognitive ability, inability to do even simple constructional tasks, and a language disorder characterized by severe word-finding difficulty. His personality was warm and outgoing, happy, and carefree. He moved normally with no motor, sensory, or coordination problems. The EEG was mildly abnormal (widespread 6–7 hertz) and the X-ray CT showed mild ventricular enlargement and suggestion of cortical atrophy. On the basis of clinical and laboratory findings, a diagnosis of Alzheimer's disease (AD) was made. [18]FDG positron CT (Figure 6) revealed grossly decreased cortical metabolism, almost exclusively involving the frontal and parietal–temporal association cortices. The primary motor–sensory cortex and the calcarine cortex showed greater metabolic activity. Similarly, subcortical structures such as the striatum and the thalamus showed active metabolism.

5. A 58-year-old male with a strong family history (siblings, father, uncles, grandfather) of Huntington's disease had a 2-year history of progressively worsening choreiform movements with a notable decrease in mental competency for at least 1 year. Examination showed chorea, facial grimacing, abnormal posture, and an irregular, slow, poorly articulated verbal output. He was forgetful but could learn new material; cognition was limited but successful for simple manipulations of knowledge and, although severely dysarthric, he showed no significant language loss. Both the movement disorder

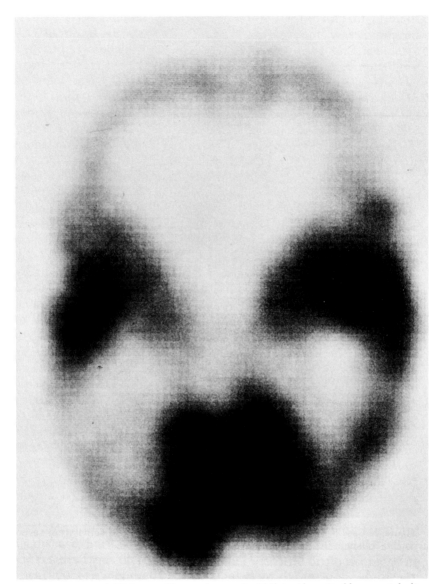

Figure 6. Case 4. FDG scan illustrating marked bilateral cortical hypometabolism except for the rolandic motor–sensory strip and the calcarine region.

and the dementia were consistent with a diagnosis of Huntington's disease. Positron CT with ¹⁸FDG (Figure 7) demonstrated considerable metabolic activity in the cortex in contrast to sharply decreased activity in the caudate nuclei bilaterally.

ing subcortical degeneration (e.g., Huntington's disease). In addition, early studies of positron CT images in a number of additional varieties of dementia (normal pressure hydrocephalus, multi-infarct dementia, Jakob–Creutzfeldt disease, Pick's disease) suggest that rather characteristic metabolic patterns can be demonstrated. Many additional parameters of cerebral metabolism can be studied in varieties of dementia by use of positron CT. For instance, focal hypometabolism in various areas of the cortex in AD and Pick's disease may be correlated with the specific onset of symptoms. Similarly, both cortical and subcortical focal hypometabolism may prove useful in understanding the varying dementia characteristics of other types of dementia.

POTENTIAL USES FOR POSITRON EMISSION TOMOGRAPHY IN NEUROPSYCHOLOGIC RESEARCH

Only limited investigations of neurologic functions and neurobehavioral problems have been performed to date, but it is not difficult to envisage considerable usefulness for the metabolic PECT technique in future research. For instance, in the normal subject, the dynamic qualities of this technique allow demonstration of asymmetrical metabolic activity during selected psychological functions. Early investigations demonstrated the anticipated increase in metabolic activity in the visual cortex following complex visual stimulation (Phelps, Kuhl, & Mazziotta, 1980). More recent work has demonstrated hemispheric asymmetry and increased metabolic activity in the temporal auditory cortex, dependent on whether the auditory stimulus had a verbal or nonverbal connotation (words or melodies) (Mazziotta, Phelps, Carson, & Kuhl, 1982).

Future metabolic studies may demonstrate asymmetrical increases in metabolism in appropriate cortical and subcortical segments during specific language activities. Appropriate manipulation of the stimulus input may demonstrate important asymmetries in cerebral activation. For instance, the occipital and parietal areas may be more metabolically active during the act of reading whereas the temporal and parietal areas may show greater activity when the subject attends to verbal discourse. Similarly, increased activity in the anterior language areas may be anticipated with prolonged verbal output. Studies of cerebral blood flow utilizing [133]Xenon (Ingvar & Schwartz, 1974; Larsen *et al.*, 1978) already indicate that various parts of the cortex are differently activated during different language acts. These demonstrations are preliminary, however, and future investigations with positron CT may lead to increased understanding of focal hemispheric participation in a number of language activities. In the same manner, varied areas of hypermetabolism can be anticipated during a wide variety of behavioral activities. With such a technique, studies that currently are dependent on clinical case material may be performed on healthy, psychologically normal control subjects in the future. Many additional directions for research on cerebral function during controlled psychological function can be contemplated, dependent on the properties of available radiopharmaceuticals and the technical limitations of the imaging equipment.

In the realm of abnormal brain function, useful localizing information is already available from the positron CT technique. Much more information on a wide variety of topics, including nearly all neurobehavioral abnormalities, can be anticipated from this dynamic technique. Thus, in addition to the studies of aphasia and dementia reported above, positron CT evaluation of individuals with varieties of alexia, agraphia, amnesia, apraxia, acalculia, and many more focal neurobehavioral disorders may reveal focal or specific combinations of alterations in cerebral metabolism that underlie the disturbed process. Not only does the positron CT technique appear to demonstrate areas of structural damage accurately, it also appears to indicate areas without structural abnormality that are not functioning normally. This dynamic capability makes the positron CT a valuable addition to the techniques currently used to study the neurobehavioral disorders caused by focal brain damage.

Finally—but probably of the greatest consequence for future behavioral research—it seems probable that the positron CT technique will have its highest value in searching for alterations in metabolism that underlie behavioral abnormalities, not based on focal structural damage. Thus, the organic personality alterations; the cognitive and behavioral changes of chronic epilepsy; the altered cerebral function that characterizes depression, mania, and schizophrenia; and the alterations of behavior produced by a variety of medications may all be reflected by focal alterations in cerebral metabolism even though there are no structural neuroanatomic changes in these disorders. The ability to probe for such alterations in "functional" disease states could offer entirely new horizons for the understanding of a myriad of neuropsychologic problems.

Summary

Preliminary work with Positron-Emission Computed Tomography has already demonstrated a position for this technique among the currently available neuropsychological localizing tools. It seems apparent that future improvements on the apparatus for imaging (the hardware) and the radiopharmaceuticals (the metabolic agents) will offer increasingly useful investigation techniques for neuropsychologic research. Positron CT appears not only to offer a valuable adjunct to the localization studies currently used in neuropsychology but also opens up entirely new vistas for meaningful correlation studies.

Current knowledge already indicates that valuable neuropsychological information will come from cerebral positron CT studies in three areas: (1) assessment of focal cerebral metabolic alterations accompanying specific psychological functions in the normal; (2) assessment of structural and related dynamic alterations of cerebral function in structural disease states; (3) assessment of alterations of cerebral functions occurring with nonstructural behavioral changes including the site of action of the behaviorally active drugs.

References

Alavi, A., Ferris, S., Wolf, A., Reivich, M., Farkas, T., Dann, R., Christman, D., MacGregor, R. R., & Fowler, J. (1980). Determination of cerebral metabolism in senile dementia using F-18-deoxyglucose and positron emission tomography. *Journal of Nuclear Medicine, 21,* 21. (Abstract)

Huang, S. C., Phelps, M. E., Hoffman, E. J., Sideris, K., Selin, C. E., & Kuhl, D. E. (1980). Non-invasive determination of local cerebral metabolic rate of glucose in normal man with (F-18)2-fluoro-2-deoxyglucose and emission computed tomography: Theory and results. *American Journal of Physiology, 238,* E69–E82.

Ingvar, D. H., & Schwartz, M. S. (1974). Blood flow patterns induced in the dominant hemisphere by speech and reading. *Brain, 97,* 274–288.

Kuhl, D. E., Phelps, M. E., Markham C. H., Metter, E. J., Riege, W. H., & Winter, J. (1982). Cerebral metabolism and atrophy in Huntington's disease determined by [18]FDG and computed tomographic scan. *Annals of Neurology, 12,* 425–434.

Kuhl, D. E., & Edwards, R. Q. (1963). Image separation radioisotope scanning. *Radiology, 80,* 653–662.

Kuhl, D. E., Edwards, R. Q., Ricci, A. R., & Reivich, M. (1973). Quantitative section scanning using orthogonal tangent correction. *Journal of Nuclear Medicine, 14,* 196–200.

Kuhl, D. E., Engel, J., Phelps, M. E., & Selin, C. (1980). Epileptic patterns of local cerebral metabolism and perfusion in man determined by emission computed tomography of [18]FDG and [13]NH$_3$. *Annals of Neurology, 8,* 348–360.

Kuhl, D. E., Hoffman, E. J., Phelps, M. E., & Ricci, A. B. (1977). Design and application of the Mark IV scanning system for radionuclide tomography of the brain. In *Medical radionuclide imaging* (Vol. 1). Vienna: IAEA, 1977, pp. 309–320.

Kuhl, D. E., Phelps, M. E., Kowell, A. P., Metter, E. J., Selin, C., & Winter, J. (1980). Effects of stroke on local cerebral metabolism and perfusion: Mapping by emission computed tomography of [18]FDG and [13]NH$_3$. *Annals of Neurology, 8,* 47–60.

Larsen, B., Skinhøj, E., & Lassen, N. A. (1978). Variations in regional cortical blood flow in the right and left hemispheres during automatic speech. *Brain, 101,* 193–210.

Mazziotta, J. C., Phelps, M. E., Carson, R. E., & Kuhl, D. E. (1982). Tomographic mapping of the auditory cortex during auditory stimulation. *Neurology, 32,* 921–937.

Metter, E. J., Wasterlain, C. G., Kuhl, D. E., Hanson, W. R., & Phelps, M. E. (1981). [18]FDG positron emission computed tomography in a study of aphasia. *Annals of Neurology, 10,* 173–183.

Ojemann, G. A. (1975). Language and the thalamus: Object naming and recall during and after thalamic stimulation. *Brain and Language, 2,* 101–120.

Phelps, M. E. (1977). Emission computed tomography. *Seminars in Nuclear Medicine, 7,* 337–365.

Phelps, M. E., Hoffman, E. J., Huang, S. C., & Kuhl, D. E. (1978). ECAT: A new computerized tomographic imaging system for positron-emitting radiopharmaceuticals. *Journal of Nuclear Medicine, 19,* 635–647.

Phelps, M. E., Hoffman, E. J., Mullani, N. A., & Ter-Pogossian, M. M. (1975). Application of annihilation coincidence detection to transaxial reconstruction tomography. *Journal of Nuclear Medicine, 16,* 210–224.

Phelps, M. E., Huang, S. C., Hoffman, E. J., Selin, C., Sokoloff, L., & Kuhl, D. E. (1979). Tomographic measuring of local cerebral glucose metabolic rate in humans with (F-18)-2-fluoro-2-deoxy-D-glucose: Validation of method. *Annals of Neurology, 6,* 371–388.

Phelps, M. E., Kuhl, D. E., & Mazziotta, J. C. (1980). Tomographic mapping of the metabolic changes in the visual cortex during visual stimulation of volunteers and patients with visual defects. *Journal of Nuclear Medicine, 21,* 21. (Abstract)

Reivich, M., Kuhl, D. E., Wolf, A. Greenberg, J., Phelps M. E., Idom, T., Casella, V., Fowler, J., Hoffman, E., Alvia, A., & Sokoloff, L. (1979). The (^{18}F) fluorodeoxyglucose method for the measurement of local cerebral glucose utilization in man. *Circulation Research, 44,* 127–137.

Sokoloff, L., Reivich, M., Kennedy, C., Des Rosiers, M. H., Patlak, C. S., Pettigrew, K. D., Sakurada, O., & Shinohara, M. (1977). The (^{14}C) deoxyglucose method for the measurement of local cerebral glucose utilization: Theory, procedure, and normal values in the conscious and anesthetized albino rat. *Journal of Neurochemistry, 28,* 897–916.

5

Localization of Cognitive Function with Cerebral Blood Flow

*Niels A. Lassen
and Per E. Roland*

Introduction

The concept of each primary sensory cortical area projecting separately to its own neighboring modality specific secondary "association" cortex is well established for the visual, auditory, and tactile–proprioceptive senses (Jones & Powell, 1970). But where is the information integrated from these or other sense modalities? We may see a match, touch it, and hear the characteristic sound when striking it. Clearly, each sense modality adds to and makes up the familiar event perceived—the striking of a match. Indeed, if one of the sense inputs differed from that expected by previous experience and that set up by the other senses, one is startled to discover that something very unusual is at hand. Imagine, for example, that a loud whistling sound is elicited when striking the match. Thus, the sense modalities often are blended; it is the combined multi-modal message that constitutes the perception.

Neuropsychologists traditionally hold that important supramo-dal—so-called tertiary—association functions allowing us to add in-puts from vision, audition, and touch are located *in the posterior part of the brain*, in cortical areas between the three secondary cor-tices mentioned (Figure 1). In particular, the late A. R. Luria ex-presses this concept in many of his texts. He locates the supramodal cortex to extensive regions of the parietal, temporal, and occipital lobes (Luria, 1973).

The present chapter endeavors to challenge this concept. The evi-dence we discuss is based on studies of regional cerebral blood flow (rCBF) in man performed in our laboratory during various visual, auditory, and tactile tests. These tests augment rCBF in the modal-ity-specific primary and secondary cortical areas in the posterior part of the brain. So far, we have not succeeded in finding posterior cortical areas where rCBF increases regardless of the sense modal-ity stimulated. The results of these tests are illustrated.

This contribution to the understanding of the localization of func-tions within the human brain is made with the further aim of il-lustrating the type of information yielded by isotope-imaging techniques applied to normal intact man performing various types of cognitive function.

Subjects

The study is based on observations made of a group of patients in whom carotid angiography was performed for diagnostic reasons, but without evidence of neurological or mental impairment present at the time of study. The clinical history gave indication for the an-giography involving catheterization of the internal carotid artery with a thin, heparin-coated plastic catheter. After informed consent, the session was extended by approximately 1 hour with the aim of further elucidating the integrity of the brain by a series of 5 to 6 intracarotid injections of sterile saline with dissolved Xenon-133, allowing measurement of rCBF during various states of brain func-tion.

In this group of patients further evidence of the normality of the brain's function during the tests included a normal neurological status, technetium-99m isotope scan or CT scan. A tentative diagnosis of epilepsy was made (on supportive electroencephalographic evidence) in a few of the patients, although most of the remaining cases were classified as normal.

Methods

The rCBF measurements were carried out in a quiet room with the subjects in the supine position on a couch and in a relaxed mental state.

The catheter in the internal carotid artery caused no discomfort as local anesthesia was used. The injections of approximately 2 ml saline with Xenon-133 caused only minimal sensations and noise on the injected side of the neck. In fact, the entire rCBF study is so undramatic that, if left to do as they wish, many patients doze off or even fall asleep. Considering also the excellent cooperation of subjects during the tests, the rCBF observations constitute only a minimal perturbation of the states studied. In particular, tenseness and anxiety (known to be able to increase rCBF diffusely in all regions of the brain) were on a fairly low level.

rCBF was measured by a computer-based multidetector 254-channel digital gamma camera (Sveinsdottir, Larsen, Rommer, & Lassen, 1977; Sveinsdottir & Lassen, 1973). The collimator is a slightly curved 4 cm-thick lead slab with one hole for each detector. For each detector, the spatial resolution is in the order of one cm² in the plane of the surface of the brain. In depth, the truncated cone of the field of vision is broader. However, due to tissue absorption, the contribution of counts from the deeper parts of the injected hemisphere is attenuated. About 8 mCi of Xenon-133 was used per injection, giving a maximal counting rate of approximately 1000 cps for detectors over the middle part of the hemisphere. rCBF is calculated by the initial slope method, using a least square linear fit on the background-corrected and logarithmically transformed data from 14 to 60 sec after the injection (Olesen, Paulson, & Lassen, 1971). The results are displayed on a television monitor using a 16-level color code. Within the first minute after each Xenon-133 injection, an arterial blood sample is collected for arterial carbon dioxide (pCO_2) measurement and rCBF corrections of 4% per mm Hg $aPCO_2$ change was used in all detectors.

The relationship between the rCBF map and known brain struc-

tures on the lateral surface of the hemispheres is determined as follows: In all subjects, the position of the head was so adjusted that
the lowest row of detectors corresponds to the orbito–meatal line
with the middle detector overlying the external auditory meatus.
During the first few seconds after the isotope injection, the distribution of counts throughout the arterial system is noted. This angio-
graphic effect (isotope angiogram) allows an approximate
localization of the lateral (Sylvian) fissure so as to assess the outline
of the labeled part of the hemisphere. The proportional system of
Talairach and Szikla (1967) allow us to determine the location of the
main cortical sulci. These are sketched on the rCBF map as described by Larsen, Skinhøj, and Lassen (1978) and Roland and Larsen (1976).

THE RESTING STATE

With the patients at rest in a quiet room (with eyes closed and
ears plugged), the normal rCBF pattern is almost the same in both
hemispheres (Larsen et al., 1978). The highest flow is found in the
frontal lobe, in particular, in its anterior–superior part (prefrontal
cortex) where rCBF is in average 15% above the hemispheric mean
value.

In many subjects, an increase of rCBF above the mean hemispheric value is seen in the part of the superior temporal gyrus (see
also Lassen, Ingvar, & Skinhøj, 1978). It corresponds to the area
activated during sound perception and probably reflects the fact that
the subjects listen despite the precautions mentioned.

In a few subjects studied, the posterior cerebral artery was filled
from the carotid system. These subjects show—even with closed
eyes—an area of relative hyperemia over the most posterior part of
the hemisphere. This is the primary visual cortex, an area with high
rCBF even in absence of visual stimulation as shown by rCBF studies tomographically by Xenon-133 inhalation (Henriksen, Paulson,
& Lassen, 1981).

The CBF pattern during rest is highly reproducible. When CBF is
expressed in percentage of the mean hemispheric flow, the coeffi-
cient of variation of the mean flow in cortical subareas each covered
by 10 detectors is only 3.3% during repeated measurements. Yet,
the mean hemispheric flow decreases by about 5% when a repeated
rest measurement is made (with an interval of 20–40 min). This sys-

tematic decrease of flow—and by inference, also of oxydative metabolism—implies that, unless one is very careful to habituate the patients, the rest condition *cannot be considered a well-defined cerebral state.* Apparently, one tends to rest (relax) better than usual in the course of a series of CBF studies.

VISUAL PERCEPTION

Simple visual perception consisting of opening the eyes and looking at a black cross increases rCBF by 21% in the *occipital and adjacent posterior–inferior temporal regions* (Melamed & Larsen, 1979). More complex forms of visual perception involving the recognition of familiar objects or a reading test increase rCBF to about the same degree and in the same area (Larsen, Orgogozo, Rougier, Sageaux, & Cohadon; 1979 see also Figure 1, lower panel). The activations during visual perception do not extend into the areas *showing rCBF increase* during auditory or tactile perception.

The visual perceptual tasks also increase rCBF in the *frontal eye field* (Figure 1, lower panel) The increase is greatest when the eyes are following a moving object; in this case, the supplementary motor areas show increased rCBF (Melamed & Larsen, 1979). The frontal eye fields also show a marked increase of rCBF during auditory perception (Figure 1, upper panel). In addition, the more complex visual perception tasks—looking at objects or reading—also increases rCBF in the upper *prefrontal cortex* (Larsen et al., 1979), an area also showing rCBF increase during auditory or tactile discrimination tasks.

The *posterior parietal regions* show an increase of rCBF in a visual perception task involving the solution of a difficult-shape discrimination task: the discrimination between elipses of almost the same shape (Roland & Skinhøj, 1981). The upper part of this area also shows rCBF increase during complex movements of the hand in a maze test and in a spiral pattern (Roland, Larsen, Lassen, & Skinhbj, 1980), but not during tactile discrimination by the hand. The lower part of this area, too, shows rCBF increase during auditory stimulation. Additionally, the complex visual discrimination task increased rCBF in the lower part of the frontal lobe, namely, in the same or nearly the same area as seen during auditory discrimination tests. This area, presumably, is involved in the verbal answers given during the test.

AUDITIVE PERCEPTION

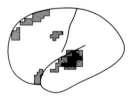

TACTILE PERCEPTION

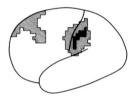

VISUAL PERCEPTION

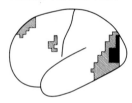

▨ 10 to 20% incr. of rCBF

■ 20 to 50% incr. of rCBF

Figure 1. Simple sensory perception performed by one neurologically intact (normal) subject during measurement of regional cerebral blood flow by intracarotid Xenon-133 injection on left side. The maps show the percentage increase in flow above the resting level.

Upper panel: Auditive perception. Shows the areas of blood flow increase during monaural (right ear) listening to simple words. Areas showing an increase comprise primary and secondary auditory cortex in temporal lobe, orbitofrontal cortex just below Broca's area, the frontal eye field just anterior to central sulcus, and upper prefrontal cortex.

Middle panel: Tactile perception. Shows the areas of blood flow increase during tactile perception of small objects with contralateral (right) hand. The objects are pressed into the palm of the motionless hand at a rate of one every 5 sec. The areas showing up are the sensorimotor hand area and the prefrontal cortex.

Lower panel: Visual perception looking with both eyes open at objects presented at a distance of approximately $\frac{1}{2}$ m. The objects were presented at the rate of one new object every 5 sec. The areas showing up comprise the secondary visual area (area 19 of Brodmann) but not the primary visual area as it filled from the noninjected basilar artery, the frontal eye field, and the prefrontal cortex.

This figure only serves to illustrate with one single study the thesis presented. The argument presented is not based on this study but on the series of studies of each type published in the literature and summarized in the text.

AUDITORY PERCEPTION

Listening to onomatopoeic words such as "splash," "crack," "bang," and so on increases rCBF by 10–20% in the *temporal region* (Larsen, Skinhøj, Soh, Endo, & Lassen; 1977 see also Figure 1, upper panel). The increase is localized to the superior and middle temporal gyrus and stretches to the *inferior posterior parietal region* on the left side where the response to words is most marked (Nishizawa, Skyhøj Olsen, Larsen, & Lassen, 1982). During a well-defined nonverbal sound discrimination task, rCBF increases in the same areas. In this case, the response is most intense on the right side, on which the extension into the *inferior posterior parietal* lobe also is seen (Roland, Skinhøj, & Lassen, 1981).

Auditory perception also increases rCBF in the *frontal eye fields* and in the *upper prefrontal cortex,* namely, in the same areas seen during visual perception (Nishizawa *et al.,* 1982; Roland *et al.,* 1981; Figure 1 upper panel). An area in the *lower posterior part of* the frontal lobe, namely, the Broca area and its right-sided homologue, also is seen (Nishizawa *et al.,* 1982; Roland *et al.,* 1981).

TACTILE PERCEPTION

Simple rhythmical movements of the mouth, hand, or foot augment rCBF in the corresponding contralateral hand and foot sensorimotor area. Thus the sensorimotor homunculus can be outlined (Lassen *et al.,* 1978; see also Orgogozo & Larsen, 1979; Roland, Larsen, Skinhøj, & Lassen, 1977.

Simple tactile perception was studied by Roland and Larsen (1976; see also Figure 1, middle panel). The test involved the discrimination of the shape of objects placed in the hand, mouth or foot. rCBF was found to increase in the contralateral sensorimotor areas. Tactile perception also increased rCBF in the prefrontal cortex (the same area as during visual or auditory perception), but not in the frontal eye fields or in the posterior superior part of the parietal lobe. This latter region showed, however, an increase of rCBF during complex movement of the hand in a maze or in a spiral pattern (Roland, Larsen, Lassen, & Skinhøj, 1980).

TRIMODAL PERCEPTION (SIMULTANEOUS VISUAL, AUDITORY, AND TACTILE PERCEPTION)

In a recently completed study, we studied the effect of a voluntary effort to discriminate the sensory signals perceived in one sensory modality during a trimodality stimulation paradigm. The subjects were stimulated simultaneously with pairs of objects pressed against their palms, pairs of ellipses projected on a screen, and pairs of tone rhythms presented to one ear. The subjects discriminated the stimuli from one modality and ignored the stimuli from the two other modalities. Three tests were performed in random sequence. During each test, the subject was asked to concentrate and discriminate stimuli from one of the three modalities. In these tests, large areas of the posterior part of the brain showed a CBF increase. The response looked like a simple addition of the single-modality stimulation rCBF patterns. A minor accentuation of rCBF increase was found in the association cortex of the modality being actively discriminated. In relationships to the problem analyzed in the present study, it should be noted that no area in the posterior part of the brain showed a larger increase of CBF during trimodality perception than during the single-modality tests. In contrast, the area of the brain that showed the larger increase of rCBF during trimodal perception was the frontal supramodal area. This suggests that, if there is a convergence of information from these three sensory modalities, it is located in the frontal lobe and more specifically in the posterior superior prefrontal cortex.

Discussion

The fact that large areas of brain cortex show increase in flow and metabolism during increased neuronal activity should be commented on first. There can be no doubt that this is the basis for the changes in the rCBF. Both studies in experimental animals and in man point unequivocally to this conclusion. Here the classical study of Raichle, Grubb, Gado, Eichling, and Ter-Pogossian (1976) may be recalled. They also reproduced in man the finding of Olesen in our laboratory, that movements of the hand increased the contralateral primary sensorimotor hand area's flow (Olesen, 1971). Raichle and co-workers (1976) found that the oxygen uptake of the same area was increased almost in proportion to the flow increase. Recently, the same basic result has been reported using Fluorine-18-labeled deoxyglucose. As reported, visual perception increases the glucose uptake of the primary and secondary visual cortex (Phelps, Mazziotta, Kuhl, Nuwer, Packwood, Metter, and Engel, 1981).

In all these as well as in our own studies, the modality-specific areas showing an increase in rCBF *are large and seem to compose the cortical areas involved in the corresponding modality in their full extent.* This is very surprising. Consider, for example, the test in which the tip of one finger is touched by a von Frey hair (Roland, Larsen, Skinhøj, & Lassen, 1977). We would not have expected that this would increase activity–metabolism–blood flow in the same fairly large sensory area as when moving the hand. Even when the finger is not touched at all, but the subject only is awaiting a touch, there is an increase of rCBF in what appears to be the entire primary sensorimotor hand area (Roland, 1981), an effect only slightly less intense than during the actual sensory stimulation. This result suggests a specific enhancement mechanism, namely, that the intense expectation of a touch on a given finger enhances (by thalamocortical circuits?) the activity level of the area—a state of depolarization with enhanced readiness for firing—amplifying so to speak—any sensory input to a maximum. The threshold is apparently lowered so that the noise level becomes an appreciable factor cf., the subjects falsely reported about 2–3 touches of the hair in a 1-minute interval although no touch was being performed (Roland *et al.*, 1981).

The observations are clear-cut: Entire cortical systems, and not subelements thereof, increase neuronal activity–metabolism–flow during the sensory types of brain activity we are discussing. The responses are graded in intensity but not in extension. On this basis—having observed that entire systems become active—the lack of *common* areas in the posterior parts of the brain is noteworthy.

The posterior part of the parietal cortex was the only region showing a rCBF increase during sensory perception involving two different sense modalities: The superior posterior part both during the difficult visual discrimination test and the complex proprioceptive perception of finger–hand–arm movements (maze test, spiral test); the inferior posterior part both during the difficult visual discrimination test and during auditory perception of verbal sounds (on the left side) or of nonverbal sounds (on the right side).

These areas (presumably Brodmann's areas 7 and 39) thus seem to serve as bimodal association areas. It is uncertain, however, whether the sensory inputs from the two senses reach these areas directly from the corresponding secondary cortices or the two inputs are actually compared and jointly analyzed in these regions to form a complete multimodal mental image. The posterior parietal lobe could be involved in hypercomplex analysis of events in extrapersonal space (Roland, Skinhøj, Lassen, & Larsen, 1980 with the supramodal synthesis being performed in other cortical areas (in frontal areas?). However, it should be stressed that simple tactile stimulation of discrimination of objects touched by the hand did *not* activate the posterior parietal lobe, nor does a simple visual perception such as looking at an object or reading a text. Only auditory analysis extends to the lower posterior parietal cortex (only on one side). Thus, with these simple tests, no overlap of rCBF increase areas is seen. To give a familiar example, consider taking a match-box, opening it, and striking a match. This is a typical four-modality perception (sound and smell also being involved) in which—according to our data—no overlap of posterior areas exist. It is our contention, therefore, that the perceptual synthesis is not taking place in posterior parts of the brain.

No attempt will be made to review the basis for the traditional concept of extensive parieto–occipito–temporal "tertiary" multi-modal cortical areas. Indeed, our observations cannot be taken as definite evidence overruling the traditional method of lesions. A rel-atively small increase of rCBF might be difficult to detect. Also it can be conceived that a given area might be involved in multimodal sensory perception *without* this necessarily involving an increase in *overall* neuronal functional activity. It should be emphasized, how-ever, that our method did allow us to find multimodally activated areas in the frontal lobe. The *frontal eye fields* showed an increase of rCBF with both visual and auditory perception. (Perhaps this area is involved in orientation in external space; it is noteworthy that it lies as part of the premotor cortex close to the motor area for the ears and neck.) The superior–anterior part of the frontal lobe (pre-frontal cortex) also is typically activated in terms of rCBF increase in complex sensory or motor tasks of various types. This, along with the fact that man has an exceptionally large frontal lobe—and also unusual faculties for complex types of perception—leads us to sug-gest that the supramodal synthesis is mainly localized there.

The intra-arterial Xenon-133 injection method used in this study offers an adequate spatial resolution of about 2.3 cm² on the super-ficial cortex. The method suffers, however, from several obvious limitations: (1) it is traumatic; therefore, it can be used only in con-junction with diagnostic angiography; (2) it is two-dimensional and limited to the area of supply of the injected artery. These limitations are, in principle, circumvented by the tomographic methods. In par-ticular, positron emission tomography holds much promise, based on the use of the metabolic-marked Fluor-18-deoxyglucose (Phelps, *et al.*, 1981). The radiation exposure to the target organ (the bladder) is, however, not entirely negligible. The cost and clumsiness of the procedure (demanding a 40-minute-steady-state period) should also be mentioned. Since photon emission tomography of inhaled Xenon-133 allows more ready repetition of the studies that last 4 min, the radiation exposure to the target organ (the lung) is less and the costs and clumsiness of the procedure is reduced (compared to the positron technique). On the other hand, the spatial resolution of the positron method is superior.

These comments touch but a few of the most promising avenues. We do not attempt to review the widely used Xenon-133-inhalation rCBF method based on a battery of stationary detectors. In principle, this method shows the same as the intra-arterial Xenon-133 method we use. But because the spatial resolution is much inferior, one cannot demand it to yield as specific an answer to localization problems. However, taken together, all methods based on radioisotopes promise to advance our understanding of the function of specific brain areas substantially.

References

Henriksen, L., Paulson, O. B., & Lassen, N. A. (1981). Regional cerebral blood flow response to visual activation recorded by emission computerized tomography of inhaled Xenon-133. *Journal of Cerebral Blood Flow and Metabolism, Supplement 1, 1,* 23–24.

Jones, E. G., & Powell, T. P. S. (1970). An anatomical study of converging sensory pathways within the cerebral cortex of the monkey. *Brain, 93,* 793–820.

Larsen, B., Orgogozo, J. M., Rougier, A., Sageaux, J. C., & Cohadon, F. (1979). Regional cortical blood flow with the 254 Channels gamma-camera. A stereo-tactic study. *Acta Neurologica Scandinavica, Supplementum 72, 60,* 234–235.

Larsen, B., Skinhøj, E., & Lassen, N. A. (1978). Variations in regional cortical blood flow in the right and left hemispheres during automatic speech. *Brain, 101,* 193–209.

Larsen, B., Skinhøj, E., Soh, K., Endo, H., & Lassen, N. A. (1977). The pattern of cortical activity provoked by listening and speech revealed by rCBF measurements. *Acta Neurologica Scandinavica, Supplementum 64, 56,* 268–269.

Lassen, N. A., Ingvar, D. H., & Skinhøj, E. (1978). Brain function and blood flow. *Scientific American, 239,* 62–71.

Luria, A. R. (1973). *The working brain.* Middlesex, England: Penguin Press.

Melamed, E., & Larsen, B. (1979). Cortical activation pattern during saccadic eye movements in humans: Localization by focal cerebral blood flow increases. *Annals of Neurology, 5,* 79–88.

Nishizawa, Y., Skyhøj Olsen, T., Larsen, B., & Lassen, N. A. (1982). Left-right cortical asymmetries of regional cerebral blood flow during listening to words. *Journal of Neurophysiology, 48,* 458–466.

Olesen, J. (1971). Contralateral focal increase of cerebral blood flow in man during arm work. *Brain, 94,* 635–646.

Olesen, J., Paulson, O., & Lassen, N. A. (1971). Regional cerebral blood flow in man determined by the initial slope of the clearance of intra-arterially injected ^{133}Xe. *Stroke, 2,* 519–540.

Orgogozo, J. M., & Larsen, B. (1979). Activation of the supplementary motor area during voluntary movement in man suggests it works as a supramotor area. *Science, 206,* 847–850.

Phelps, M. E., Mazziotta, J. C., Kuhl, D. E., Nuwer, M., Packwood, J., Metter, J., & Engel, J., Jr. (1981). Tomographic mapping of human cerebral metabolism: Visual stimulation and deprivation. *Neurology, 31,* 517–529.

Raichle, M. E., Grubb, R. L., Gado, M. H., Eichling, J. O., and Ter-Pogossian, M. M. (1976). Correlation between regional cerebral blood flow and oxidative metabolism. *Archives of Neurology (Chicago), 33,* 523–526.

Roland, P. E. (1981). Somatotopical tuning of postcentral gyrus during focal attention in man. A regional cerebral blood flow study. *Journal of Neurophysiology, 46,* 744–754.

Roland, P. E., & Larsen, B. (1976). Focal increase of cerebral blood flow during stereognostic testing in man. *Archives of Neurology (Chicago), 33,* 551–558.

Roland, P. E., Larsen, B., Lassen, N. A., & Skinhöj, E. (1980). Supplementary motor area and other cortical artas in organization of voluntary movements in man. *Journal of Neurophysiology, 43,* 118–136.

Roland, P. E., Larsen, B., Skinhøj, E., and Lassen, N. A. (1977). Regional cerebral blood flow increase due to treatment of somatosensory and auditory information in man. *Acta Neurologica Scandinavica, Supplementum 64, 56,* 540–541.

Roland, P. E., & Skinhøj, E. (1981). Extrastriate cortical areas activated during visual discrimination in man. *Brain Research, 222,* 166–171.

Roland, P. E., Skinhøj, E., Larsen, B., & Lassen, N. A. (1977). The role of different cortical areas in the organization of voluntary movements in man. *Acta Neurologica Scandinavica, Supplementum 64, 56,* 542–543.

Roland, P. E., Skinhøj, E., & Lassen, N. A. (1981). Focal activations of human cerebral cortex during auditory discrimination. *Journal of Neurophysiology, 45,* 374–386.

Roland, P. E., Skinhøj, E., Lassen, N. A., & Larsen, B. (1980). Different cortical areas in man in organization of voluntary movements in extrapersonal space. *Journal of Neurophysiology, 43,* 137–150.

Sveinsdottir, E., Larsen, B., Rommer, P., & Lassen, N. A. (1977). A multidetector scintillation camera with 254 channels. *Journal of Nuclear Medicine, 18,* 168–174.

Sveinsdottir, E., & Lassen, N. A. (1973). A 254-detector system for regional cerebral blood flow. *Stroke, 4,* 365.

Talairach, J., & Azikla, G. (1967). *Atlas of stereotaxic anatomy of the telencephalon.* Paris: Masson.

6

Localization of Language and Visuospatial Functions by Electrical Stimulation

Catherine A. Mateer

Introduction

As this volume attests, observations about the functional localization of cognitive functions in the human brain are derived from a variety of techniques. Each technique is inherently associated with both advantages and disadvantages that define and limit the theories and models of functional brain organization derived from the observations. This chapter considers a body of data and the models those data have suggested for the intrahemispheric organization of cognitive functions that have been derived from the technique of electrical stimulation mapping. We review data based on both language and language-related functions in reference to left dominant hemisphere organization and visuospatial functions in reference to right nondominant hemisphere organization. A body of data derived from stimulation of subcortical structures, particularly the thalamus, is not discussed in this chapter as recently it has been the subject of several reviews (Mateer & Ojemann, 1983; Ojemann, 1982).

The Technique of Electrical Stimulation Mapping for Functional Localization

Historical Perspectives and Working Hypotheses

It has long been known that cortical function in animals and man can be altered by focal application of small electrical currents (Cushing, 1909; Fritsch & Hitzig, 1870). Extensive use of the technique in man developed in conjunction with the development of surgical techniques for cortical resection of epileptic foci under local anesthesia (Penfield & Jasper, 1954; Penfield & Perot, 1963; Penfield & Roberts, 1959). Identification of sensorimotor cortex and of cortex important to language by the stimulation mapping procedure allows these areas to be spared, greatly increasing the margin of safety associated with cortical resection. Continued experience with stimulation mapping of cortical function has identified minimal if any additional risk to surgical patients specific to cortical stimulation (Ojemann, in press).

Application of an alternating electrical current to neural tissue in general and to cortical tissue in particular has a variety of excitatory and inhibitory effects both locally and at a distance from the stimulation site. (See review by Ranck, 1975.) Neither specific predictions nor detailed descriptions of the physiological effects of stimulation are available at this time. Observations of the effects of electrical stimulation thus are approached empirically.

Specific movements or reports of sensation are commonly evoked by focal cortical application of electrical stimulation in awake patients. The sensory reports specific to auditory and visual as well as to somesthetic sensations, and the motor responses are commonly associated with stimulation at discrete sites and are very repeatable over multiple stimulations. With few exceptions, the stimulation sites associated with motor and sensory responses are located in areas one might predict for them on the basis of classic neuroanatomical organization. In contrast, in the quiet patient who is not engaged in task-specific behavior, stimulation of cortex outside of these areas, at the same level of current, usually has no observable or reported effects. These areas of cortex are said to be silent.

If, however, the patient is engaged in a specific task, for example, a measure of spoken language such as naming, application of the current to one or more sites in the silent region may disrupt performance on the ongoing task. If care is taken so that the level of stimulation used is below that generating afterdischarges, recovery of normal function resumes the instant the current is removed. This disruptive effect of stimulation on behavior has been modeled as a reversible temporary lesion similar to the transient disruptive effect on isolated function seen in focal seizures. The exact nature and extent of functional neuronal disruption caused by the stimulating current is not well documented; empirically, the stimulation effects at a particular site are often both repeatable and quite different from the repeated effects of stimulation at sites only a few millimeters away (Ojemann & Whitaker, 1978a). Stimulation effects thus are modeled as temporary lesions localized in both space and time.

ADVANTAGES AND DISADVANTAGES

The limitations to understanding functional brain organization derived from this technique are, in many respects, similar to those inherent to models of functional organization based on spontaneously occurring cerebral lesions. What both techniques identify are areas essential for some facet or facets of a cognitive or behavioral process. This is not necessarily the area that primarily participates in or generates the process. In some circumstances, the function of a disrupted area may be only to provide access to fibers in passage between more directly involved cortical regions. One major advantage over lesion studies that the stimulation mapping technique provides is the small size of the involved area at any one time, providing a greater degree of spatial resolution for localization. A second advantage is the sudden onset and immediate reversibility of the effect. It is unlikely that observations attained in stimulation mapping studies are as affected by recovery of function and compensatory reorganization as are observations made in studies based on spontaneous brain lesions.

A third advantage of the stimulation mapping technique is that stimulation effects on multiple behaviors can be assessed at multiple cortical sites in an individual patient. The resultant pattern of changes not only provides evidence for the involvement of particular areas in aspects of cognitive functions, but can provide valuable insights into the relative dependence and/or independence of different language related functions. Spontaneous lesions involving a much broader cortical area usually result in a wide variety of symptoms and are thus far more likely to mask these important interrelationships. Dissociation of functions by their disruption at different sites, as well as association of functions by their mutual disruption at common sites, is critical to a better understanding of neurolinguistic organization. Indeed, the double dissociations of stimulation-related disruption of separate language functions provide the bases for our development of a model of brain organization for language that is different in several respects from those derived from lesion data.

The major limitations of the stimulation mapping technique include the population available for investigation and the testing constraints. Patients undergoing these neurosurgical procedures obviously have neurological abnormalities which predate the clinical procedures. Aside from the sodium amytal determination of language localization and the data regarding probable conditions for interhemispheric reorganization (Rasmussen & Milner, 1977), the effects of the disease process on cerebral organization in general and functional intrahemispheric localization in particular are essentially unknown. Preliminary data (Ojemann & Whitaker, 1978) does not support a correspondence between the extent of the epileptic cortex as determined by electrocorticography and language localization as identified by stimulation mapping, suggesting that the disease process may have little effect on the intrahemispheric localization of language, but further observations of this nature are necessary.

Another limitation, the nature of test procedures, relates to the requirements of task design and administration. The need for comparable test items for testing across sites and for repeated measures of intraoperative baseline test performance without stimulation requires that multiple test items of comparable difficulty be prepared. A further limitation is that test items be of a level of difficulty and length that each item can reasonably be completed within 12 sec, the upper limits of stimulation duration at any one site at any one time. Difficulty level must be set so that baseline control nonstimulation error rates are near zero and yet that tasks are demanding enough to engage various levels of linguistic or cognitive involvement.

GENERAL METHODS

The bulk of this chapter reviews results from cortical stimulation studies carried out in the Department of Neurological Surgery at the University of Washington. All studies are conducted during craniotomies for resection of medically intractable epileptic foci under xylocaine or bupivacaine local anesthesia. In most cases, the focus is in the anterior temporal lobe with the surgical exposure encompassing not only all of the lateral surface of the temporal lobe but portions of the posterior frontal and inferior parietal cortex adjacent to the Sylvian fissure. Preoperative assessments include a neuropsychologic battery for epilepsy (Dodrill, 1978) and determination of language lateralization by intracarotid Amytal (WADA) testing. Almost all patients come to surgery with a history of pharmacologic intervention for the seizure disorder. Most are on one or more of the common anticonvulsants including phenytoin, carbamazepine, valproate, primidone, and phenobarbital.

The design of the intraoperative stimulation studies has involved obtaining multiple samples of performance on a number of different tasks assessing related behaviors in conjunction with stimulation of multiple sites on the lateral cortical surface in each patient. Whether language related behaviors or visuospatial functions are tested depends on the side of operation and the known language lateralization. Frequent samples of task performance on which no stimulation occurs are pseudorandomly interspersed with stimulation trials. The performance on trials without stimulation serves as the measure of intraoperative control performance. Multiple samples of a particular behavior obtained during stimulation at a particular site (commonly at least three) are evaluated with respect to a large corpus of performance on nonstimulation control trials (commonly 70–80 trials) to statistically evaluate whether performance with stimulation at a particular site is different from control performance. A binomial single-sample test in which the control performance serves as the estimator of error probability is utilized for the statistical assessment (Siegel, 1955).

Stimulation studies are carried out after electrocorticographic

identification of the epileptic focus and identification of sensorimotor cortex by cortical stimulation. Multiple sites at the posterior
margins of the identified epileptic focus and in nonepileptic brain
in the temporal, inferior parietal, and posterior frontal cortex are
selected and marked by placement of sterile numbered tickets. The
threshold current for afterdischarge is identified for each site and
all stimulation during mapping is at a current level just below the
lowest of these thresholds. Trains of 60 Hz, 2½ msec total duration
biphasic square wave pulses from a constant current stimulator are
delivered through bipolar silver ball electrodes, 5 mm apart. The
threshold for afterdischarge using these stimulation parameters is
variable across patients (3–8 mA between peaks of biphasic pulses);
within patients, it is both consistent across sites outside of Rolandic
cortex and remarkably stable for repeated stimulation of a particular site. Stimulation outside Rolandic cortex generally produces no
movement or detectable sensation so that patients are unaware of
when current is applied. All testing is carried out using repetitive
trials. Stimulation is applied at the onset of a trial or segment of a
trial and is maintained for the duration of the segment, typically
4–12 sec depending on the function being tested. Patients' responses
and markers indicating both trial and stimulation onset and offset
are recorded on audio and, where appropriate, videotape for subsequent analysis.

Localization of Language-Related Behavior
in the Dominant Left Hemisphere

Concepts about the neurological organization of human communication is divided into two broad areas. The first area involves identification of cortex concerned with language on the basis of
alterations in naming. Two general principles, discrete localization
and individual variability, are well demonstrated in the analysis of
evoked disruption of naming. In addition, the large body of data on
naming has allowed analysis of the relationship of other variables
such as sex and general verbal ability to cortical organization of
naming as determined by this technique. The second area involves
the identification of subdivisions of language function and their interaction using the cortical stimulation mapping paradigm. These
subdivisions include—in addition to naming—articulatory accuracy, integrity of grammatic and semantic aspects of linguistic

structure in sentence level productions, short term verbal memory, nonverbal oral praxis, and speech sound identification. Localization of these subdivisions and an analysis of their patterns of interaction will be used to suggest a model of neurolinguistic organization.

LANGUAGE AND LANGUAGE-RELATED MEASURES

Three language tests measuring five different language functions have been used in these stimulation mapping studies. One test measures naming, reading of simple sentences, and short-term verbal memory, the latter in a single-item paradigm patterned after the Peterson and Peterson (1959) measure. This test consists of a series of consecutive trials presented visually as slides. The first segment of each trial is a slide of an object whose name is a common word with a carrier phrase such as "this is a—" printed above it. The patient is instructed to read the carrier phrase and name the object. The second segment of each trial is a slide with an 8–10-word sentence which the patient is to read aloud. The verb in the second clause of each sentence is left blank, and is to be completed by the patient. The sentences are constructed so they must be completed with one of a small number of inflected verb forms. The third segment of each trial is a slide with the word "recall" printed on it. This acts as a cue for the patient to state aloud the name of the object pictured on the first slide of this trial, a name retained across the distraction produced by reading the sentences. Stimulation occurs during the naming segment on some trials, the reading segment on others, and the recall segment on still others. Control trials are pseudorandomly interspersed with stimulation trials. The sequence of site and test conditions is so arranged that no site is stimulated consecutively and stimulation at each site on each condition is distributed throughout the testing period. Performance of this test is analyzed for stimulation effects on naming and reading, and for the effects of stimulation at the time of input (naming), storage (reading), or retrieval (recall) on short-term verbal memory. Trials with errors in naming are excluded from analysis of memory performance to ensure that the information to be remembered has been adequately perceived.

A second test of language-related functions assesses the ability to mimic single or sequential oral–facial postures. The patient is shown a series of slides, each with three simple oral–facial postures such as protrusion of the tongue or pursing of the lips. One series of slides shows the same posture repeated three times; the second series shows three different postures. The patient is instructed to mimic the postures. Stimulation occurs on a randomly selected half of each series. The patient's facial movements are recorded onto videotape together with markers identifying onset, offset, and location of stimulation. These tapes are initially evaluated without knowledge of whether stimulation has occurred.

The final language test measures the ability to identify phonemes embedded in a carrier phrase. A stop consonant, /p/, /b/, /t/, /d/, /k/, or /g/, is embedded in the nonsense disyllable /ae___ma/ on pre-recorded tapes in live voice. The carrier phrase with the embedded consonant is presented in a two-second period followed by a two-second quiet period during which the patient responds. Stimulation occurs only during the two seconds when the disyllable with its embedded consonant is presented and not during the response period to avoid any confounding of effects of stimulation on speech output. For all tests, markers indicating that stimulation has or has not occurred are recorded on a separate channel so off-line scoring can be done blindly as to the presence or absence of stimulation.

GENERAL CHARACTERISTICS OF LANGUAGE ORGANIZATION SUGGESTED BY STIMULATION MAPPINGS

DISCRETE LOCALIZATION

The discreteness of effects evoked by stimulation is a striking feature of the electrical mapping studies. Stimulation of one cortical site will alter a language function, such as naming, on every trial, whereas stimulation at the same current at another site within a half cm along the same gyrus may have no effect whatsoever (Ojemann & Whitaker, 1978). This discreteness of effect is found not only in relationship to the specific cortical site that is stimulated but also to the particular language-related task used. With a constant stimulating current, one frequently finds sites where only one of the multiple language functions tested is altered with stimulation.

Different cortical sites in an individual seem primarily concerned with different language-related functions. Of three behaviors (for example, naming, reading, and short-term verbal recall), only one may be disrupted at a particular cortical site; performance on the others may be unaffected by stimulation. Indeed, as will be discussed in the results from analysis on sentence-reading performance, only one aspect of performance on a task may be disrupted. Grammatical usage may be disrupted in the context of otherwise fluent, well articulated, and semantically correct productions with stimulation at one site, whereas stimulation at another may selectively alter only articulatory or semantic aspects.

INDIVIDUAL VARIABILITY

Although separate and often isolated functional changes can be discretely associated with stimulation of a particular cortical site in individual patients, the exact cortical localization of the sites showing these changes seems to be highly variable across patients, who, nevertheless, all show the usual pattern of left brain dominance. Because of its easy administration and scoring and the very low baseline error rates it generates, naming is the language task which has, at this point, proved most fruitful in characterizing and understanding the degree and nature of this individual variability in cortical organization of language. These studies are discussed, describing results on the naming task.

IMPLICATIONS ABOUT CORTICAL ORGANIZATION OF LANGUAGE SUGGESTED BY EVOKED DISRUPTION OF NAMING

Naming errors, including total speech arrest, inability to name with retained ability to speak (anomia), and misnaming have been found with stimulation of a broad area of lateral dominant cortex. Some of the individual sites where naming changes have been evoked extend well beyond the traditional limits of the lateral cortical language areas, into middle and superior portions of the frontal lobe (Ojemann & Whitaker, 1978), anteriorly in temporal lobe (Ojemann & Mateer, 1979), and well back almost to the parieto-occipital junction (Van Buren, Fedio, & Frederick, 1978). Even with respect to the traditional language areas, there is considerable individual variability in the extent of cortex related to naming by stimulation mapping. Stimulation of a small area in the left posterior inferior frontal cortex immediately in front of face motor cortex almost invariably produces speech errors, usually in the form of speech arrest. Outside of this area, however, disruption of naming by stimulation in any of seven arbitrarily identified zones in the frontal, temporal, and parietal cortex, including all of the posterior superior temporal gyrus, the traditional Wernicke's area, is seen in less than two-thirds of the patients (Ojemann, 1979; Ojemann & Whitaker, 1978).

The degree of individual variability in location of sites related to several types of language change on the reading task and to the memory task appear to be as great as that for naming. (These data are discussed later in this chapter in relationship to Figure 2.) With a broad sampling of linguistic behavior, as is provided by the multiple functions tested, most, though not quite all patients, do show some kind of language change with stimulation of the traditional language zones, the inferior posterior frontal cortex and the middle to posterior superior temporal gyrus. This suggests that the overall areas related to language may be relatively uniform, but with individual variability of sites related to specific language functions. Such a proposal is not inconsistent with the data from spontaneous lesions. Aphasias resulting from what may appear as nearly identical cortical lesions may have quite variable linguistic characteristics. And indeed, variable behavioral correlates of cortical areas should not be so surprising in view of the high degree of individual variability in both gross morphological structure (Rubens, Mahowald, & Hutton, 1976) and cytoarchitectonic patterns (Galaburda, Sanides, & Geschwind, 1978) in human cortex.

Although individual variability of cortical organization of language functions by the stimulation mapping technique thus is not unexpected, we attempt to use it to further explore what may be important underlying correlates of cortical organization of language functions. Not all individuals use language with the same degree of facility and across groups of individuals, a variety of investigative techniques yield different patterns of neurolinguistic organization. We correlate two independent patient characteristics, the patient's sex and their preoperative verbal IQ with patterns of stimulation related naming changes. We used sex as a correlate because recent data suggest differential patterns of aphasia in males and females following anterior versus posterior left hemisphere lesions (Kimura, 1980). Verbal IQ was selected as an independent measure of general verbal facility.

SEX DIFFERENCES IN VARIABILITY

Distribution of sites on the left lateral cortex involved in naming by the stimulation mapping technique varied significantly between a sample of eight males and 10 females (Mateer, Polen, & Ojemann, 1982). Overall, naming errors were evoked from 63% of the total sites sampled in males (32 of 51) but from only 38% of the total sites in females (16 of 68) (.025 $p < .05$). When the lateral cortex was divided into eight zones (Figure 1) the percentage of sites in a zone related to naming change was significantly higher for males than females in two of the zones, an anterior frontal zone (80% of males versus 22% of females, $p < .05$) and a posterior parietal zone (males 57%, females 0%, $p < .05$). Proportionately, males were also at least twice as likely to demonstrate evoked naming errors with stimulation of an anterior parietal zone and two middle temporal gyrus zones, though these differences did not reach significance. Males

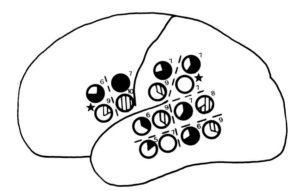

Figure 1. Sexual variability in language localization in dominant left lateral cortex. Dashed lines separate eight arbitrary zones established in anterior and posterior language areas. The numbers adjacent to each circle indicate the number of patients with one or more sites of stimulation mapping in each zone. The circle graphs, given separately by sex, show the proportion of patients making *naming* errors on a statistically significant portion of trials with stimulation at one or more sites in that zone (black filled areas for males, stripe filled areas for females). Stars indicate the two zones for which the sex difference in proportion was significant ($p < .05$) (From Mateer, Polen, & Ojemann, 1982).

appeared to use a broader overall area of left cortex for naming. Thus, sex may to some degree determine not only interhemispheric patterns of language organization, but the extent and pattern of intrahemispheric representation of language.

Verbal IQ was also correlated with patterns of stimulation evoked naming change (S. Polen & G. Ojemann, unpublished observations). A series of 21 patients ranging in preoperative IQ from 69 to 115 was divided into two groups on the basis of verbal IQ. Of 10 patients with verbal IQs at or below 96, 7 demonstrated naming changes with stimulation in the posterior parietal region, only 1 of 10 patients with verbal IQ's greater than 96 demonstrated evoked changes in naming with stimulation in that area ($p < .025$). They have hypothesized that the presence of language functions in the parietal lobe, at least for purposes of naming, may reflect a less advantageous pattern of cortical language organization.

MAPPING THE BILINGUAL BRAIN

A final area in which the issue of variability in functional representation has been addressed has involved measurement of a single language function such as naming in two different languages. These studies were done in a small group of bilingual patients undergoing awake craniotomy with stimulation mapping (Mateer & Rapport, 1983; Ojemann & Whitaker, 1978b; Rapport, Tan, & Whitaker, in press). In all cases, there have been some dissociated sites implicated in each language, cortical sites where stimulation altered naming in one language but not in the other. At other sites, naming in both languages was disrupted with stimulation. This dissociation of cortical sites involving different languages is consistent with dissociated recovery of different languages seen in cases of polyglot aphasia (Paradis, 1977). Another striking feature of the stimulation mapping in two languages: Naming in the language in which patients were less competent was altered from a greater number of sites and thus a broader area of cortex than naming in the language in which they were familiar. It has been hypothesized that the area of cortex utilized for a particular language process may be larger for functions of greater unfamiliarity and/or less automaticity.

We have also had the opportunity to extend these bilingual investigations into the area of manual communication systems in two patients and found results similar to that seen with two oral languages (Mateer, Polen, Ojemann, & Wyler, 1982; Mateer, Rapport, & Kettrick, in press). One patient was tested in both oral language and finger spelling, the other in oral language and American Sign Language. Both patients were normally hearing and acquired the manual systems within the preceding 3 years. In both patients, some common and some dissociated cortical sites were identified with disruption of expression in each language. In both cases, the manually based system of expression, the more recently learned and less automatic, was disrupted at a greater number of sites.

In conclusion, individual variability in localization of language function appears not to be simply an artifact of the mapping technique. Variability in extent of language related cortex, at least as identified by naming, is consistent with results from studies using other methods of functional localization and with known anatomic variability. In addition, the variability is correlated with independent measures such as sex, verbal IQ, general facility with a language system, and probably with a host of other variables we have yet to identify.

ORGANIZATION OF LINGUISTIC FUNCTIONS DERIVED FROM SENTENCE READING

Object naming has traditionally been used as the behavioral measure of language. It is obvious from studies of aphasia, of course, that many other aspects of linguistic behavior can be specifically disrupted in association with brain dysfunction. Indeed, interest in the linguistic analysis of aphasia has significantly impacted the study of acquired language deficit in the last decade (Blumstein, 1981). A procedure, therefore, was devised to evoke sentence level expressive productions, using a reading task in conjunction with the cortical stimulation mapping procedure. Of interest was the analysis of disturbances of phonologic, semantic, and syntactic features of language use in relationship to transient focal brain disruption via the stimulation mapping techniques.

The subjects on which the analysis of reading disruption was based were 14 native English-speaking monolingual adult patients (10 female, 4 male), age 18–46 years ($x = 28.1$ years) (Mateer, 1982).

characteristics between patients with Broca's and Wernicke's aphasia, although such errors were more frequent in patients with the former. (In contrast, phonetic dissociation, an acoustic distinction not measurable in our study, did differentiate patients in the Blumstein study.)

NEOLOGISMS

Ten sites were associated with neologisms, that, by criteria, were normally articulated, had acceptable phonologic form, and either were not associated with target or had less than 50% of the phones of target words. Some multisyllabic, phonetically varied neologisms often occurred in the context of extensive semantic and grammatic breakdown (e.g., If next *winzer* is worth and sucks . . .). In these cases, patients often started a sentence correctly with neologisms appearing only when content words were required, suggesting a possible semantic basis for the disturbance. Other neologistic productions occurred in the context of severe articulatory breakdown. Although coarticulated, these "phonetic neologisms" occurred in a context of articulatory breakdown characterized by production of isolated grouping sounds and absence of phonologic form (e.g., if the secretary will *dai* tencils, I will /zətəb/, I /bədətvit/, /pətətoz/these neologisms appeared to bear a greater relationship to overall phonologic and articulatory breakdown than the previous examples, there was a similar tendency for functor words to be better preserved than the content words.

OVERLAP OF ERROR TYPES

Of the 9 sites representing articulatory errors, 6 (67%) were associated only with articulatory change. When these sites were associated with another kind of change, it was always with grammatical change. The sites associated with articulatory change were in inferior frontal, superior mid-temporal, and inferior parietal cortex in all cases but one within one gyrus of the Sylvian fissure. In contrast to this pattern of isolated articulatory change, only 3 of 15 grammar sites (20%) and 4 of 14 semantic sites (29%) were isolated changes in one category. Ten sites representing 71% of semantic sites and 67% of grammatic sites had both kinds of error. All three isolated grammar sites and two of the four isolated semantic sites were at least one gyrus away from the Sylvian fissure.

Of the 12 mixed sites (83%) where both grammar and semantics were disrupted, 10 were in the immediate periSylvian cortex. In summary, sites associated with grammatical error overlapped with articulation-related sites to a small extent, and with semantically related sites to a greater extent. Articulation and semantic sites overlapped only once and then with grammar as well. It may be that grammatical function serves as the interface between the articulatory–phonologic and the semantic system. Articulatory and overlapping grammatic-semantic functions are represented in the periSylvian region. Isolated grammatically and semantically related sites appeared to have a more distal representation.

INDIVIDUAL VARIABILITY IN EVOKED ALTERATIONS
ON SENTENCE READING

As in naming, there is a substantial degree of individual variability in the distribution of sites associated with stimulation evoked alterations in reading. The numbers of Figure 2 represent the percentage of patients in whom sites located in 1 of 16 designated areas

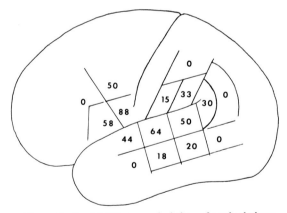

Figure 2. Variability in probability of evoked alterations in sentence reading. Numbers represent the percentage of patients for whom sites in each of the 16 arbitrarily designated regions on the left lateral cortex are associated with significant alterations in reading. Areas most strongly implicated include the posterior and inferior frontal zones and the middle and posterior portions of the superior temporal gyrus. Data is based on 14 patients. All zones were not sampled in all patients.

was associated with significant reading disruption (errors in one or more categories relative to baseline performance). The areas most often involved across patients include, in order of frequency: the inferior posterior frontal zone (88%), the middle superior temporal gyrus zone (64%), and the inferior anterior frontal zone (58%) followed by the posterior mid-frontal and the posterior superior temporal gyrus zones (50% each). With stimulation of other regions surrounding these zones, only between 0–44% of patients demonstrated significant reading disruption.

Examples of distribution of errors are seen in the maps for two individual patients (Figure 3). Some sites are associated with multiple error types. These are almost invariably located in the immediate periSylvian region. Articulatory or phonologic disruption is also only seen with stimulation in this region. Isolated disruption of a single aspect of linguistic production such as grammatic or semantic usage or of naming is usually found at some distance from the periSylvian cortex.

THE RELATIONSHIP BETWEEN ERRORS OF NAMING
AND ERRORS ON THE READING TASK

One of the reasons for developing the reading task was to evaluate more complex aspects of linguistic production in order to sensitize our measure of language function. The distribution and overlap of naming and reading errors is diagrammed in Figure 4. In the 14 patients whose results on the reading task were presented in the previous section, 26 sites were associated with evoked naming errors. Of these sites, 88% were also associated with significant alterations in at least one error category on the reading task. Of the 53 total sites associated with evoked changes in reading, 28 (63%) were not associated with naming errors. Thus, whereas most sites associated with naming errors were also associated with reading errors, many sites are associated only with what appears to be the more sensitive reading task. Two of the three sites involved with naming only were located in the posterior portion of the middle temporal gyrus. These findings are strikingly consistent with the lesion data. Although naming deficits are ubiquitous with almost all aphasic types and usually overlap to some extent with other kinds of linguistic disruption, anomic patients in whom the naming deficit is prominent and often isolated have been reported to have re-

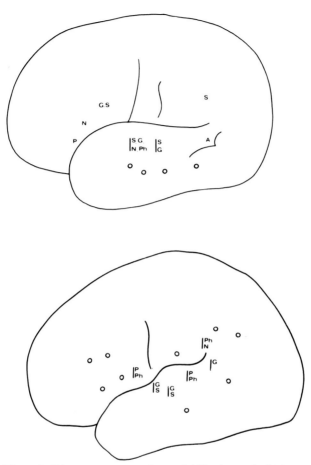

Figure 3. Diagrams representing variability in cortical stimulation mapping results for naming and sentence reading in two patients. Each circle or cortical location marked by letter(s) represents a site which was stimulated in a standard mapping paradigm. Letters indicate significant changes in performance from baseline performance in the form of speech arrest (A), anomia (N), articulatory perseveration (P), articulatory or phonologic errors (Ph), semantic errors (S), grammatical errors (G). Letters next to a vertical line represent multiple functions disrupted from stimulation at a single site.

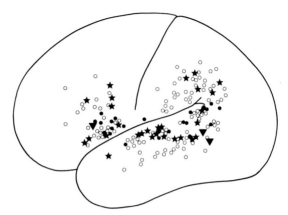

Figure 4. Composite map for 14 patients. Each circle or symbol represents a stimulation site. Inverted triangles represent three sites at which only naming was altered, one in the anterior frontal region, two in the posterior portion of the mid–temporal gyrus. Stars represent sites where only one or more aspects of sentence reading was altered. Filled circles represent sites at which both naming and reading were altered.

stricted lesions in this same region involving the posterior mid-temporal gyrus (Mazzocchi & Vignolo, 1979).

EVOKED ALTERATION IN SHORT-TERM VERBAL MEMORY

Disruption of recall, using the previously described Peterson and Peterson (1959) short-term postdistractional recall task, has been associated with stimulation of sites on the dominant lateral cortex. Often, stimulation of a particular site is effective in disrupting recall only when it is applied during one of the phases, that is, during the input to short-term memory (naming slide), the distraction phase (reading slide), or the retrieval from short-term memory (recall slide) (Ojemann, 1978). How do these memory-related sites overlap with other language related functions? Seventeen memory-related sites were identified in a subsample ($n = 10$) of the 14 patients discussed previously in relationship to reading performance. Of those 17 sites, 13 (76%) were associated only with evoked memory changes, not with naming or reading disruption. Memory sites have consistently been characterized by this largely separate cortical representation across several series of patients (Ojemann, 1979, 1982; Ojemann & Mateer, 1979). The locations of these memory-related sites are usually at some distance from but surrounding the periSylvian cortex in high- to mid-frontal, mid-temporal, and especially parietal cortex. Indeed, evoked changes in memory are the most common change seen with parietal stimulation. Again, this localization is consistent with the data from lesion studies. Although, some degree of short-term verbal memory impairment is seen in nearly all aphasic syndromes, conduction aphasia, an aphasic syndrome that a number of authors argue is fundamentally related to short-term verbal memory impairment, is most commonly localized by anatomical locus of lesion to parietal cortex (Warrington, Logue, & Pratt, 1971).

Oral Movement Sequencing and Phonemic Identification

EVIDENCE FOR BROAD PERISYLVIAN REPRESENTATION

Historically, oral apraxia, an impairment in producing single, voluntary, nonverbal oral movements, has been associated only with nonfluent, so-called motor aphasias. In a study of patients with spontaneous lateralized lesions, however, it was found that the ability to imitate a sequence of nonverbal oral–facial movements was impaired, not only in nonfluent aphasic patients, but also in fluent aphasic patients (Mateer & Kimura, 1976). It was hypothesized that a general impairment of motor control for complex, sequenced movement underlay, to some extent, the expressive impairments observed in aphasia. Oral movement-sequencing studies were developed for use with the cortical stimulation mapping paradigm to further identify the extent of left cortex involved in complex oral motor behavior.

Using the imitation tasks described in a previous section, we found that repetition of the same movement was disrupted with stimulation of sites only in a small region of posterior inferior frontal cortex just anterior to the face motor cortex, a region corresponding roughly to, but smaller than, the traditional motor speech area. In Figure 5, based on data from eight patients, six such sites are indicated by filled triangles. In all cases, these sites were also associated with arrest on naming and reading, suggesting they represent

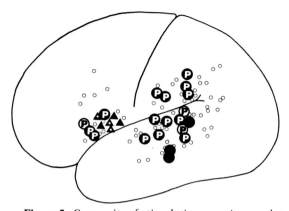

Figure 5. Composite of stimulation mapping results on the mimicry of nonverbal oral–facial postures and the identification of phonemes in eight patients. All sampled sites are indicated by a circle or triangle. The triangles indicate sites where repeated production of the same movement was altered. Large filled circles indicate sites where repeated production of a single movement was intact but production of sequences of three different movements was impaired. Evoked alterations in phonemic identification are indicated by white squares at repeated movement sites and by large P's at all other sites. The overlap in sites where oral movement production and phonemic identification overlap is significant at the .01 level. (From Mateer, 1983).

part of a cortical motor pathway for oral–facial movement that is critical for speech. It is not part of face motor cortex per se since no oral or facial movements were evoked. At three of these six sites (50 percent), stimulation was associated also with significant errors on the Stitt consonant identification task. Involvement of inferior frontal cortex in or near the motor face area with phonemic identification has previously been documented by Darwin, Taylor and Milner (1975) and Taylor (1979) in cases with discrete surgical resections in this region.

Disruption of the imitation of three different postures, a sequence of oral movements, was disrupted over a much broader area, from sites throughout the extent of periSylvian cortex in the frontal, temporal, and parietal lobes. Seventeen such sites, marked by filled circles, were associated with such alterations of sequenced oral movement as production of incorrect movements and incorrect sequencing of movements. Oral motor-sequencing behavior appears to involve a broad band of dominant periSylvian cortex well outside the classical sensorimotor areas.

Disruption of identification of imbedded consonants using the Stitt consonant identification task was also evoked from a broad range of periSylvian cortex. Surprisingly, a high degree of overlap was found between sites associated with disrupted phonemic identification and disrupted oral-movement production. Indeed, in the patient sample represented in Figure 5, 14 of the 17 sites (82 %) associated with disruption of sequential oral movements were also associated with disruption of phonemic identification. No disruption of either of these functions was found with nondominant right hemisphere stimulation. The overlap between production and perception of speech is widely documented both clinically and in the experimental literature. (See review by Mateer, 1983.) Indeed, models such as the motor theory of speech perception were developed on the strength of apparent interactions between these systems (Liberman, Cooper, Shankweiler, & Studdert–Kennedy, 1967). We have hypothesized that these areas of periSylvian cortex which are involved in both the production of movement sequences and the perception of phonemes provide the neural basis for much of the basic production and perception of speech. This notion is not inconsistent with findings from spontaneous lesion studies. The extent of lesions that give rise to a permanent motor aphasia as identified by Mohr (1976) encompasses the same periSylvian areas of cortex where these sites are located. Of the sequential oral movement sites identified in Figure 4, 72% were also associated with speech-related disruption. Remember that in the analysis of alterations on the reading task, articulatory alteration was associated with stimulation of sites only throughout this same broad periSylvian region.

SUMMARY OF THE MODEL FOR CORTICAL ORGANIZATION
OF LANGUAGE

The model of dominant hemisphere language organization in lateral cortex developed from stimulation mapping studies lends itself more easily to a concentric organization around the Sylvian fissure than it does to the more classical anterior–posterior distinctions. A small posterior inferior frontal region just anterior to motor face cortex appears to be critical to voluntary oral motor responses. Surrounding this area anteriorly, posteriorly, and inferiorly in the periSylvian cortex of frontal, temporal, and parietal lobes is a broad region with sites important to the sequencing of oral movement and the decoding of speech sounds as well as to accurate articulatory selection and production. This system is surrounded frontally, temporally, and parietally by a short-term verbal memory system that is largely separate from any of the other measured language functions. Specific features of linguistic usage such as naming and the generation and use of grammatic and semantic structures also appear to have localized representation. These linguistic functions all have some periSylvian representation where they often overlap with each other and, at least in the case of grammar, overlap with areas important for articulatory phonologic functions. Further away from periSylvian cortex in all three lobes, sites specific to grammatical accuracy, to semantic appropriateness, or to naming are identified.

This model is consistent with the major findings from clinical studies of aphasia. A few aphasias are characterized predominantly by one kind of linguistic disruption, agrammatic aphasia, anomic aphasia, conduction aphasia, and semantic jargonaphasia. These syndromes usually involve not only smaller lesions, but lesions that do not involve the immediate periSylvian cortex (Mazzocchi & Vignolo, 1979). In the context of results from stimulation mapping, they might be seen as disrupting aspects of language function which are more separately represented outside of periSylvian cortex. In contrast, most patients with persisting aphasia present with a broad array of expressive and receptive deficits involving multiple linguistic, memory, and motoric deficits. Lesions underlying these more common aphasias typically involve large portions of the periSylvian cortex and/or its underlying connections (Mazzocchi & Vignolo, 1979; Mohr, 1976). This is the area of cortex that we have suggested, on the basis of stimulation-related disruption, is critical to oral motor sequencing, articulatory production, and phonemic perception as well as to multiple aspects of linguistic function. Indeed, there is some suggestion it is the area where linguistic aspects are encoded and decoded via motor and perceptual mechanisms. Finally, fluency is one of the best predictors of the relative anterior/posterior extension of lesion (Benson, 1967). Our model would predict that nonfluency, usually characterized by halting, effortful production, represents extension of the lesion into or undercutting of the inferior posterior frontal region we have identified as critical to discrete oral motor output.

Localization of Nonverbal Functions
in the Nondominant Hemisphere

Although right hemispheric specialization for visuospatial function is a well-documented feature of functional lateralization of the brain in man, discrete localization of nonverbal visuospatial functions within the right hemisphere is less well established. Over the last 3 years, we have used the electrical stimulation mapping procedure to determine intrahemispheric localization of several visuospatial functions on the nondominant lateral cortex in a series of patients undergoing right-sided craniotomies for treatment of seizure disorders (Fried, Mateer, Ojemann, Wohns, & Fedio, 1982; Mateer, in press-b).

TESTS AND METHODS

The report of initial findings from these studies was based on a series of 10 adult patients (7 male, 3 female), age 16–42 years ($x = 24.3$) (Fried, Mateer, Ojemann, Wohns, & Fedio, 1982). Two different tasks, each designed to assess both perception and delayed postdistractional recognition of visuospatial material, were used. As described in the preceding section on language testing, tasks consisted of series of consecutive trials. Each trial had three phases, a target stimulus presentation with direct match to sample as a measure of perception, a distraction, and a delayed recognition of the target stimulus from a multiple choice array. Electronically timed stimulus presentations were made via achromatic slides using vertical arrays. The first of the two tasks required, in the first phase, that one of three faces be matched with the target face. The second phase, requiring the patient to count backward by threes from a two-digit number for 8 sec served as a distractor. In the third phase, the initial target face was to be selected from a field of three faces, two that were not previously presented. In the second task, the first or perceptual phase required that one of three lines be matched on the basis of orientation to a target line. The distractor for this task was a judgment of the emotion or mood depicted by a facial expression. The faces were selected from a series of photographs of posed facial expressions (Ekman & Friesen, 1976). In the final recognition phase, the orientation of the initial target line was to be selected from three differently oriented lines (examples of stimulus items are presented in Fried *et al.*, 1982). Stimulation was applied during only one phase of a trial on experimental trials, on no phase during control nonstimulation trials. At least three samples of performance on perceptual matching, the distractor task, and the delayed recognition were obtained with stimulation at each site in each patient. Significance of stimulation effects was determined by statistical comparison to nonstimulation control trials. Due to different levels of ability on these tasks across patients, the statistical requirements for acceptable baseline performance, and the constraints imposed by time and patient fatigue, not all tasks were given to nor reported for all patients.

RESULTS OF VISUOSPATIAL MAPPING

A summary of the results is presented in Figure 6 which is a composite map of individual sites across all patients. Perceptual errors represent statistically significant errors on the matching portion of either the face or line orientation task (incorrect matches or failures to respond). Seven sites representing 6 of the 10 patients were associated with stimulation related perceptual errors. They were located in the parieto-occipital junction, the posterior–superior and mid-temporal gyri, and the posterior–inferior frontal lobe. Multiple errors at single sites, suggesting greater perceptual involvement, were seen only with stimulation at the parieto-occipital sites and one of the frontal sites.

On those trials in which perception was ascertained by correct matching, delayed recognition performance was analyzed. In five of the patients, nonstimulation control trial performance on recognition of line orientation met criterion level for statistical determination of stimulation-related significance effects. One of these patients—and one other patient—met criterion level for determination of significance on the face recognition task. At 14 sites in these six patients, a statistically significant number of recognition errors was evoked. Most of the sites (79%) cluster in the posterior portion of the superior temporal gyrus, extending into the parietal lobe. Across recognition tasks, significant effects were seen only when stimulation was applied during one phase of the memory task (input, storage, or output) at all but 3 of the 14 sites. In the one patient

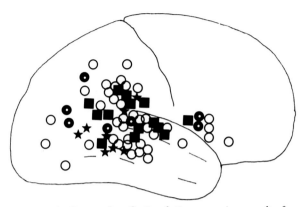

Figure 6. Composite of stimulation mapping results for visuospatial functions in the nondominant right lateral cortex of 10 patients. Each symbol represents a site. Black circles (more easily distinguished from the black squares by their white centers) represent sites where perception (direct match) of faces or line orientation was disrupted with stimulation. Black squares represent sites where memory (delayed post-distractional recognition) for line orientation and/or faces was significantly disrupted relative to control trial performance. Black stars represent sites where judgments of emotions depicted by facial expressions were altered relative to judgments of the same faces made during control trials. All sites are significant at between p < .05 and p < .14. Not all tests were administered nor reported in association with stimulation at each site. (See Fried, Mateer, Ojemann, Wohns, & Fedio, 1982.)

in whom both recognition memory on both kinds of stimuli could be measured, memory for line orientation was disturbed at 3, face memory at 2 of these 3. Preliminary observations thus suggest an overlap in sites where stimulation alters memory for either faces or lines and a strong dissociation of sites on the basis of participation in a particular memory stage (input, storage, output).

The effect of stimulation on one of the distractor tasks, the labeling of emotional expression was assessed in eight of the patients. Isolated changes in the way a given face was labeled in association with stimulation were considered as errors. Statistically significant changes in labeling were found with stimulation at six sites in four patients ($p < .05$) and an additional two sites in one patient ($p < .14$).

Six of eight (75%) of these sites are in the posterior part of the middle temporal gyrus. Where tested, these sites were not associated with errors in the perception of faces per se or in their delayed recognition. Changes in the labeling of facial expressions were not seen with stimulation of the posterior mid-temporal gyrus in the *left* dominant hemisphere of a patient in a series of left craniotomies.

Figure 6 clearly illustrates that changes in different visuospatial functions were evoked from different cortical sites. Considering perception of either faces or line orientation, recognition of either faces or line orientation and emotional face labeling, no site showed change on more than one of the three functions. Although substantial individual variability exists across patients in the exact area of cortex involved in different functions, the same general cortical area commonly altered the same function (perception, memory) when measured across different spatial input (faces, lines).

Electrical stimulation mapping during perception and short-term memory for line orientation and faces, and labeling of facial emotional expressions has provided evidence for discrete localization in the right nondominant hemisphere. These visuospatial functions in the nondominant hemisphere appear to be as discretely localized as verbal functions in the dominant hemisphere.

CONCLUSIONS

Models of brain organization for both language and visuospatial functions derived from the electrical stimulation mapping studies reviewed in this chapter indicate quite discrete functional localization within all cortex, including those areas commonly known as association cortex. The models would predict that the effects of brain damage are very dependent on the location of injury, with increasing area of injury relating to greater impairment primarily because of the greater likelihood of damage to multiple yet discrete functional areas. Within a general framework, there appears to be considerable individual variability in the exact location of areas related to a particular task. To some degree, however, the individual patterns of localization appear to be related to other variables. In the case of naming, these variables include overall language ability and sex of the individual. Finally, a strong suggestion emerges from this work that, even in adults, there is considerable plasticity of cortical function. Cortical involvement appears to change with time, ability level, and experience.

Models should provide a departure point for and guide to further studies. We are developing procedures to specifically test many of the hypotheses the models have generated. Advances in knowledge about brain-behavior relationships will, as always, critically depend on use of a broad range of approaches, techniques and theories. The perspective provided by electrical stimulation mapping has, and will, continue to be important in that effort.

Acknowledgments

Supported by NIH Grant NS 1805 17111 and by NIH Teacher Investigator Development Award HK97 NS 00505, both awarded by the National Institute of Neurological and Communicative Disorders and Stroke, PHS/DHHS. The author is an affiliate of the Child Development and Mental Retardation Center of the University of Washington. Operative studies were carried out in conjunction with Drs. G. A. Ojemann, R. L. Rapport, A. A. Ward, and A. R. Wyler.

References

Benson, F. D. (1967). Fluency in aphasia: Correlation with radioactive scan localization. *Cortex, 3,* 373-394.

Blumstein, S. (1973). *A phonological investigation of aphasic speech.* The Hague: Mouton.

Blumstein, S. (1981). Neurolinguistic disorders: Language-brain relationships. In D. B. Filskov & J. J. Boll (Eds.), *Handbook of clinical neuropsychology.* New York: Wiley.

Cushing, H. (1909). A note upon the faradic stimulation of the post-central gyrus in conscious patients. *Brain, 32,* 44-54.

Darwin, C., Taylor, L., & Milner, B. (1975). Proceedings of the seventeenth international symposium of neuropsychology. *Neuropsychologia, 13,* 132.

Dodrill, C. (1978). A neuropsychological battery for epilepsy. *Epilepsia, 19,* 611-623.

Ekman, P., & Friesen, W. V. (1976). *Pictures of facial affect.* Palo Alto, California: Consulting Psychologists Press.

Fried, I., Mateer, C., Ojemann, G., Wohns, R., & Fedio, P. (1982). Organization of visuospatial functions in human cortex: Evidence from electrical stimulation. *Brain, 105,* 349-371.

Fritsch, G., & Hitzig, E. (1870). Uber die elektrische erregbarkeit des Grosshirns. *Archiv fuer Anatomie, Physiologie und Wissenschaftliche Medicin, 37,* 300-332.

Galaburda, A., Sanides, F., & Geschwind, N. (1978). Human brain: Cytoarchitectonic left-right asymmetirics in the temporal speech region. *Archives of Neurology (Chicago), 35,* 812-817.

Goodglass, H. (1976). Agrammatism. *Studies in Neurolinguistics, 1,* 237-260.

Kimura, D. (1980). Sex differences in intrahemispheric organization of speech. *Behavioral and Brain Sciences, 3,* 215-263.

Liberman, A., Cooper, F., Shankweiler, D., & Studdert–Kennedy, M. (1967). Perception of the speech code. *Psychological Review, 74,* 431–461.

Mateer, C. (1982). Cortical organization of language: Evidence from electrical stimulation studies. *University of Washington Working Papers in Linguistics: Proceedings of the 1981 Western Conference on Linguistics, 7,* 32–38.

Mateer, C. (1983). Functional organization of the right nondominant cortex: Evidence from electrical stimulation. *Canadian Journal of Psychology, 37,* 36–58.

Mateer, C. (1983). Motor and perceptual functions of the left hemisphere and their interaction. In S. J. Segalowitz (Ed.), *Language functions and brain organization.* New York: Academic Press.

Mateer, C., & Kimura, D. (1976). Impairment of nonverbal oral movements in aphasia. *Brain and Language, 4,* 262–276.

Mateer, C., & Ojemann, G. A. (1983). Thalamic mechanisms in language. In S. J. Segalowitz (Ed.), *Language functions and brain organization.* New York: Academic Press.

Mateer, C., Polen, S., & Ojemann, G. (1982). Sexual variation in cortical localization of naming as determined by stimulation mapping. *Behavioral and Brain Sciences, 5,* 310–311.

Mateer, C., Polen, S. B., Ojemann, G. A., & Wyler, A. R. (1982). Cortical localization of finger spelling and oral language: A case study. *Brain and Language, 17,* 46–57.

Mateer, C., & Rapport, R. (1982). Organization of language cortex in two bilinguals. Paper presented at meetings of the American Neurosurgical Society, Washington, D.C.

Mateer, C., Rapport, R. L., & Kettrick, C. (in press). Cerebral organization of oral and signed language responses: Case study evidence from amytal and cortical stimulation studies. *Brain and Language.*

Mazzocchi, F., & Vignolo, L. A. (1979). Localization of lesions in aphasia: Clinical CT scan correlations in stroke patients. *Cortex, 15,* 627–654.

Mohr, J. (1976). Broca's area and Broca's aphasia. *Studies in Neurolinguistics, 1,* 201–236.

Ojemann, G. A. (1978). Organization of short-term verbal memory in language areas of human cortex: Evidence from electrical stimulation. *Brain and Language, 5,* 331–348.

Ojemann, G. A. (1979). Individual variability in cortical localization of language. *Journal of Neurosurgery, 50,* 164–169.

Ojemann, G. A. (1982). Subcortical aphasias. In H. Krishner & F. Freeman (Eds.), *Neurology of aphasia.* Swets & Zeitlinger B. V.: Lisse, 127–137.

Ojemann, G. A. (in press). Brain organization for language from the perspective of electrical stimulation mapping. *Behavioral and Brain Sciences.*

Ojemann, G. A., & Mateer, C. (1979). Human language cortex: Localization of memory, syntax and sequential motor-phoneme identification systems. *Science, 250,* 1401–1403.

Ojemann, G. A., & Whitaker, H. A. (1978). Language localization and variability. *Brain and Language, 6,* 239–260. (a)

Ojemann, G. A., & Whitaker, H. A. (1978). The bilingual brain. *Archives of Neurology (Chicago), 35,* 409–412. (b)

Paradis, M. (1977). Bilingualism and aphasia. *Studies in Neurolinguistics, 3,* 65–122.

Penfield, W., & Jasper, H. (1954). *Epilepsy and the functional anatomy of the human brain.* Boston: Little, Brown.

Penfield, W., & Perot, P. (1963). The brain's record of auditory and visual experience: A final summary and discussion. *Brain, 86,* 595–696.

Penfield, W., & Roberts, L. (1959). *Speech and brain mechanisms.* Princeton, N.J.: Princeton University Press.

Peterson, L., & Peterson, M. (1959). Short term retention of individual verbal items. *Journal of Experimental Psychology, 58,* 193–198.

Ranck, J., Jr. (1975). Which elements are excited in electrical stimulation of mammalian central nervous system: A review. *Brain Research, 98,* 417–440.

Rapport, R. L., Tan, C. T., & Whitaker, H. A. (in press). Language function of dysfunction among Chinese and English speaking polyglots: Cortical stimulation, Wada testing and clinical studies. *Brain and Language.*

Rasmussen, T., & Milner, B. (1977). The role of early left brain injury in determining lateralization of cerebral speech functions. *Annals of the New York Academy of Sciences, 299,* 355–369.

Rubens, A., Mahowald, M., & Hutton, J. (1976). Asymmetry of the lateral (Sylvian) fissures in man. *Neurology, 26,* 620–624.

Siegel, S. (1955). *Nonparametric statistics for the behavioral sciences.* New York: McGraw-Hill.

Taylor, L. (1979). Psychological assessment in neurosurgical patients. In T. Rasmussen and R. Marino (Eds.), *Functional Neurosurgery.* New York: Raven Press.

Van Buren, J., Fedio, P., & Frederick, G. (1978). Mechanism and localization of speech in the parieto-temporal cortex. *Neurosurgery, 2,* 233–239.

Warrington, E. K., Logue, V. C., & Pratt, R. T. C. (1971). The anatomical localization of selective impairment of auditory verbal short-term memory. *Brain, 92,* 885–896.

7

Localization of Lesions
in Broca's Motor Aphasia

*David N. Levine
and Eric Sweet*

The precise topography and extent of cerebral damage required
to produce Broca's aphasia is still unknown. Despite the fact that
the history of modern cerebral localization began with this question
over 100 years ago (Broca, 1861), the answers are not yet complete.
This does not mean that progress has not been made. Some questions have been answered. Yet others, although in principle quite
straightforward, still elude our grasp.

The Clinical Syndrome

Before we can discuss the localization of a syndrome intelligently,
we must define the syndrome we intend to localize. To the extent

185

that there is disagreement about what constitutes Broca's aphasia, there will be controversy about its localization.

Fortunately, this problem is not a major one. There exists a large core of aphasic patients whose set of clinical characteristics, although showing some variation, is sufficiently uniform and distinct that to virtually all investigators of aphasia it stands apart as a specific syndrome. Whether the label is *aphemia* (Broca, 1861), *motor aphasia* (Wernicke, 1874), *verbal aphasia* (Head, 1926), *expressive aphasia* (Weisenburg & McBride, 1935), *nonfluent aphasia* (Howes & Geschwind, 1964), or *Broca's aphasia*, these patients tend to be categorized similarly by all investigators despite major differences in theoretical views and interpretations of the symptoms.

SPEECH

The major feature distinguishing this group of patients from other aphasics is a severe nonfluency of speech. Often, they are mute at the onset of the stroke that renders them aphasic. Subsequently, speech returns to a limited and variable degree. Occasionally, a patient will remain mute for months or years. More often, speech is limited to a few stereotyped expressions that generally occur in situations where speech is an appropriate behavior. The expressions, often uttered quite clearly, may consist of a phrase ("Jesus Christ"), a word ("fine," "yes"), or nonsense. In some patients, the speech consists of brief, poorly differentiated mumbling in which an intelligible word or two may be embedded. Less severely affected patients have a greater number of words and expressions that are used more discriminately, so that simple one-word answers are possible for many questions. Substantive nouns and verbs may be preserved in contrast to a lack of grammatical modifiers, auxilliaries, prepositions, etc. This is also called agrammatism or telegraphic speech. Some patients, when attempting to utter a sentence, begin with one or a few words, but then, after pauses and at times much effort, begin to utter verbal paraphasias or express frustration at an inability to continue. Those patients capable of longer utterances speak slowly and with effort, often at a measured, monotonous pace, frequently misarticulating and stumbling over words. Though all speech is severely affected, those utterances involving repetition or reading aloud are more readily accomplished than those involving spontaneous or conversational speech.

OTHER ORAL–LINGUAL MOVEMENTS

A large number of these patients suffer from inability to utilize lips, tongue, and pharynx for a variety of voluntary acts other than speech. Some patients have difficulty swallowing their food and saliva for days or even weeks following the stroke that rendered them aphasic, but recovery is usually complete. Severely affected, speechless patients may be unable to protrude the tongue, either to verbal request or in imitation of the examiner. Patients not as severely affected (such as those uttering some single words or phrases) may be able to protrude the tongue but be slow or uncoordinated in moving it from side to side. Even when this can be done at reasonable speed, acts such as whistling or clucking are poorly done. The degree of speech loss of these patients is highly correlated with the degree of such oral apraxia (DeRenzi, Pieczuro, & Vignolo, 1966).

WRITING

Writing with the unparalyzed left hand is almost always nonfluent and inaccurate. Spontaneous writing or writing to dictation is usually more impaired than copying, but severely affected patients may have trouble with all of these tasks. The correct letters may be poorly formed, incorrect letters appear with frequent perseverations, and letters may be written atop one another or at uneven heights.

COMPREHENSION

Language comprehension is also impaired to a variable degree. Often, comprehension of simple requests is intact or becomes so with the passage of time from the onset of stroke. However, the deficit in comprehension can then be brought out by increasing the number of steps in a request. It is rare to find a patient with severe Broca's aphasia who is able to perform a three-commission request, even though the average 4- or 5-year-old is capable of such a task.

Such deficits in comprehension are often interpreted as manifestations of "apraxia." However, the deficit can be brought out not only by augmenting the number of serial acts required of the patient, but also by increasing the syntactic complexity of the command, retaining the request for only a single act. Difficulty in comprehending the syntactical elements of speech has been contrasted with facility in comprehending the substantives (Zurif, Caramazza, & Myerson, 1972). Furthermore, the comprehension deficits are manifest in tests requiring matching phrases to pictures and in tests requiring only binary (yes–no) responses to questions. Thus, the deficit is augmented not only by increasing the complexity of the required response, but also by increasing the complexity of the language input, keeping the response requirements constant.

The comprehension deficits often follow a particular order of severity with regard to the modality and nature of the input. In general, imitation of the examiner's movements (oral or limb gestures) is superior to obeying a spoken request, which is in turn superior to obeying a written request. Thus, a patient may protrude his tongue in imitation of the examiner but not to a spoken request. Later, when successful with the latter, he may still be unable to obey the printed command "STICK OUT YOUR TONGUE."

Finally, the comprehension deficits involve semantic systems other than ordinary spoken and written language. For example, comprehension of numbers and signs of arithmetic operations are also impaired.

GENERAL BEHAVIOR

The patient is usually alert and reacts promptly to the presence and speech of the examiner. Nonverbal memory usually is well preserved, the patient having little difficulty learning to recognize his physicians or nurses, to identify his hospital room, and to abide by a simple daily schedule. Emotional lability is common. The patient is often easily angered or reduced to tears, although the lability rarely reaches the degree seen in patients with bilateral lesions resulting in pseudobulbar palsy.

OTHER NEUROLOGIC DEFICITS

Associated neurologic signs include a right hemiparesis, which is almost invariable at the outset of the aphasia when it results from stroke. Usually, the hemiparesis persists, especially in the arm, or improves along with the patient's speech capacity. Rarely, the speech may remain severely impaired, but the right hemiparesis nearly completely disappears. A right-sided sensory loss may or may not be present, and a visual field defect is usually absent after the acute phase.

Such "core" cases, although encompassing a wide variety of aphasic patients, rarely evoke substantial disagreement with regard to classification. Disagreements, however, do arise with regard to patients at the fringes of this nuclear group. The following questions are occasionally asked: (1) How much of a deficit in comprehension of speech is allowed before a patient is considered a "global" rather than a "Broca's" aphasic, and is this distinction of any predictive value with regard to neuropathology? Or, at the opposite extreme, at what point does nonfluency of speech become so mild that it is indistinguishable from the pauses that mark the word-finding difficulties of otherwise fluent dysnomic aphasics? (2) At what point in the evolution of the clinical picture is the classification to be carried out? Should we confine the term *Broca's aphasia* to patients, like Broca's, in whom the syndrome has been present for months or years? Should we include the patient who, in 8 weeks, progresses from mutism through a stage of halting word-by-word speech, completing only some sentences, to a stage of effective speech communication that is fluent except for mild word-finding difficulty? What about the patient who does this in days or hours?

These questions are of value in illustrating that the term "Broca's aphasia" is still not used unambiguously and may include more or less of the aphasic population, depending on the investigator's preference. Doubtless, the range of neuropathology in Broca's aphasia will be wider if the range of the syndrome is greater. In this review, we apply the term more narrowly to the noncontroversial "core" cases with long-standing, severely nonfluent speech, resembling the patients studied by Broca.

Pitfalls in Inferences about Localization

Erroneous inferences about localization may occur for several reasons. The most important of these is a failure to study lesions that do *not* produce Broca's aphasia as well as those that *do*. Errors also may arise from failure to consider the nature and speed of evolution of a lesion, the existence of a previous lesion, and anomalies of cerebral lateralization.

Examination only of positive cases—that is, those with Broca's aphasia—can lead to false conclusions. One must also examine the lesion in negative cases—those without Broca's aphasia. Suppose that a lesion of Area *B* is necessary for Broca's aphasia to occur. Suppose, too, that because of the vascular topography, a lesion of Area *B* is nearly always accompanied by a lesion of Area *A*. One might mistakenly conclude that a lesion of Area *A* is necessary for Broca's aphasia, unless one also examined those negative cases where lesions affected Area *A* but not Area *B*. Indeed, it has been claimed repeatedly that the third frontal gyrus has served as such an Area *A* with regard to Broca's aphasia. Only by synthesizing the evidence from both the positive and the negative cases can we ascertain the lesions that are both necessary and sufficient to produce the syndrome.

One's conclusions about localization also may be influenced by the nature of the lesion, especially by its speed of evolution, although insufficient attention has been devoted to this potential source of error. A sudden insult, such as occurs with infarction, hemorrhage, or contusion, may present a different picture from a slowly progressive lesion such as infiltrating tumor (Hécaen, 1972; von Monakow, 1914). In general, we concern ourselves with cases of sudden damage arising in the context of cerebral stroke or trauma.

The existence of prior lesions, especially during childhood, may also influence one's conclusions. It is well known (Rasmussen & Milner, 1977) that substantial lesions of the language areas of the left hemisphere during early childhood may result in right hemisphere dominance for speech. In such patients, a second lesion of the left hemisphere in adult life may have substantially less effect on speech than in patients with no prior left hemisphere damage. In our discussion, we will confine ourselves to patients with no history of cerebral damage early in life.

Similar remarks apply to differences in handedness—namely, to variations in cerebral lateralization not attributable to early lesions. Most right-handed patients have speech controlled by the left hemisphere, but a small minority may have a speech-dominant right hemisphere (e.g., see Trojanowski, Green, & Levine, 1980). Approximately one-third of lefthanders, however, may show right hemisphere speech dominance, and some evidence indicates that lateralization of speech control may not be as pronounced in some left-handed patients as it is in right-handed patients (Hécaen & Sauguet, 1971). In lefthanders with either right hemisphere speech dominance or incomplete lateralization, the effects of a given left hemisphere lesion on speech will not duplicate the effects of the same lesion in a patient with left hemisphere speech dominance.

Techniques of Delineating Cerebral Lesions

The techniques utilized to determine the size and location of cerebral lesions are discussed in other chapters, and will not be reviewed here. Computerized tomography (CT) has increased the accuracy of localization beyond previous techniques such as conventional gamma scanning after radioisotope injection. However, with regard to Broca's aphasia, CT in its present form still leaves unanswered many questions that can only be satisfactorily approached by careful postmortem examination. For example, to decide the relative importance of the inferior frontal gyrus and the precentral gyrus is very difficult with CT alone, because the two gyri are adjacent, and there is often uncertainty as to the relative involvement of each. The CT is also relatively insensitive to lesions that are confined to the cerebral surface (i.e., cortex) even if these extend over a wide area of the brain. Future technical refinements may enhance resolution and at least partially alleviate these problems.

The Roles of Deep and Superficial Lesions in Broca's Aphasia

An assumption in many of the early studies of the localization of Broca's aphasia was that the lesion had to destroy or completely isolate a specific region of the cerebral cortex. Broca felt that this region was the left third frontal gyrus, which stored the "motor memories" necessary for speech. Likewise, Wernicke (1874) called Broca's aphasia "cortical" motor aphasia and distinguished it from "subcortical" motor aphasia. The latter differed from Broca's aphasia clincially (preserved writing, reading, and speech comprehension) and anatomically (a deep lesion separating the cortex of the third frontal gyrus from the brainstem, but preserving the integrity of the third frontal gyrus and its cortico–cortical connections to other parts of the hemisphere). For both Broca and Wernicke, Broca's aphasia required a superficial lesion that destroyed the cortex of the third frontal gyrus directly, or (by involving the immediately subjacent white matter) isolated this cortex not only from the brain stem but from its cortico–cortical connections to Wernicke's areas and to other parts of the left hemisphere.

It is clear that this view must be modified in at least two ways. First, Broca's aphasia may result not only from a lesion of cortex and its immediately subjacent matter. It may also result from a lesion of the deeper portions of the left hemisphere. There are no consistent differences currently known between Broca's aphasia caused by deep lesion and that resulting from a superficial lesion. Second, the area of cortex critical to the production of Broca's aphasia—if a critical area exists—may not be the third frontal gyrus. There is considerable controversy regarding the cortical areas involved in Broca's aphasia resulting from superficial lesions and the subcortical structures involved in Broca's aphasia resulting from deep lesions. The following discussion considers each of these controversies.

Broca's Aphasia Resulting from Deep Left-Hemisphere Lesions

Marie (1906) first drew attention to a role for deep lesions of the left hemisphere in Broca's aphasia. He claimed that patients with Broca's aphasia invariably had a lesion in the "Lenticular zone," shown in Figure 1. This zone was defined precisely in the anteroposterior dimension by the anterior and posterior borders of the insula. In the lateromedial dimension, the boundaries were less well specified but extended at least from the insular cortex laterally to the ventricular system medially. The dorsal–ventral boundaries were never specified. This region contains many gray-matter structures (insula, claustrum, putamen, caudate, globus pallidus) and white-matter tracts (extreme capsule, external capsule, internal capsule, possibly some of corona radiata superiorly). The relative roles of each were not clear, but Marie, in his earlier writings, favored an important role for the putamen.

Despite his emphasis on the importance of deep lesions, Marie was unwilling to attribute the occurrence of Broca's aphasia to a deep lesion alone. Instead, he ascribed the motor speech difficulty (anarthria) to the deep lesion but claimed that the "genuine" aphasic disturbances, which included paraphasia and impaired comprehen-

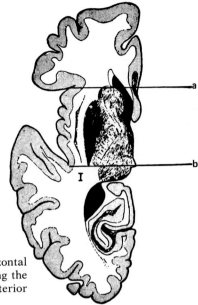

Figure 1. Pierre Marie's schematic horizontal section of a cerebral hemisphere, illustrating the lenticular zone with its anterior (a) and posterior (b) boundaries.

sion, required a concomitant lesion of Wernicke's area (temporo-parietal cortex). Thus Marie, too, considered aphasia as primarily a cortical phenomenon.

Foix and Levy (1927) demonstrated, in their studies of the pathology of middle cerebral artery occlusion, that Broca's aphasia could result from a deep lesion alone, without concomitant lesions of the cortex and the immediately subcortical white matter on the convexity of the cerebral hemisphere. They found that the severity of the aphasia was related to the size of the deep lesions. Only large lesions resulted in the full syndrome of Broca's aphasia.

The conclusions of Foix and Levy have been borne out by modern studies employing computerized tomography. Mazzocchi and Vignolo (1979) found that deep lesions alone can result in Broca's aphasia. We too have observed this repeatedly, as is illustrated by the following case:

Case 1: R. B., a 75-year-old right-handed man suddenly became mute with a right hemiparesis. His strength on the right improved quickly, and he soon walked without assistance, although his grip was weak. Four weeks after his ictus, examination showed him to be completely mute. He was unable to repeat even single vowel sounds. There was significant oral and facial apraxia: He could not protrude his tongue or shut his eyes on spoken request and was only partially successful on imitation. He was able to match single spoken words to the appropriate object in an array, but failed when two words were spoken and he was required to point to each object in turn. He obeyed some but not all single-step commands. Reading comprehension was poor, even at the single-word level. He was unable to write to dictation with either hand, but successfully copied his name. His right arm was mildly weak, but his leg was spared, and his face moved symmetrically. There was no visual field deficit. CT scan showed a deep lesion in the lenticular zone, extending upward into the corona radiata (Figure 2).

Ten months after his stroke he was re-examined. He had improved significantly, although he remained severely aphasic. Speech was low in volume and dysarthric, often sounding like an undifferentiated mumble. Hesitation and stammering were frequent, but occasional words, often paraphasic, could be discerned. He was able to write a few short words to dictation but not a complete sentence. Writing was small; many letters were no more than unintelligible loops and spelling was poor. He refused to write with the left hand. He obeyed two-step but not three-step commands. Reading comprehension had improved to the point of obeying one- and two-step written commands and selecting the correct printed word to complete a simple sentence. However, he took an inordinately long time and erred on the more difficult sentences.

Although it is now clear that a large lesion of the lenticular zone can result in Broca's aphasia, the crucial structures within the lenticular zone are still unknown. Several hypotheses have been advanced, but the evidence is scanty.

INSULAR CORTEX HYPOTHESIS

This hypothesis attempts to reconcile the fact that lesions *deep* within the left hemisphere may result in Broca's aphasia with the assumption that cortical damage (or total isolation) is necessary. The insula lies deep within the hemisphere, hidden in the depths of the Sylvian fissure, and covered externally by the operculated portions of the frontal and temporal lobes. In Broca's aphasia, a role for the cortex of the insula, especially its anterior portions, has been suggested repeatedly (Bernheim, 1900; Dejerine, 1914), usually as part of a more extensive area, including the third frontal gyrus. Recently, Mazzocchi and Vignolo (1979) again have drawn attention to the insula on the basis of CT findings in Broca's aphasics. The insula

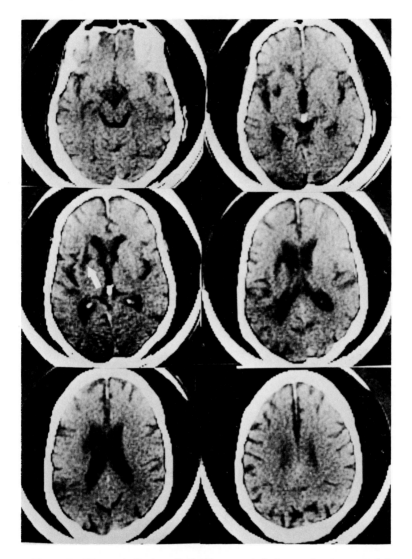

Figure 2. CT scan in Patient R. B. The most inferior section is at top, left; the most superior section is at bottom, right. A low density area, consistent with infarction, is situated in the left lenticular zone. It appears to involve portions of putamen and internal capsule at middle left (arrow) where its extent is greatest. It also extends superiorly to involve the corona radiata adjacent to the body of the left lateral ventricle, deep to the central gyri.

hypothesis suffers, however, from exclusive attention to positive cases and neglect of negative ones. Many patients with small lesions confined to insular cortex are not aphasic (von Monakow, 1914). A case of Moutier (1908) and Marie is a good example.

Jacquet, a 55-year-old, right-handed man, entered Bicetre because of blindness from glaucoma and remained there for 9 years—until his death. There had been no history of stroke although examination showed some atrophy of the legs, more marked on the right. His speech was fluent with no articulatory difficulty. In fact, he tended to logorrhea. While polite with friends, he was often verbally and physically aggressive with strangers. He was considered demented, but never a Broca's aphasic. The brain was studied in serial section. There was destruction of nearly the entire posterior half of the third frontal gyrus (F3) and complete destruction of the anterior insula of the left hemisphere by an old infarct. An old, left temporoparietal lesion was also present. The precentral gyrus was only mildly affected.

Conversely, in patients with Broca's aphasia and primarily deep lesions, other structures in addition to the insula are invariably involved. In fact, in several of the cases presented by Moutier (1908), studied in serial section, the insular cortex was either entirely or nearly entirely spared. More work is required in which both negative and positive cases are considered before accepting the insular cortex as all or part of the site whose destruction produces Broca's aphasia.

PUTAMEN HYPOTHESIS

Marie's early emphasis on putaminal damage in Broca's aphasia has not been borne out by subsequent evidence, although appropriate cases bearing on this hypothesis are rare. What is required are cases of unilateral lesions of the dominant hemisphere, occurring in adulthood, and confined to the putamen, sparing adjacent white matter tracts.

Damage *restricted to the putamen* occasionally occurs, but is usually bilateral. It may occur gradually in such conditions as Wilson's hepatolenticular degeneration or the nigrostriatal degeneration of Adams, van Bogaert, and van der Eecken (1964). It may also occur more abruptly, as in anoxia following strangulation or poisoning (Dooling & Richardson, 1976). When bilateral damage is severe, the patient may be mute as part of a generalized rigidity or akinesia. Comprehension rarely has been tested extensively in such patients, but the patient of Dooling and Richardson was said to "select colors, objects, and numbers; follow multi-step commands; add simple sums; and write words and short phrases to command." It appears that putaminal disease may result in mutism, but only with extensive bilateral disease and in the context of generalized rigidity or akinesia.

Unilateral lesions of the putamen are more common but are rarely restricted to this structure. They occur after infarction or hypertensive hemorrhage, and Broca's aphasia often results when the lesion involves the left hemisphere. However, the damage almost invariably extends beyond the putamen to involve the adjacent white matter tracts, and the resulting aphasia cannot be attributed to lesion of the putamen alone. (More recent CT evidence concerning putaminal lesions in aphasia are discussed in Chapter 3.) Dooling and Adams (1975) studied several cases of post-hemiplegic athetosis in which the damage heavily affected the putamen with relative sparing of the internal capsule. Aphasia was not a part of the clinical syndrome, but the lesions in their cases all were incurred during childhood. Carpenter (1950) reviewed the literature of hemiathetosis, including cases with lesions occurring in adulthood. Although many of the cases involved extensive unilateral damage to the putamen with relative sparing of the internal capsule, most were unsuitable for localization of aphasia either because the right hemisphere was the one affected or, if the left hemisphere was involved, there was inadequate documentation of speech deficit and/or handedness to ascertain whether the left hemisphere was speech dominant.

An exception is the case of Ringer (1879). The patient at age 28 developed sudden right hemiplegia, hemianesthesia, and loss of speech. He quickly recovered speech, sensation, and finally right-sided movement, but, as his strength improved, right hemiathetosis developed. At autopsy a cystic softening occupied the posterior two-thirds of the left putamen, extending posteriorly into the infero-medial portion of the internal capsule. The presence of transient aphasia suggests that the involved left hemisphere was speech-dominant, but the rapid recovery of speech suggests that the heavily damaged putamen did not participate in mediation of his recovered speech.

In summary, it is highly unlikely that a unilateral lesion confined to the putamen of the dominant hemisphere will result in a severe, long-lasting Broca's aphasia. The latter is almost invariably accompanied by hemiplegia, suggesting the need for involvement of the corticospinal tract.

CAPSULO-COMMISSURAL HYPOTHESIS

The capsulo-commissural hypothesis emphasizes the white rather then the gray matter structures of Marie's lenticular zone. It is assumed that there is a particular region of cerebral cortex (see next section) of the left hemisphere required for control of speech. Information from this cortex must reach the bulbar nuclei innervating the oral–lingual–pharyngeal musculature, and two main routes are available: (1) the corticobulbar fibers of the left internal capsule; and (2) the commissural fibers of the corpus callosum, activating homologous cortex of the right hemisphere (followed by the corticobulbar fibers of the right hemisphere). Lesions of either of these pathways alone is insufficient to cause severe, lasting Broca's aphasia. However, involvement of both pathways by a large, deep lesion would isolate the speech-dominant left hemisphere from the bulbar nuclei and Broca's aphasia would ensue.

There is considerable evidence that lesion of either pathway alone does not result in Broca's aphasia. A lesion of the left internal capsule alone frequently results in right hemiplegia without aphasia (e.g., Fisher, 1979). Transection of the corpus callosum alone, although often resulting in transient mutism, does not result in severe, long-lasting aphasia, whether the transection is performed surgically in patients with childhood brain damage (Gazzaniga & Sperry, 1967) or is the result of infarction of the anterior cerebral artery territory in patients with previously normal brains (Liepmann & Maas, 1907).

The evidence that lesions of both pathways are sufficient to produce Broca's aphasia is understandably meager. Both pathways are indeed interrupted in most, if not all, of the deep lesions resulting in Broca's aphasia, but these lesions are usually extensive enough to involve other structures as well. Isolated lesions of both pathways (i.e., a lesion of the left internal capsule and a callosal transection) are rare. The well-known case of Bonhoeffer (1914) is one example, and it provides some support for the capsulo-commissural hypothesis.

The patient was a 51-year-old man who, after several days of headaches, suddenly developed moderate speech difficulty. The following day he suffered another attack resulting in right hemiparesis and complete inability to speak. The right hemiparesis quickly improved, but examination 4 months later disclosed no spontaneous speech except an occasional "yes." Even recitation of overlearned series (such as counting) was impossible and repetition was poor, even for single words or syllables. Reading aloud was no better.

Comprehension of speech was tested only for simple commands, which were usually performed successfully, the failures being ascribed to apraxia. Comprehension of print was poor, even for matching single words with the correct object. A severe apraxia, involving the face and limbs, left more than right, affected movements to verbal command or imitation. He was severely agraphic with either hand.

At autopsy, 9 months after the ictus, there was a large infarction in the territory of the left anterior cerebral artery. It involved the anterior two-fifths of the second frontal gyrus, the anterior four-fifths of the first frontal gyrus, most of the cingulate gyrus, and all but the splenium of the corpus callosum. There was a second lesion, involving the anterior limb of the left internal capsule, sparing putamen, external capsule, and insula. Finally, there was a small left parieto-occipital lesion.

Bonhoeffer felt that the first two lesions provided a capsulo-commissural isolation of the left hemisphere speech areas from the bulbar nuclei, confirming Heilbronner's (1910) hypothesis that (1) the internal capsule and (2) the callosum-opposite capsule are the two main routes for speech impulses to reach the brain stem from the left hemisphere.

The capsulo-commissural hypothesis is, at this time, the most attractive of the three hypotheses relating Broca's aphasia to deep lesions of the left hemisphere. Cases such as that of RB are assumed to have a single deep lesion interrupting *both* the capsular and the commissural outputs from a critical area of the left cerebral cortex. It is important to study the pathological anatomy of deep left cerebral lesions postmortem in patients both with and without Broca's aphasia. However, before such evidence can be fully evaluated, it is necessary to localize the critical area of cortex where commissural and capsular outflows are interrupted by the deep lesion. This is discussed in the following section.

Broca's Aphasia Resulting from Superficial Left-Hemisphere Lesions

Broca's aphasia may also result from "superficial" lesions that spare the lenticular zone of Marie. Commonly, such lesions are infarctions in the superficial territory of the left middle cerebral artery that spare the territory irrigated by the deep penetrating lenticulostriate branches. Although, in keeping with the terminology of Foix and

Levy (1927), we refer to these lesions as "superficial," they are by no means exclusively cortical. Invariably, the white matter subjacent to the cortex is involved to some degree. But the even deeper white matter tracts and gray matter of the lenticular zone are spared.

In principle, sorting out the relevant from the irrelevant areas in Broca's aphasia should be an easier task in the superficial zone— where the origins and the terminations of projection and association fibers are widely separated—than deeper in the hemisphere, where they run as compact bundles. There remains, however, considerable controversy over the location and size of superficial lesions required to produce Broca's aphasia. The major hypotheses are presented as follows:

THE THIRD FRONTAL GYRUS (F3)

Broca first postulated that F3 was the seat of "motor speech memories" which were lost in Broca's aphasia. Later, Liepmann (1915) and Dejerine (1914) postulated that the neurons of this "mnestic center" activated the more purely "executive" cortex of the precentral gyrus to produce speech. A lesion of F3 would produce the entire complex of speechlessness and variable comprehension disturbances referred to as Broca's aphasia. The precentral gyrus was not considered to be part of the "language area."

The third frontal gyrus is a complex structure with three major subdivisions according to surface topography (Figure 3). Posteriorly, immediately anterior to the precentral gyrus, is the pars opercularis. Anterior to this opercular portion of F3 is the pars triangularis, an inverted triangle whose sides are formed by the ascending rami of the anterior Sylvian fissure, and whose base is formed by the inferior frontal sulcus. Anterior to the pars triangularis is the pars orbitalis, much of which, as the name suggests, is on the orbital surface of the frontal lobe.

The classical Broca's area includes the pars opercularis according to everybody. Some investigators, such as Liepmann, included the pars triangularis, but others, such as Goldstein, did not (Isserlin, 1936). Many included other, adjacent structures as well: the inferior portion of the precentral gyrus, posteriorly; the anterior convolutions of the insula, inferiorly; and the middle frontal gyrus, superiorly. The focus, however, remained at the pars opercularis of F3.

In support of this localization, Henschen (1922) collected from the

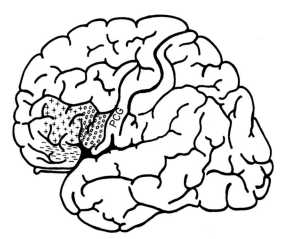

Figure 3. Lateral view of a cerebral hemisphere. The third frontal gyrus is denoted by cicles (pars opercularis), crosses (pars triangularis), and horizontal lines (pars orbitalis). PCG denotes the precentral gyrus immediately posterior to the third frontal gyrus.

literature 49 cases with aphemia or mutism associated with lesions restricted to F3. More recently, Hécaen and Consoli (1973) presented 19 cases with lesions of F3; 10 had articulatory difficulties and all had pauses and hesitation in spontaneous speech. Kertesz, Lesk, and McCabe (1977) used isotope scans to localize recent Broca's aphasia defined by standardized test scores. The images were overlapped, and most covered F3.

Against the F3 hypothesis is an equally impressive body of evidence. The supporting proof cited previously is weakened when critically scrutinized. Of Henschen's 49 cases, 29 had hemiplegia or hemiparesis, suggesting that the lesions extended beyond F3. In 11 others, aphemia was only transient. Another 3 had only mild aphasia or a syndrome quite distinct from Broca's aphasia. Three others showed lesions extending beyond F3 on postmortem exam, in two no lesion of F3 was actually found, and in one, a surgical case, the localization was uncertain. No case unequivocally supported the F3 hypothesis. In Hécaen and Consoli's study, F3 lesions included not only involvement of the third frontal gyrus, but of more anterior and superior areas of cortex as well as the precentral gyrus. Finally, in the study of Kertesz et al. (1977), as many lesions included the precentral gyrus as included F3.

Stronger evidence against the F3 hypothesis comes from cases in which, despite a lesion of F3, there was either only mild aphasia or no aphasia at all. Niessl von Mayendorf (1926) collected several cases from the literature of right-handed subjects with autopsy-proven lesions of F3—including the pars opercularis—in whom no aphasia was present. Goldstein (1948) noted that good recovery was compatible with destruction of Broca's area on the left. Mohr, Pessin, Finklestein, Funkenstein, Duncan, and Davis (1978) found that focal lesions of F3 may produce transient mutism, progressing to mild paraphasia and word-finding difficulty in hours to weeks. The extent to which even this mild dysphasia resulted from lesion of structures adjacent to F3, rather than to F3 itself, is not clear. Such negative cases have often been explained by postulating that in some patients the nondominant F3 takes over the mediation of speech when the left F3 is destroyed. (Henschen, 1922) Contradicting this view is the finding that even bilateral destruction of F3 is consistent with only mild aphasia (Levine & Mohr, 1979). There is no known case of a lesion of F3 alone which produced a lasting, severe Broca's aphasia. (See Levine & Sweet, 1982.)

THE PRECENTRAL GYRUS

The precentral gyrus (consisting of agranular cortex) is situated immediately anterior to the central sulcus and immediately posterior to the first, second, and third frontal gyri, which consist of granular cortex. As previously mentioned, the precentral gyrus was excluded from the language area by Dejerine (1914) and Liepmann (1915) on theoretical grounds. They postulated that F3 was a center for motor speech memories, whereas the precentral gyrus, receiving commands from F3, had only an executive rather than a mnestic motor function. There is, however, no evidence to support this model (Levine & Sweet, 1982). Rather, there is much evidence implicating the precentral gyrus in Broca's aphasia. Niessl von Mayendorf (1926), studying cases of cerebral infarction, concluded that the precentral gyrus was invariably affected. Penetrating missile wounds resulting in motor aphasia are centered around the central sulcus rather than F3 (Conrad, 1954; Schiller, 1947). Stimulation of the precentral gyrus may produce mouth, lip, and tongue movements and elementary vocalization more easily than stimulation anywhere else (Penfield & Roberts, 1959). Finally, Trojanowski et al. (1980) recently have presented a patient with severe, lasting Broca's aphasia who, at postmortem examination, had infarction limited to the cortex and subcortical white matter of the precentral gyrus, sparing the deep territory of the lenticular zone and almost completely sparing F3.

However, there is negative evidence. Penfield and Roberts (1959) reported resection of the inferior portion of the precentral gyrus in several patients with only transient aphasia. Mohr *et al.* (1978) noted no difference between patients with small lesions of the Rolandic operculum and patients with lesions of F3; neither group developed severe, lasting Broca's aphasia.

A possible resolution of this seeming contradiction is that the cases of Penfield and Mohr *et al.* involved damage to a far smaller portion of the precentral gyrus than the lesion in the patient of Trojanowski *et al.* We are accustomed to think of the precentral gyrus as a mosaic, composed of motor representations of distinct body parts, forming the familiar inverted homunculus (Penfield & Boldrey, 1937) in which rostral body parts—including tongue and lips—are located inferiorly. According to this view, a lesion of the inferior precentral gyrus where facial, lingual, and pharyngeal movements are represented would affect these movements as severely as a lesion of the entire precentral gyrus. Yet, extensive work, summarized by Phillips (1966), indicates that the pattern of motor representation is not such a mosaic. Instead, the representations of different body parts overlap extensively. Each body part has an extensive representation in the precentral gyrus, with the area on the homunculus representing only the center of gravity of a wider distribution. Thus, it is possible that only extensive lesions of the left precentral gyrus, including all but the upper third, will produce a lasting and severe Broca's aphasia.

It must also be remembered that the surgical excisions of Penfield involved regions of the brain that had previously been damaged, often as far back as early childhood. Since each body part has an extensive rather than a highly focal representation in the precentral gyrus, it is possible that areas adjacent to the injured inferior precentral region compensated for highly focal damage and that such compensation was even more marked when the damage occurred in childhood. Glees and Cole (1950) provided evidence in the monkey for compensation of motor deficits in the macaque by areas of motor cortex adjacent to focal lesions.

The importance for speech of areas of precentral gyrus superior to the inferior peri-Sylvian region may be illustrated by the following case:

C. T., a 62-year-old woman—with a history of transient jaundice

5 years previously—was admitted with chills and fever. Blood cultures grew *Staphylococcus aureus* and liver function tests were abnormal. She was treated with antibiotics and intravenous fluids and survived for 17 days. Three days prior to admission, her speech had become slurred and she seemed to have hallucinations of music. Two days later she stopped speaking entirely and was less responsive. On admission to the hospital, there was no vocalization. She raised a hand or a leg to spoken request but obeyed no other commands. Her eyes roved from side to side but did not fixate the examiner. With treatment, she improved dramatically. By the third hospital day, she was quite alert but unable to vocalize. She obeyed requests to hold up one finger, to hold up four fingers, and to touch her nose. There was severe right facial weakness. She remained in this state for the next 10 days. The only vocalization was an occasional grunting or moaning sound. She was unable to swallow. She obeyed one-step commands but only occasional two-step commands and often nodded inappropriately to yes–no commands. She was unable to spell her name by pointing to an alphabet card.

Subsequently, she became lethargic, stuporous, and finally comatose with progressive hepatic and renal failure. Postmortem examination showed bacterial endocarditis involving the aortic valve with infarcts of the spleen and kidney and cirrhosis of the liver.

Externally, the brain showed a collection of blood in the Rolandic fissure with swelling and softening of the precentral and postcentral gyri (Figure 4). On horizontal section, a hematoma extended from the middle portion of the left Rolandic fissure into the precentral and postcentral gyri, involving both the cortex and the immediately subcortical white matter. The diameter of the roughly spherical hematoma was approximately 2.5 cm.

Microscopic examination of serial sections through the hematoma showed marked destruction of a large segment of the Rolandic branch of the left middle cerebral artery consistent with a diagnosis of hemorrhage from a mycotic aneurysm. The remainder of the brain was normal except for several small infarcts no greater than 2–3 mm in greatest dimension. These involved the cortex of the superior portion of the right precentral gyrus, the left dentate nucleus, and the left cerebellar hemisphere.

In this patient, a highly focal hemorrhage, involving the midportion of the left precentral and postcentral gyri, produced total loss of speech and moderate comprehension and spelling deficits, which lasted 2 weeks until the patient's death. The short survival does not

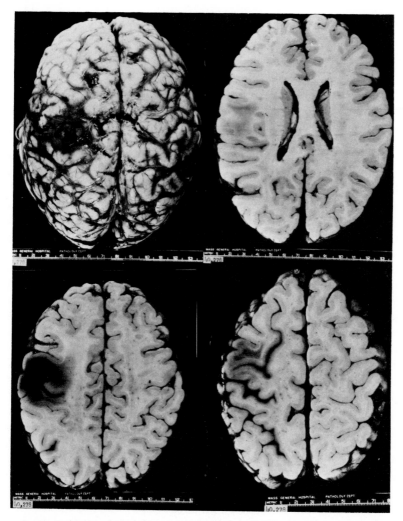

Figure 4. Photographs of the external surface of the brain (top left dorsal view) and of three horizontal brain slices in Patient C. T. The circumscribed superficial hematoma over the middle third of the left Rolandic fissure (top left) involves the precentral gyrus, and to a lesser extent, the postcentral gyrus (bottom left). Sections below (top right) and above (bottom right) the hematoma show some edema of the central gyri but no hemorrhage.

allow any conclusions as to the degree of recovery one might expect with such a lesion. Nevertheless, it appears that the precentral gyrus, even the middle third, has a role in speech and other language activities.

THE EQUIPOTENTIALITY (SIZE) HYPOTHESIS

Recently Mohr *et al.* (1978) have demonstrated that severe, lasting Broca's aphasia is often associated with extensive lesions involving the third frontal gyrus, frontal operculum, insula, and often areas of cortex and white matter superior and posterior to these regions—encompassing the entire territory of the superior division of the left middle cerebral artery. The authors suggested the possibility that no area within this complex is of primary importance for producing the syndrome. The analogy is drawn of a team that is only weakened but still able to function when one or two players are missing (mild dysphasia with small infarcts) but is completely disrupted and unable to function when too many players leave and only one or two remain (severe dysphasia with large infarcts).

This hypothesis requires further proof. The data, although consistent with the hypothesis, are also consistent with the precentral gyrus hypothesis. The larger lesions affect more of the precentral gyrus and/or its brain stem and commissural outflow. It may be for this reason that severe Broca's aphasia ensues. Furthermore, the equipotentiality hypothesis cannot explain the persistent Broca's aphasia in the case of Trojanowski *et al.* (1980) in which the lesion was confined to the precentral gyrus. Aphasia, like hemiplegia, may have a focal area of primary importance surrounded by a fringe, and that nuclear area may be the precentral gyrus.

The recent CT studies of large aphasic populations (Barat, Constant, Mazoux, Caillé, & Arné, 1978; Kertesz, 1979; Mazzocchi & Vignolo, 1980; Mohr *et al.*, 1978; Naeser & Hayward, 1978) have unfortunately not resolved the controversy over localization. In most cases, lesions are large and involve both the superficial and deep territories. But it is not at all clear that the lesions must be large, and careful attention must be given to the more circumscribed lesions, confined either to the superficial or the deep territories that result in Broca's aphasia. It is hoped that the careful laying out of alternative hypotheses, and future refinements in CT localization will finally resolve the still unanswered questions.

References

Adams, R. D., van Bogaert, L., & van der Eecken, H. (1964). Striato-nigral degeneration. *Journal of Neuropathology and Experimental Neurology, 23*, 584–608.

Barat, M., Constant, P., Mazoux, J. M., Caillé, J. M., & Arné, L. (1978). Corrélations anatomo-cliniques dan l'aphasie. Apport de la tomodensitométrie. *Revue Neurologique, 134*, 611–617.

Bernheim, F. (1900). *De l'aphasie motrice.* Thèse de Paris.

Bonhoeffer, K. (1914). Klinischer und anatomischer Befund zur Lehre von der Apraxie und der motorischen Sprachbahn. *Monatschrift fuer Psychiatrie und Neurologie, 35*, 113–128.

Broca, P. (1861). Nouvelle observation d'aphemie produite par une lesion de la partie postérieure des deuxième et troisième circonvolutions frontale. *Bulletin de la Societe Anatomique de Paris, 6*, 398–407.

Carpenter, M. D. (1950). Athetosis and the basal ganglia. *Archives of Neurology and Psychiatry, 63*, 875–901.

Conrad, K. (1954). New problems of aphasia. *Brain, 77*, 491–509.

Dejerine, J. (1914). *Sémiologie des affections du système nerveux.* Paris: Masson.

DeRenzi, E., Pieczuro, A., & Vignolo, L. A. (1966). Oral apraxia and aphasia. *Cortex, 2*, 50–73.

Dooling, E. C., & Adams, R. D. (1975). The pathologic anatomy of posthemiplegic athetosis. *Brain, 98*, 29–48.

Dooling, E. C., & Richardson, E. P. (1976). Delayed encephalopathy after strangling. *Archives of Neurology (Chicago), 33*, 196–199.

Fisher, C. M. (1979). Capsular infarcts—the underlying vascular lesions. *Archives of Neurology (Chicago), 36*, 65–73.

Foix, C., & Levy, M. (1927). Les ramollissements sylviens. *Revue Neurologique, 2*, 1–51.

Gazzaniga, M. S., & Sperry, R. W. (1967). Language after section of the cerebral commissures. *Brain, 90*, 131–148.

Glees, P., & Cole, J. (1950). Recovery of skilled motor function after small repeated lesions of motor cortex in macaque. *Journal of Neurophysiology, 13*, 137–148.

Goldstein, K. (1948). Language and Language Disturbances. New York: Grune and Stratton.

Head, H. (1926). *Aphasia and kindred disorders of speech.* London & New York: Cambridge University Press.

Hécaen, H. (1972). *Introduction à la neuropsychologie.* Paris: Larousse.

Hécaen, H., & Consoli, S. (1973). Analyse des troubles du langage au cours de lésions de l'aire de Broca. *Neuropsychologia, 11*, 377–388.

Hécaen, H., & Sauguet, J. (1971). Cerebral dominance in left-handed subjects. *Cortex, 7*, 19–48.

Heilbronner, K. (1910). Aphasische Storungen. *In* M. Lewandowsky (Ed.), *Handbuch der neurologie* (Vol. 1). Berlin: Springer-Verlag, p. 1074.

Henschen, S. E. (1922). *Klinische und anatomische Beitrage zur Pathologie des Gehirns* (Vols. 5–7). Stockholm: Nordiska Bokhondel'n.

Howes, D., & Geschwind, N. (1964). Quantitative studies of aphasic language. *Research Publications—Association for Research in Nervous and Mental Disease, 42*, 229–244.

Isserlin, M. (1936). Aphasia. *In* O. Bumke & O. Foerster (Eds.), *Handbuch der neurologie* (Vol. 6). Berlin: Springer-Verlag, pp. 627–806.

Kertesz, A. (1979). *Aphasia and associated disorders. Taxonomy, localization and recovery.* New York: Grune & Stratton.

Kertesz, A., Lesk, O., & McCabe, P. (1977). Isotope localization of infarcts in aphasia. *Archives of Neurology (Chicago), 34,* 590–601.

Levine, D. N., & Mohr, J. P. (1979). Language after bilateral cerebral infarctions: Role of the minor hemisphere in speech. *Neurology, 29,* 927–938.

Levine, D. N., & Sweet, E. (1982). The neuropathologic basis of Broca's aphasia and its implications for the cerebral control of speech. *In* M. Arbib, D. Caplan, & J. Marshall (Eds.), *Neural models of language processes.* New York: Academic Press.

Liepmann, H. (1915). Diseases of the brain. *In* C. W. Burr (Ed.), *Curschmann's textbook on nervous diseases.* New York: McGraw-Hill (Blakiston).

Liepmann, H., & Maas, O. (1907). Fall von linkseitiger Agraphie und Apraxie bei rechtsseitiger Lahmung. *Journal fuer Psychologie und Neurologie, 10,* 214–227.

Marie, P. (1906). Revision de la question de l'aphasie: La troisième circonvolution frontale gauche ne joue aucun role spécial dans la fonction du langage. *Semaine Medicale, 26,* 241–247.

Mazzocchi, F., & Vignolo., L. A. (1979). Localization of lesions in aphasia: Clinical CT scan correlation in stroke patients. *Cortex, 15,* 627–654.

Mohr, J. P., Pessin, M. S., Finklestein, S., Funkenstein, H. H., Duncan, G. W., & Davis, K. R. (1978). Broca aphasia: Pathologic and clinical aspects. *Neurology, 28,* 311–324.

Moutier, F. (1908). *L'aphasie de Broca.* Paris: G. Steinheil.

Naeser, M. A., & Hayward, R. W. (1978). Lesion localization in aphasia with cranial computerized topography and the Boston Diagnostic Aphasia Exam: *Neurology, 28,* 545–551.

Niessl von Mayendorf, E. (1926). Uber die sog. Brocasche Windung und ihre angebliche Bedeutung fur den motorischen Sprachakt. *Monatsschrift fuer Psychiatrie und Neurologie, 61,* 129–146.

Penfield, W., & Boldrey, E. (1937). Somatic motor and sensory representation in the cerebral cortex of man as studied by electrical stimulation. *Brain, 60,* 389–443.

Penfield, W., & Roberts, L. (1959). *Speech and brain mechanisms.* Princeton, N.J.: Princeton University Press.

Phillips, C. G. (1966). Changing concepts of the precentral motor area. *In* J. C. Eccles (Ed.), *Brain and conscious experience.* New York: Springer-Verlag, pp. 389–421.

Rasmussen, R., & Milner, B. (1977. The role of early left-brain injury in determining lateralization of cerebral functions. *Annals of the New York Academy of Sciences, 299,* 355–369.

Ringer, S. (1879). Notes of a post-mortem examination on a case of athetosis. *Practitioner, 23,* 161–176.

Schiller, F. (1947). Aphasia studies in patients with missile wounds. *Journal of Neurology, Neurosurgery and Psychiatry, 10,* 183–197.

Trojanowski, J. Q., Green, R. C., & Levine, D. N. (1980). Crossed aphasia in a dextral: A clinicopathological study. *Neurology, 30,* 709–713.

von Monakow, C. (1914). *Die Lokalisation im Grosshirn.* Wiesbaden: Bergmann.

Weisenburg, T., & McBride, K. E. (1935). *Aphasia—A clinical and psychological study.* New York: Commonwealth Fund.

Wernicke, C. (1874). *Der aphasische Symptomenkomplex.* Breslau: Cohn & Weigert.

Zurif, E. B., Caramazza, A., & Myerson, R. (1972). Grammatical judgements of agrammatic aphasics. *Neuropsychologia, 10,* 405–417.

8

Localization of Lesions in Wernicke's Aphasia

Andrew Kertesz

Review of the Anatomical Studies

Wernicke (1874) expanded our knowledge of brain and language by throwing light on the sensory variety of aphasia. His model was inspired by his short stay with Meynert who promoted the concept of the motor–sensory, anterior–posterior dichotomy of cerebral cortex. Meynert (1866) himself described a case with lack of comprehension and paraphasic speech, without hemiplegia, associated with an infarct of the posterior insular artery. Wernicke adapted the sensory–motor dichotomy to the concept of language mechanisms. In his influential first article on the subject, he detailed ten cases, only four with autopsy data, none of them illustrated. One of them, an infarct in the temporal lobe, had a great deal of atrophy; the other had a cerebral abscess occupying much of the temporal lobe. The other two had global aphasia with large peri-Sylvian infarcts. Al-

209

though he described paraphasias, he did not draw the distinction between neologistic jargon and circumlocutory speech with mainly semantic paraphasias.

Soon after the publication of Wernicke's "aphasische symptomen-complex," more autopsied cases of sensory aphasia appeared in the literature and the concept of *word deafness,* a term coined by Kussmaul (1877) to denote central comprehension disturbance, began to take hold. Lichtheim (1885) distinguished several varieties of sensory aphasia, in his scheme of speech disorders, giving credit to Wernicke for some of them.

1. Speech deafness with impaired repetition and writing to dictation but preservation of reading and voluntary (spontaneous) writing. He described auditory inattention and inability to recognize melodies in his patient, who also considered music that he formerly enjoyed, as "too much noise."
2. Wernicke's type, in addition to word deafness, featured paraphasia, agraphia, and alexia. He also recognized that pure speech deafness may be seen in the course of evolution from Wernicke's aphasia.
3. Transcortical sensory aphasia with poor comprehension and preserved repetition
4. Conduction aphasia with poor repetition, paraphasias, and relatively good comprehension.

A substantial series of sensory aphasics was reviewed by Starr (1889) in New York. From the literature, he collected 50 cases where Broca's area was not involved. Many of them were taken from Seppili's (1884) and Amidon's (1885) series. Seven of these cases were considered "pure word deafness" and their lesion was limited to the posterior two-thirds of the first and second temporal convolutions. Paraphasias were present in 27 cases but he could not be sure of any difference in the localization between the cases with or without paraphasia. He thought the limits of the area where sensory aphasics have lesions included the superior temporal, the inferior parietal, and the occipital convolutions. Word blindness was found in five cases limited to the angular gyrus and the cortex of the inferior parietal lobule, but also in four cases where other structures were also involved. Starr recognized the limitations of contemporary localizationists when he wrote, "The pathology of Sensory Aphasia rests more upon forcible assertion and the analysis of ingenious diagrams than it does upon the collation of reliable evidence." He also perceived that "a considerable modification of symptoms occurred after the first few weeks and conclusions would be unreliable from pathology which is obtained very soon after the onset."

Henschen (1920–1922) collected the most extensive series of localized cases of sensory aphasia in his Volume VI of the monumental *"Pathologie des Gehirns."* The descriptions of the clinical features are very uneven as they were abstracted from many sources in the literature. Often, there is no detail about fluency or repetition although word deafness usually is mentioned as a feature of these protocols. Autopsy material is illustrated only in less than one-third of the cases, and although there are a few excellent photographs or drawings—even myelin-stained sections—the majority are in one dimension only and some of the specimens are badly distorted or mutilated. He summarizes the clinical descriptions in a telegraphic style and adds his own comments. Several tables are constructed such as those with involvement of the first temporal gyrus (T_1) only, those with T_1 and T_2 involvement as well, and so on. In addition to anatomical groupings, there are tables of jargonaphasia and amusia based on a somewhat arbitrary behavioral classification. He drew some conclusions which seem to be justified, nevertheless, on the basis of the number of his cases, as well as in view of subsequent evidence:

1. Word deafness is part of the paraphasic language disorder but it may exist by itself
2. Heschl's gyrus (Q), the first temporal (T_1), and second temporal (T_2), gyri are involved as a rule in pure word deafness
3. In case of paraphasic jargon, the temporal operculum (planum temporale) behind Heschl's gyrus is damaged as well. This, in addition to posterior T_1 and T_2, is Wernicke's area, according to common usage.

It was around that time that Cecil and Oscar Vogt (1910) made their contribution by investigating in detail the myelination of various cortical regions. Kleist, in his studies (1934, 1962), continued to promote the idea of the myeloarchitectonic divisions of the temporal lobes. These were presented in detail in his monograph on sensory aphasia and amusia. Several different cases were described with autopsy correlations, and Kleist was forced to conclude there were no obvious clinical differences among cortical, subcortical, and transcortical lesions. One patient (Case Papp) with a lesion of the planum temporale as well as T_1 and T_2 had word deafness, and a second lesion on the right side apparently prevented recovery. Word sense deafness (case Bayr) appeared to be equivalent to semantic jargon with verbal paraphasias and comprehension deficit and was produced by a small lesion between the first and second temporal gyrus. Sentence deafness (case Seuf) was described as severe semantic jargon with long, irrelevant but syntactically normal replies to questions. The quality of musical tones were appreciated but melodies could not be reproduced. Repetition tests were not described in this case report. The posterior portion of the first temporal convolution and the supramarginal gyrus were affected. Two of his cases had neologisms (cases De and Dol) and both had similar lesions of the transverse gyri, the regio paratransversalis in the planum temporale, and the posterior third of the temporal lobes in addition to other areas of the temporal lobes that were involved less consistently. Another (case Rit) with a deep temporal lesion extending to the ventricles had almost complete speech deafness, but it is not clear from the linguistic detail given what exactly was meant by this term. The clinical descriptions were often incomplete in this study; in some cases, for instance, repetition was used to classify patients as conduction aphasics; in others, it was not documented. The distinction among sentence, word, and word sense deafness appeared arbitrary, although conformed somewhat to output patterns—what we now describe as semantic, phonemic and neologistic jargon. Kleist also concluded that the "same clinical pictures of sensory aphasia can be brought about by lesions in different situations in relation to the cerebral cortex."

Is Wernicke's Aphasia a Single Entity?

Although *Wernicke's aphasia* is defined as "a fluent paraphasic speech disturbance with severely impaired comprehension and repetition," further subdivisions of the syndrome have been attempted ever since it was described. These are based on the features of the speech output (Huber, Stachowiak, Poeck, & Kerschensteiner, 1975; Lecours & Rouillon, 1976) or the modalities involved, mainly the presence or absence of the verbal–visual dissociation (Hier & Mohr, 1977). Lecours, Osborn, Travis, Rouillon, and Lavallee-Huynh (1981) distinguished at least eight kinds of jargon including: phonemic jargon with conduction aphasia, semantic jargon, neologistic jargon, derived morphemic paraphasias, dyssyntactic jargon, homonymic jargon, psychotic jargon of language, and glossolalia. They did not believe that the nature, localization, and extent of the lesion or functional lateralization of language explained the differences. Some would argue that this is overclassification to an impractical degree and that minor differences between jargon outputs are related more to day-to-day fluctuations, stages of recovery, the context of discourse, and the individual involved. Others may not be convinced that glossolalia should be considered a variety of jargon, instead of restricting the term to the religious phenomenon of "speaking in tongues." The continuous, almost total, replacement of lexical items in a discourse was designated undifferentiated jargon by Alajouanine (1956). A similar case was presented by Perecman and Brown (1981) which they called "phonemic jargon," but this is easily confused with the French terminology that uses the same for conduction aphasia. This patient had bilateral (temporal–parietal on the left and parietal on the right) lesions on CT.

The following classifications of Wernicke's aphasia, based on the characterization of speech output, in order of frequency of their occurrence, represent clinical distinctions agreed to by most clinicians. They all have poor comprehension and repetition in common:

1. Paraphasic output with severe comprehension and repetition disturbance—the original Wernicke's aphasia. The discourse is fluent with phonemic and semantic substitutions; yet, most of it is understandable. Reading and writing are similarly affected. Paragrammatism occurs but the syntax is, by and large, preserved.

2. Semantic jargon, where the substitutions are mostly semantic, but to such an extent that the discourse is unintelligible. Reading is comparably affected. It is seen with poor repetition in Wernicke's aphasia in the acute stage, or in the course of recovery from neologistic jargon. Semantic jargon also occurs with good repetition in transcortical sensory aphasia.

3. Neologistic jargon with mostly neologistic substitutions. Reading is similar. At times, writing is graphorrheic, but at other times, almost absent. Anosognosia is often present. A particularly severe variety is undifferentiated jargon (almost all words are substituted or the lexical items are not clearly separated by pauses, auxilliary words, pronouns, etc.). Low-volume mumbling jargon probably is related to this category also, because the few cases we had the opportunity to follow developed into neologistic jargon, and had temporal lesions.

4. Pure word deafness, with significant comprehension and repetition defect but relatively preserved discourse with only a few or no paraphasias. Reading and writing are relatively intact. It occurs

de novo but also during recovery from neologistic, semantic, or paraphasic speech patterns.

Pure Word Deafness, Auditory Agnosia, and Cortical Deafness

The relationship of pure word deafness, auditory agnosia for sounds, and cortical deafness is complex. These entities are relatively rare; therefore, only a few cases are available with localization. Munk (1881) used the term "mind" (psychic) deafness for dogs following the bilateral removal of auditory cortex. The clinical experience accumulating throughout the last 100 years indicated that word deafness is rarely, if ever, pure and the term should be used less frequently.

Liepmann and Storch (1902) reported a case of word deafness with a subcortical lesion in the left temporal lobe, apparently isolating the auditory association area from auditory input from either side. Unfortunately, that patient was illiterate so reading and writing could not be tested. Most patients with word deafness were unable to identify melodies, which is called "sensory amusia" although this also appears occasionally without aphasia (Quensel & Pfeifer, 1923). Schuster and Taterka's (1926) case of word deafness also had a left-sided-only lesion, with associated sound agnosia and amusia. These symptoms, taken together, are described as cortical deafness in other reports, especially if the subjective complaint is hearing loss. Occasionally, auditory inattention is marked, and the patient fails to turn toward the sound stimulus (Hemphill & Stengel, 1940; Wohlfart, Lindgren, & Jernelius, 1952). Severe auditory inattention may be mistaken for deafness. Pure tone audiometry (Mahoudeau, Lemoyne, Foncin, & Dubrisay, 1958) supported that word deafness and auditory agnosia are independent from hearing loss.

Agnosia for sounds is common with Wernicke's aphasia, according to Vignolo's (1969) review, but at least one case documents its existence without aphasia with a right temporal lesion (Spreen, Benton, & Fincham, 1965). Delayed perception and distorted sound appreciation (unpleasant sound) has been reported for thalamic lesions (Arnold, 1946). Patients with perceptual discriminating defects had right hemisphere lesions; others with semantic associative defects, had left hemisphere lesions in an analysis of auditory agnosia by Vignolo (1969). Cortical deafness is described in the acute stages of lesions affecting both temporal lobes. Cortical deafness is considered a separate condition by some, but others regard it as a combination of auditory verbal and nonverbal agnosia related to destruction of both Heschl's gyri and adjacent temporal tissue. There are variably sophisticated descriptions of this condition in the literature, but only a few with pathology.

Kanschepolsky, Kelly, and Waggener (1973) had a patient with bilateral temporal infarction proven on autopsy who complained of deafness for speech but could read well and hear the tuning fork bilaterally. His spontaneous speech, writing, and naming were intact but he could not enjoy music. Pure tone audiogram, sound localization, and temporal order identification were normal for his age, but threshold–duration function and loudness discrimination were impaired. Sophisticated auditory testing in other cases (Jerger, Weikers, Sharbough, & Jerger, 1969) also supports the finding that unilateral temporal lesions result in little or no loss of primary auditory function. Bilateral lesions show some loss of perceptual function, such as the temporal patterns of sounds, but some, such as pure tone discrimination, are well preserved. Therefore, the concept of cortical deafness needs to be modified toward a variable combination of central auditory disorders.

Michel, Peronnet, and Schott (1980) defined cortical deafness on the basis of absent cortical auditory-evoked potentials in a case with bilateral lesions. However, the late evoked potentials are variably impaired in other reported cases. Auerbach, Allard, Naeser, Alexander, and Albert (1982) investigated a patient with bilateral, but predominantly right temporoparietal lesion who had difficulty with "prephonemic" consonant feature discrimination for placing, partial word deafness, amusia, and sound recognition. The older, smaller, left temporal infarct was clinically "silent" and the larger, recent, right temporal infarct seemed to produce all the symptoms in this right-handed man. Cortical evoked potentials to auditory clicks were abnormal in the right hemisphere only. He also had moderate deficit in pure tone audiometry and abnormal click fusion and counting which was interpreted as an apperceptive disorder of "temporal auditory acuity." The authors concluded that their case was different from a higher disorder in linguistic discrimination that is a fragment of Wernicke's aphasia, but it was not cortical deafness as the evoked potentials and audiometry were normal on the left side.

We had a case that qualifies as "pure" word deafness because of well-preserved spontaneous speech and reading. He presented us

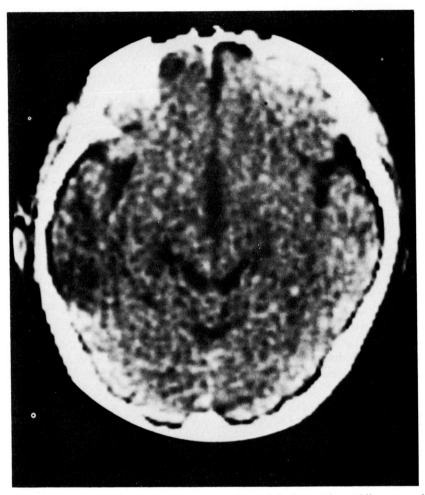

Figure 1. The lowermost cut in a patient with word deafness. The middle temporal gyrus is affected.

with the complaint that is typical of many of these patients—he could not hear words as speech but only as meaningless noise. He could talk without obvious errors and, to most observers, his spontaneous speech appeared normal. He had some paraphasias, mostly verbal substitutions, and also the occasional phonemic errors. He understood very little, not even at the simple word level and his repetition was very poor initially. He had people write down what they wanted because his reading comprehension was quite good. After a

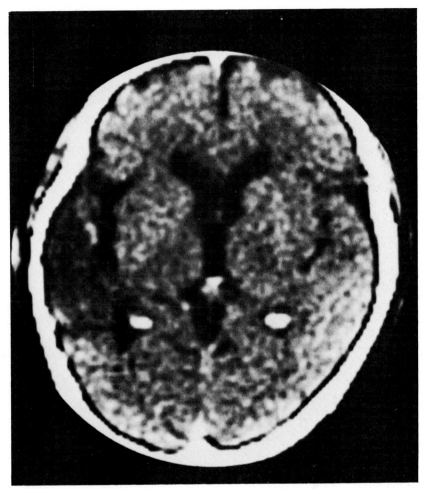

Figure 2. The second cut in Case 1 indicates involvement of the superior temporal gyrus and the middle portion of the temporal operculum.

few weeks, his repetition improved to a great extent and, at times, he was echolalic without understanding what he was repeating. He recognized 8 out of 12 environmental sounds correctly. He could not identify the crowing of a rooster, the noise of water pouring into a glass, a car horn, or a crying baby, mismatching the pictures representing these sounds.

The CT scan (Figures 1–4) shows the extent of the lesion in the left temporal lobe.

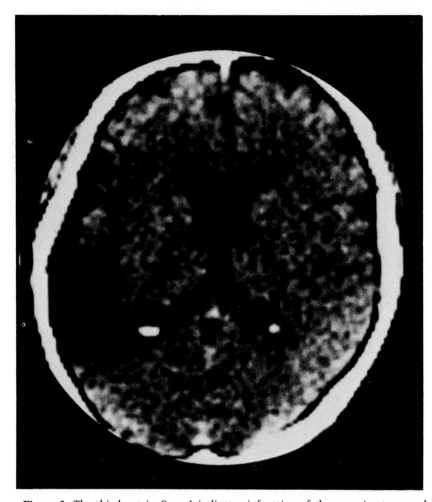

Figure 3. The third cut in Case 1 indicates infarction of the superior temporal gyrus, posterior portion of the temporal operculum, and the anterior portion of the supramarginal gyrus. The isthmus of the temporal lobe and the optic radiation probably is spared as the infarct does not reach the lateral ventricle.

In summary, the term "pure word deafness" should be used when the patient complains of not understanding speech but hearing everything else; when reading, writing, and spontaneous speech are well preserved; and environmental sounds are recognized. The lesions are usually unilateral in the speech-dominant hemisphere. Auditory agnosia for sounds and amusia are distinct entities although they are often present with aphasia. Cortical deafness is the result

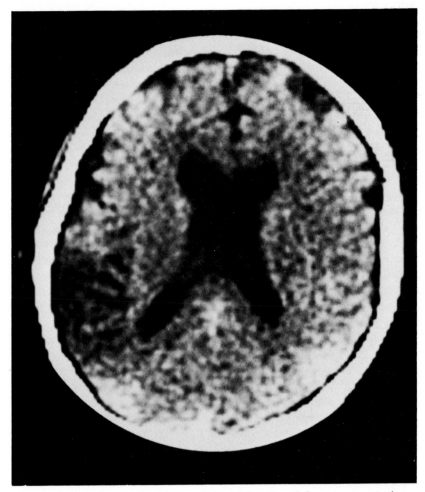

Figure 4. The upper cut in Case 1 indicates infarction of the supramarginal gyrus above the Sylvian fissure in a patchy fashion.

of bilateral lesions and the patient appears clinically deaf with preserved primary hearing but impaired central auditory processing.

Lesions in Neologistic Jargon

The localization of lesions in neologistic jargon aphasia, the most severe form of Wernicke's aphasia, was the subject of the study by Kertesz and Benson (1970). Five autopsied cases and five others localized by isotope scans and angiography were selected from a large aphasic population because of their uniform linguistic and behavioral characteristics. All had copiously produced fluent neologistic jargon, often excessive speech in relationship to the eliciting stimulus, associated with poor auditory comprehension, repetition, naming, and, in some cases, lack of recognition of their aphasia. Their speech, although resembling English syntactically, prosodically, and even phonetically, was devoid of information value by virtue of the majority of nouns and many verbs being transformed into neologisms. Neologisms are defined as unrecognizable nonwords in contrast to semantic jargon where the substitutions are recognizable words or verbal paraphasias.

It is often a matter of degree as to which of the two types of paraphasias dominate the speech output of an aphasic at a given time. We have shown (in 1970) that the initially severe neologistic jargon often recovers through semantic jargon toward anomic aphasia. We called the initial or subsequently persisting language disturbance "neologistic jargon" when at least 20% of the lexical items were neologisms, although this increased to about 80% at times. Responses to naming and repetition showed even higher evidence of neologisms than spontaneous speech.

The anatomical findings indicated that in each case the most posterior portion of the first temporal convolution, the supramarginal gyrus, and the underlying white matter were involved. Figure 5 indicates the isotope overlap of the lesions. In three cases, the lesion was limited in size and was located strategically at the posterior end of the Sylvian fissure. In two of the cases, the temporal involvement was minimal. Transverse sections showed involvement of the temporal and parietal operculum and underlying white matter, including the arcuate fasciculus in every case. The syndrome of neologistic jargon is usually seen in the larger lesions extending parietally, posteriorly, and temporally inferiorly.

A more recent anatomical study of jargon (Kertesz, 1981) confirmed these results by CT scan and isotope localization (Figures 6–8). A new autopsied case was added, again with relatively little temporal involvement (Figures 9 and 10). This lesion appears to be small on the lateral surface and involves only a centimeter of the posterior end of the first temporal gyrus (T_1). However, cross sections reveal a more extensive lesion of the temporal and parietal operculum (Figure 10).

The structure, then, that is invariably destroyed in neologistic jargon aphasia is the temporoparietal junction, the combination of the

NEOLOGISTIC JARGON-
ISOTOPE AND AUTOPSY OVERLAP

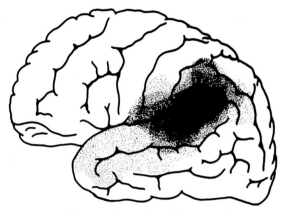

Figure 5. The overlap of an isotope and autopsy study of Kertesz and Benson (1970). The overlap of isotope and autopsied infarcts on the lateral surface indicates involvement of both the upper and the lower lip of the Sylvian fissure, the superior temporal gyrus, and the supramarginal gyrus.

NEOLOGISTIC JARGON CT OVERLAP

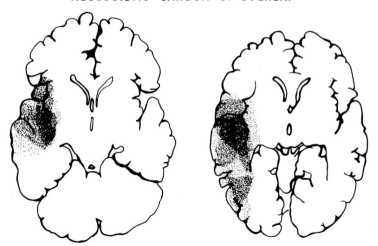

Figure 6. The overlap of lesions on the CT scan in neologistic jargon. These two lower cuts represent inferior and middle temporal portions of the lesions. The temporal operculum of the insula is involved. Reprinted with permission from Kertesz (1981).

NEOLOGISTIC JARGON CT OVERLAP

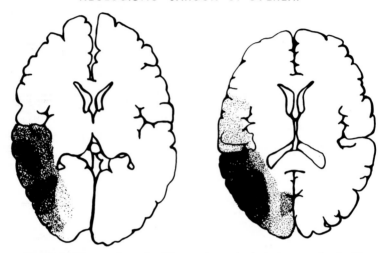

Figure 7. The overlap of a CT scan in neologistic jargonaphasia. These cuts are through Wernicke's area and supramarginal gyrus indicating involvement of the superior temporal gyrus, the temporal operculum, supramarginal gyrus, and the parietal operculum of the Sylvian fissure. Reprinted with permission from Kertesz (1981).

NEOLOGISTIC JARGON CT OVERLAP

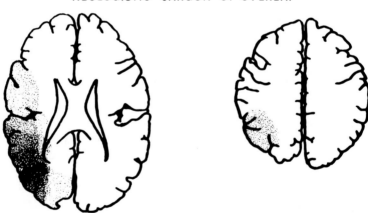

Figure 8. The CT overlap in neologistic jargon. These cuts represent the parietal region, the supramarginal gyrus, and, to some extent, the angular gyrus involvement. Reprinted with permission from Kertesz (1981).

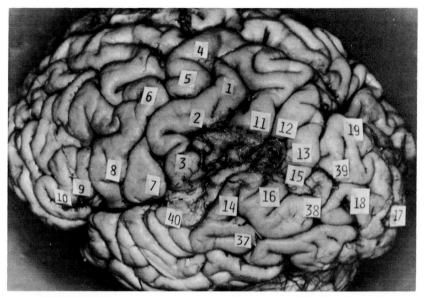

Figure 9. The lateral surface of the brain from a patient who had neologistic jargon aphasia up to the time of death. The brain is rotated slightly, so it is viewed from slightly behind and above. The superior temporal gyrus (between 40 and 14), the inferior parietal lobule (between 3 and 11), the supramarginal gyrus (under 12), and angular gyrus (in front of 39) are involved.

posterior end of the temporal (T₁) and the *supramarginal gyrus,* and the posterior ends of the temporal and parietal operculae. Since the *supramarginal* and the *inferior parietal* region is implicated in conduction aphasia as well, lesions in this area seem crucial in the genesis of phonemic errors and neologisms. The posterior–superior temporal region lesion probably contributes to the comprehension deficit as well as the anosognosia or the curious nonrecognition of the speech disturbance, possibly by the virtue of disengaging internal auditory monitoring. Anosognosia for speech, first emphasized by Alajouanine (1956), is not seen to any significant degree without comprehension deficit. However, since there are cases of severe auditory comprehension deficit without anosognosia or jargon, this is not an obligatory two-way association.

The recovery of comprehension closely parallels the recovery from neologistic output disturbance. This also supports the intrinsic relationship between the comprehension deficit and faulty output. The temporal auditory association areas likely play an important role in monitoring not only auditory input but also phonemic, syntactic,

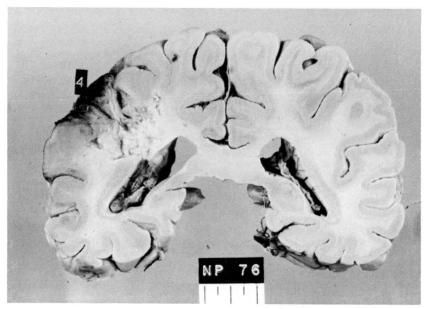

Figure 10. Cross section of the same brain as in Figure 9 at the level of the supra-marginal gyrus showing the depth of the lesion. With permission from Kertesz (1981).

and semantic selection for output. In fact, there is ample evidence from information-processing studies and cybernetics that the decoding and encoding processor are closely related. This is also plausible according to our clinical–anatomical studies. The selection of linguistic elements is likely simultaneous rather than consecutive although the primacy of semantic selection—and perhaps semantic recognition—has been advocated by some. In support of the role of auditory system in output is the experimental evidence of producing paraphasic speech with delayed auditory feedback in normals (Lee, 1950). Wernicke himself thought that it was the disordered auditory monitoring that produced the jargon. Somewhat against the importance of comprehension deficit in the production of phonemic paraphasia is the fact that conduction aphasics, on the whole, have good comprehension. It could be argued that auditory comprehension and auditory monitoring of internal speech processes are, in fact, separate mechanisms, even though the anatomical proximity suggests a close relationship.

In addition to the amount of neologisms, the degree of impairment in comprehension (and, it seems, temporal lobe involvement) separates neologistic jargon and Wernicke's aphasia from conduction aphasia. Lesions in conduction aphasia are often inferior parietal and supramarginal although there is often some temporal lobe involvement as well (Damasio & Damasio, 1980; Green & Howes, 1977; Kertesz, Harlock, & Coates, 1979). The fact that these patients have better comprehension may be related to more involvement of the inferior parietal region and the supramarginal gyrus than of the temporal lobe, that, in turn, seems to be involved more in Wernicke's and jargon aphasia.

The majority of cases with neologistic jargon aphasia (6 out of 10 in our series) have visual field defects, indirectly indicating the depth and posterior location of the lesions. Some are relatively anterior but deep central temporal lesions may also produce field defect because of the forward curve of the optic radiation (Meyer's loop).

Lesions in Semantic Jargon

This group is distinct linguistically; therefore, most investigators agree to separating them clinically. We looked at this group from the anatomical point of view (Kertesz, 1981) and found there is but a minor difference in the location of the lesions when compared to the neologistic group. The lesions of five cases of semantic jargon were slightly smaller and somewhat more temporal and inferior than those with neologisms. On the other hand, patients with transcortical sensory aphasia who have semantic jargon clearly have far more posterior lesions. (See Chapter 10 in this book.) There is, however, an overlap between the lesions of semantic and neologistic groups in the posterior inferior temporal region. These findings are compatible with the recent CT studies of Cappa, Cavallotti, and Vignolo (1981) who found that patients with semantic substitutions have lesions posterior to those with phonemic paraphasias. Brown (1981), trying to emphasize the bilaterality of these cases, had CT scans on three cases of semantic jargon. One patient with a head injury had only unilateral lesion, another had an old frontotemporal lesion on the right side in addition to a new one on the left, and the third, who had bilateral lesions of unknown etiology, extent, or timing, displayed fluctuating jargon. A fourth case without CT pictures was said to have atrophy. There is the evidence from our laboratory as is presented in this chapter and in the chapter on transcortical sensory aphasia (Chapter 10) that severe semantic jargon can be produced by unilateral temporal lesions with poor comprehension and repetition (Wernicke's aphasia) and by temporo-occipital lesions with poor comprehension but good repetition (transcortical sensory aphasia) (Kertesz, Sheppard, and McKenzie, 1982).

Patients with acute confusional or amnestic states and severe degenerative (Alzheimer's) disease often show semantic jargon which has been termed the language of confusion (Darley, 1964). This is somewhat misleading because many confused or confabulating Korsakoff's patients do not have semantic jargon. Therefore, confusion per se is not the reason for this language disturbance. The unilateral cases demonstrate, also, that bilateral or diffuse impairment is not a prerequisite in the production of this syndrome.

Anatomical Correlation of Functional Processing

The location of lesions in Wernicke's aphasia suggests the important role of the temporoparietal junction in the comprehension and production of language. Recent studies with CT scans confirmed the existence of auditory association areas for comprehension in the posterior–superior temporal lobe by demonstrating the consistent association of comprehension deficits for language, music, and nonverbal sounds with lesions in the area. Although bilateral lesions often produce severe, persisting deficits unilateral large lesions are sufficient to impair comprehension permanently.

Phonemic paraphasias are almost invariably associated with inferior parietal and supramarginal lesions, be it conduction aphasia with well-preserved comprehension or neologistic jargon aphasia with more temporal involvement and, presumably, disconnected auditory monitoring.

The combination of comprehension deficits with semantic jargon may occur with or without the preservation of the ability to repeat. Semantic jargon is often associated with some phonemic errors in Wernicke's aphasia, but not in transcortical sensory aphasia. The location of the lesions is clearly more anterior (temporal) in Wernicke's aphasia in comparison to those in transcortical sensory aphasia (temporooccipital). This indicates that comprehension can be impaired with lesions outside the auditory association area in the upper Sylvian region of the temporal lobe. In these instances, the comprehension deficit can be disassociated from repetition. On the other hand, when lesions involve Wernicke's area in the superior posterior temporal region, repetition deficit invariably occurs. The evidence supports multiple-level processing, which can be affected together and separately.

The following processes can be distinguished

1. Auditory perception followed by phonological and lexical categorization or feature analysis
2. Auditory comprehension with semantic associations
3. Auditory monitoring of phonological assembly
4. Auditory monitoring of lexical assembly
5. Word finding through semantic associations.

The deficits occurring in various combination produce the following clinical syndromes. Figure 11 illustrates the lesions and the disrupted processes.

1. *Pure Word Deafness (PWD)* The deficit is restricted to the mechanism of auditory categorization, or categorical perception and sorting. The patient has difficulty comprehending and repeating. Speech assembly continues to be driven by other association areas, and the spontaneous speech is relatively free of paraphasias. Visual input is better comprehended and reading is preserved.

2. *Transcortical Sensory Aphasia (TSA)* The deficit is in auditory comprehension and semantic association but auditory categorization and monitoring of phonemic and lexical assembly are preserved allowing repetition without phonemic paraphasias. The language area, disconnected from the semantic field, continues to elicit some spontaneous speech even though it may be semantically bizarre and irrelevant to the discourse.

AUDITORY LANGUAGE PROCESSES

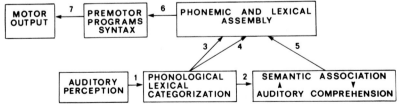

Figure 11. This processing model indicates the stages of language comprehension and the numbers indicate the clinical syndromes that may occur when these stages of auditory processing are disrupted. (Further explanation is in the text.)

were never properly challenged and, possibly, were less question-
able than the understanding of its physiological mechanism. When
the history of the anatomical localization of conduction aphasia is
reviewed, one encounters almost as much agreement as dispute.

What then, does the classical anatomical controversy consist of?
Wernicke (1874) predicted the insula would be the crucial area of
damage. He was convinced that major connecting systems between
Wernicke's and Broca's areas would course either through or underneath the insular cortex, and that damage to this area would
break apart the communication between the two major language
structures. Needless to say, there was no fine anatomical evidence
to support Wernicke's reasoning, but one can hardly take issue with
the conspicuous fact that the insula seemed to be in the middle of
the road that may have connected Wernicke's and Broca's areas.
But the case of Lichtheim (1885) gave support to Wernicke's prediction: The patient had Wernicke's *Leitungsaphasie*; at autopsy, the
core of the lesion was clearly in the insula.

The cases of conduction aphasia that Goldstein came to describe
(1911, 1948) were anatomically comparable and again fully supported Wernicke's prediction. Nevertheless, there was some conflicting evidence, best exemplified by the case of Liepmann and
Pappenheim (1914) in which the insula was intact. Wernicke by then
had revised his original proposal and considered that the crucial
connecting system coursed not in the insula but in the arcuate fasciculus, a component of the superior longitudinal fasciculus. The
physiological point was still the same, that Wernicke's and Broca's
areas were anatomically disconnected, but the site of disconnection
was different.

It must be said that this account of conduction aphasia was better
founded in anatomical evidence, for, if there had been no indication
then of the existence of temporofrontal connections underneath the
insula, there was, on the contrary, acceptable evidence of the existence of temporofrontal connections via the arcuate fasciculus (Dejerine, 1901). This fasciculus originated in auditory association
cortex and traveled caudalward and upward around the rearmost
portion of the sylvian fissure, it arched in the parietal operculum
underneath the supramarginal and somatosensory cortices, and then
traveled forward in the depth of the frontal operculum to reach
Broca's area component of the premotor region. Nevertheless, although on the basis of the Liepmann and Pappenheim (1914) case
and of anatomical knowledge of the day, Wernicke built an acceptable argument to conjoin conduction aphasia and lesions of the ar-

cuate fasciculus in the parietal operculum, he still was unable to account for cases such as Lichtheim's in which the arcuate fasciculus would not appear to be damaged. Writing extensively about conduction aphasia, which he renamed "central aphasia," Goldstein (1948) was no more able to resolve the discrepancy and in fact brushed anatomical evidence aside to fit conduction aphasia into an idealized scheme.

More recently, Benson, Sheremata, Bouchard, Segarra, Price, and Geschwind (1973) have come across this anatomical conflict in a pathological study of three cases of conduction aphasia. Two of their cases, Cases 1 and 3, had clear damage to the supramarginal gyrus. The insula was not affected, nor was there damage to Wernicke's area. The lesions were exclusively supra sylvian. Damage to the arcuate fasciculus (as previously noted runs deep underneath the supramarginal gyrus) could be inferred from the distribution of the white matter damage. However, Case 2 had lesions in the insula and in auditory cortex, with a purely subsylvian location: The supramarginal gyrus was not damaged and it could be concluded that neither was the arcuate fasciculus, at least not in the portion in which it is presumably organized as an individual bundle in the parietal operculum. Yet, it is clear that damage to auditory cortex and underlying white matter in Wernicke's area could have destroyed the arcuate fasciculus at its origin. Furthermore, it is possible that in Case 2 of Benson *et al.*, the lesion of the insula also contributed to the syndrome.

The advent of computerized tomography (CT) has permitted yet another look into the problem, and recent advances in anatomical tracing techniques provide some information helpful in the interpretation of CT scan findings.

In a recent study (Damasio & Damasio, 1980), we reported on the CT scan correlates of five cases of conduction aphasia. These patients were studied with the Multilingual Aphasia Battery (Benton, 1969, 1983), consisting of a series of standardized and validated tests of visual naming, sentence repetition, aural comprehension and reading comprehension. The diagnosis of conduction aphasia was made on the basis of results obtained in those tests and according to the Boston School of Aphasia (Goodglass & Kaplan, 1972). All patients had CT scans done on EMI scanners. Four patients had suffered thrombotic infarctions and one patient had a hemorrhagic event, all in the left hemisphere. All were studied during the first 3 months after the stroke. Three patients were women and two were men, their ages varying between 35–47 years. All but one were complete righthanders, and the left-handed subject had a family history of strong dextrality.

Initially, all four patients with thrombotic infarctions had right central facial paresis as well as right brachial paresis, along with aphasia. In all, the paretic symptoms improved while the aphasia persisted. The one patient with an intracerebral hemorrhage was more severely affected initially, with drowsiness and lack of communication which cleared within a few days. All patients had fluent speech with occasional paraphasias. Sentence repetition was very defective, characterized by omissions, phonemic paraphasias, and, occasionally, by complete blocking.

The CT scans of these patients were studied by plotting the lesions onto corresponding templates in which the cytoarchitectonic areas of Brodmann's map had been marked. In four cases, there was compromise of the insular region. Also, in four cases, there was variable degree of involvement of the superior temporal gyrus and an extension of the lesion into the inferior parietal region. In all cases, the lesions were deep and compromised the white matter underlying the previously mentioned regions. In no case was there involvement of the angular gyrus, the posterior portions of the second and third temporal gyrus, or Broca's area.

Some cases involved the insular region and the auditory cortex. An example is Case 1 (Figure 1) in which the infarct is limited to the insular cortex, to its underlying substance, and to the auditory cortex and underlying white matter. There is only minimal involvement of the large expanse of auditory association cortex (Area 22). Most of the latter lies in the planum temporale (corresponding to the core or Wernicke's area) and appears spared.

Other cases, although involving the insula and the auditory areas, also extended into inferior portions of the parietal operculum, as exemplified by Case 3 (Figure 2). Here the infarct involved insular region, auditory cortex, and extended into the more anterior and inferior portions of the supramarginal gyrus (Area 40). Compared to the previous example, there was even less involvement of Area 22 in this case.

Case 4 exemplified a case with little involvement of insular structures, but with almost complete destruction of the core of the auditory areas of the left hemisphere and minor involvement of the

---

Figure 1. CT scan and templates of Case 1. The area of decreased density in the left hemisphere involves insula, primary auditory cortex, and part of auditory association cortex.

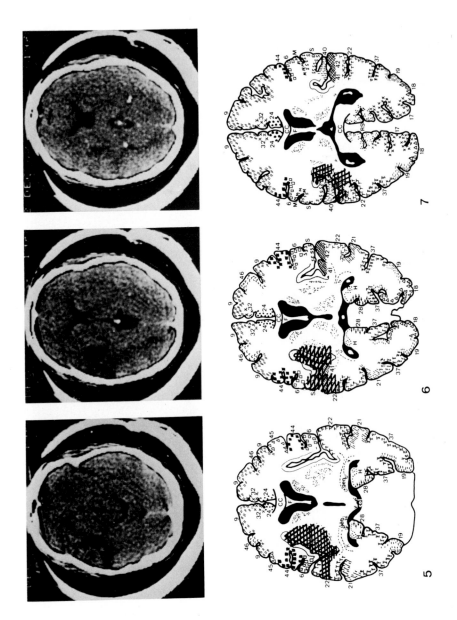

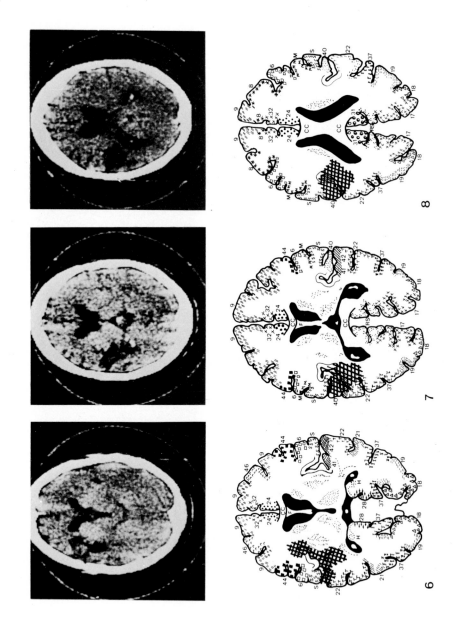

inferior portions of the supramarginal gyrus. Again, the planum temporale appears spared.

In Case 5 (the one case of intracerebral hemorrhage), damage was almost exclusively confined to the region of the insula and lateral putamen. In all likelihood, there was damage to both cortical and subcortical areas in the insular region as well as the lateral putamen, with extension into the temporal isthmus and into white matter underlying Area 40 in its more anterior and inferior portion. It is not possible to discern direct involvement of either Wernicke's or Broca's areas.

After the completion of the study, we continued seeing patients with conduction aphasia. The most remarkable recently provided us with the CT counterpart of what Benson *et al.* described in their Cases 1 and 3. H. P. was a 33-year-old woman, right-handed, with an acute hemorrhagic infarction in the left hemisphere, secondary to bleeding from an arteriovenous malformation. Other than aphasia, her one symptom was decreased dexterity in the right hand. Her speech was fluent with occasional global and phonemic paraphasias. Sentence repetition was severely impaired with word omissions and frequent phonemic and global paraphasias. Her aural comprehension was remarkably intact; so was her reading ability. As in the other patients with conduction aphasia, her memory and visuospatial abilities were intact.

The analysis of the patient's CT scan shows that the lesion involves the supramarginal gyrus (Area 40) on the left side. There is no evidence of damage to areas 41, 42, 22 or to the insula (Figures 3 and 4). A detailed report by the neurosurgeon confirms that the lesion is exclusively supra-Sylvian.

Judging from such material, there appear to be at least two fundamental anatomical patterns associated with conduction aphasia. One corresponds to lesions of the supramarginal gyrus in which the arcuate fasciculus is compromised. In the other, both auditory and insular cortices as well as underlying white matter are damaged. Some cases appear to have a combination of both patterns and have lesions that involve supramarginal gyrus and underlying arcuate fasciculus, auditory cortex and underlying white matter, and insula and underlying white matter.

There is postmortem evidence of such anatomical combinations:

Figure 2. CT scan and templates of Case 3. The area of decreased density involves insula, primary auditory cortex, and extends into inferior and anterior portions of supramarginal gyrus.

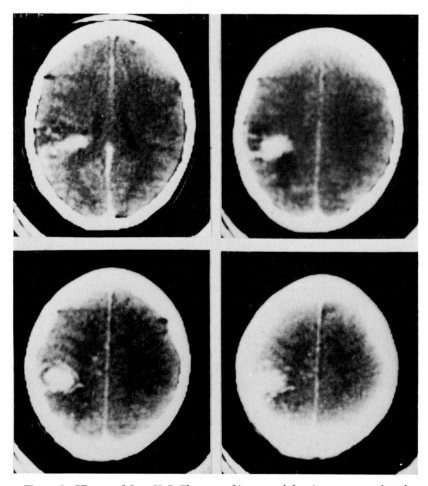

Figure 3. CT scan of Case H. P. The area of increased density corresponds to hemmorrhage and is located in the left parietal lobe. There is extensive subcortical involvement. Temporal lobe and insula are not involved.

Figure 4. Template of the CT scan in Figure 3. The lesion involves the white matter underlying the supramarginal gyrus (Area 40).

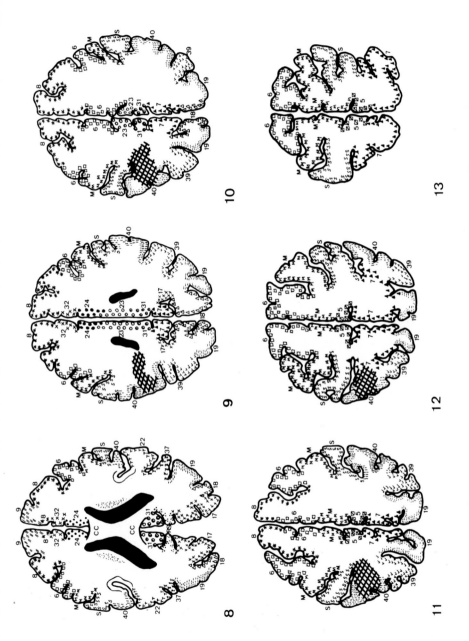

For instance, the case of Sheremata, Andrews, and Pandya (1974), in which both insula *and* arcuate fasciculus were involved, although the arcuate fasciculus was compromised at its rostral (frontal) end. Whichever the pattern, arcuate, insular, or a combination thereof, the anatomical correlates of conduction aphasia are distinct. They cannot be mistaken for those of Broca's or Wernicke's aphasias. There may be an overlap with structures that also can be damaged in Wernicke's aphasia. But it is clear that such anatomical overlap is accompanied by a behavioral overlap. Both conduction aphasia and Wernicke's aphasia have a remarkable impairment of verbal repetition. A composite diagram of cases of conduction aphasia is shown in Figure 5. The composite loci of Broca's and Wernicke's aphasias, derived from a different study (Damasio & Damasio, 1979), are also indicated. There is little question that all three syndromes have distinct localizations, as judged by CT scan (Damasio, 1981). A similar conclusion had been reached by Naeser and Hayward (1978) and by Kertesz, the latter working with both radionuclide brain scans and with CT (Kertesz, Harlock, & Coates, 1979; Kertesz, Lesk, & McCabe, 1977).

Thus, conduction aphasia can appear in relationship to two different patterns of brain damage. If in both circumstances the syndrome may be considered the result of a sensorymotor disconnection, it is necessary to postulate the existence of two separate conduction pathways (Figure 6), that is, the auditory-motor connection that supports repetition behavior can be achieved by two different channels. It is possible that they are complementary, two components of a powerful system of auditory–motor connections. Conceivably, one component might be of greater functional importance than the other but that is of little importance. Damage to either will impair repetition behavior.

There is now anatomical evidence to support the contention that the auditory–motor linkage on which repetition behavior depends can be achieved by more than one anatomical channel. Dissection work, from the time of Dejerine until today, proves the arcuate fasciculus to be an anatomical reality. But evidence of an insular channel was not available for a long time, and it is possible that its lack made Wernicke discard his original and logical proposal. However, modern anatomical tracing techniques in the rhesus monkey show that there are additional pathways between auditory–temporal and motor–frontal structures (Pandya, 1979). Such pathways take the shorter and anatomically logic route of the extreme capsule, under-

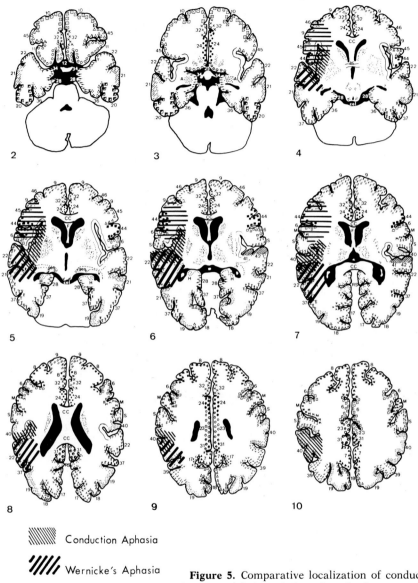

Conduction Aphasia

Wernicke's Aphasia

Broca's Aphasia

Figure 5. Comparative localization of conduction, Wernicke's and Broca's aphasias at each template level.

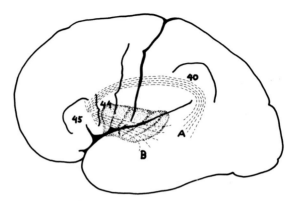

Figure 6. Temporofrontal pathways involved in conduction aphasia. *A* (arcuate fasciculus) and *B* (subin-
sular pathway) represent the extremes of a powerful
and possibly continuous connectional system.

neath the insular cortex. Their fibers can be seen beneath the insular cortex, but not, it appears, between the claustrum and the
lenticular nucleus (that is, in the external capsule). These two pathways may actually form a continuum of powerful auditory–motor
connections which utilizes several anatomical routes.

In addition, there exist connections that travel around the posterior end of the Sylvian fissure and arch in the parietal operculum,
the animal counterpart of the classical arcuate fasciculus. Granted
that the rhesus monkey is not notable for its ability to repeat words,
it is likely that such structures subserve a variety of other repetition
behaviors in which auditory input and some sort of vocal production are involved. Be that as it may, Pandya's data provide strong
evidence for the existence of heretofore unsuspected anatomical
connections between auditory and motor cortices.

In conclusion, it appears that the anatomical distinctiveness of
conduction aphasia is just as remarkable as its behavioral distinctiveness. The classical controversy regarding the anatomical patterns preferably associated with conduction aphasia is possibly a
false one. Two distinct anatomical patterns can produce the syndrome but appear to affect the same functional system. It remains
to be seen whether subtle clinical characteristics or the profile of
recovery will allow the correct prediction of the underlying anatomical pattern.

References

Benson, D. F., Sheremata, W. A., Bouchard, R., Segarra, J. M., Price, D., & Geschwind, N. (1973). Conduction aphasia: A clinicopathological study. *Archives of Neurology (Chicago)*, *28*, 339–346.

Benton, A. L. (1969). Development of a multilingual aphasia battery: Progress and problems. *Journal of the Neurological Sciences*, *9*, 39–48.

Benton, A. L., Hamden, K., Varney, N., & Spreen, O. (1983). *Contributions to neuropsychological assessment*. New York: Oxford University Press.

Brown, J. (1972). *Aphasia, apraxia and agnosia*. Springfield, Ill.: Thomas, Chapter 5.

Damasio, H. (1981). Cerebral localization of the aphasias. In M. T. Sarno (Ed.), *Acquired aphasia*. New York: Academic Press.

Damasio, H., & Damasio, A. R. (1979). "Paradoxic" ear extinction in dichotic listening: Possible anatomic significance. *Neurology*, *29*, 644–653.

Damasio, H., & Damasio, A. R. (1980). The anatomical basis of conduction aphasia. *Brain*, *103*, 337–350.

Dejerine, J. (1901). *Anatomie des centres nerveux*. Paris: Reuff.

Geschwind, N. (1965). Disconnexion syndromes in animals and man. *Brain*, *88*, 237–294, 585–644.

Goldstein, K. (1911). Uber die amnestische and centrale aphasie. *Archiv fuer Psychiatrie und Neurologie*, *48*, 408.

Goldstein, K. (1948). *Language and language disturbances*. New York: Grune & Stratton, Chapter VII.

Goodglass, H., & Kaplan, E. (1972). *The assessment of aphasia and related disorders*. Philadelphia: Lea & Febiger.

Kertesz, A., Harlock, W., & Coates, R. (1979). Computer tomographic localization, lesion size, and prognosis in aphasia and nonverbal impairment. *Brain and Language*, *8*, 34–50.

Kertesz, A., Lesk, D., & McCabe, P. (1977). Isotope localization of infarcts in aphasia. *Archives of Neurology (Chicago)*, *34*, 590–601.

Kinsbourne, M. (1971). *Conduction aphasia*. Read before the annual meeting of the American Academy of Neurology, New York.

Kleist, K. (1962). *Sensory aphasia and amusia*. Oxford: Pergamon, Chapter 3.

Lichtheim, L. (1885). On aphasia. *Brain*, *7*, 433–484.

Liepmann, H., & Pappenheim, M. (1914). Uber einem fall von sogenannter Leitungsaphasie mit anatomischem befund. *Neurologie und Psychiatrie*, *27*, 1–41.

Naeser, M. A., & Hayward, R. (1978). Lesion localization in aphasia with cranial computed tomography and the Boston Diagnostic Aphasia Exam. *Neurology*, *28*, No. 6, 545–551.

Pandya, D. N. (1979). Personal communication. Observations to be published.

Sheremata, W. A., Andrews, R., & Pandya, D. N. (1974). Conduction aphasia from a frontal lobe lesion. *Transactions of the American Neurological Association*, *99*, 249–252.

Warrington, E. K., & Shallice, T. (1969). The selective impairment of auditory verbal short-term memory. *Brain*, *92*, 885–896.

Wernicke, C. (1874). *Der aphasische Symptomencomplex*. Breslau: Cohn & Weigert.

10

The Localization of Lesions
in Transcortical Aphasias*

*Alan B. Rubens
and Andrew Kertesz*

Introduction

Lichtheim (1885) was the first to call attention to the syndrome called "transcortical aphasia." He described a patient with greatly reduced spontaneous speech and writing but with relatively preserved ability to repeat, read aloud, and to write to dictation. As he could not account for the preservation of repetition on the basis of Wernicke's (1874) model of motor, sensory, and commissural aphasia (conduction aphasia, *Leitungsaphasie*), Lichtheim proposed that the basis of transcortical aphasia is a pathological separation between an intact speech area and a diffusely represented nonlanguage cor-

*This work supported in part by the Ontario Health Research Grant #PR721 and NICDS Contract N01-NS-7-2378

245

tical area (concept center or *Begriffsfeld*) on which the speech area is dependent for activational and conceptual control. This would leave repetition intact while disrupting either spontaneous speech or auditory comprehension. Lichtheim referred to the effect of this separation as peripheral "commissural," or white matter pathway aphasia (*Leitungsaphasie*).

Wernicke (1886) accepted Lichtheim's model, but he preferred to restrict the term *Leitungsaphasie* to what is now called conduction aphasia. He introduced the term *transcortical aphasia* for those aphasias in which repetition was intact because the central language zone was spared, although separated pathologically from other nonlanguage areas. At present, transcortical aphasia is commonly divided into aphasia in which repetition is disproportionally preserved compared to reduced and simplified spontaneous speech (transcortical motor aphasia), impaired comprehension (transcortical sensory aphasia), or both (mixed transcortical aphasia).

Despite its current wide popularity, the use of the term has received much criticism over the years by many authors. Some have properly objected to the use of a pathophysiologic (explanatory) term to label a disturbance of verbal behavior, whereas others have directly questioned the transcortical explanation itself. Wernicke (1908), although arguing for its continued use on theoretical grounds, expressed reservations about the anatomical evidence supporting the transcortical model. Bastian (1897) rejected it, attributing the disproportionate sparing of repetition to mild damage of a cortical speech center. Bastian believed that subtotal cortical damage could increase cortical excitability threshold to a critical level where reaction to a strong externally generated stimulus such as heard speech would still be possible when response to a weaker internal stimulus (required in spontaneous speech) was no longer possible. This concept was adopted by Goldstein (1948) as an explanation of his own observation that in motor aphasia, particularly of the posttraumatic type, repetition tends to return before spontaneous speech. Niessl von Mayendorf (1911), on the other hand, pointed to the nondominant hemisphere as the source of repetition in transcortical patients. The occasional occurrence of right hemisphere repetition is suggested by reports in the more modern literature of patients in whom repetition despite major lesions of the speech area was preserved (Gloning, Gloning, & Hoff, 1963; Mohr, Pessin, Finkelstein, Funkenstein, Duncan, & Davis, 1978; Rubens, 1976; Stengel, 1936, 1947).

Kurt Goldstein (1917, 1948) is the author who has contributed most to the literature of transcortical aphasia. He introduced the term "isolation of the speech area" for the pathological separation of the speech zone (Wernicke's area, Broca's area, and their interconnections) from an ideational field by widespread pathology. There are several pathologically verified examples of this syndrome in the literature (Geschwind, Quadfasel, & Segarra, 1968; Whitaker, 1976). Isolation of the speech area is now used by some authors interchangeably with the term *mixed transcortical aphasia*, and by others as equivalent to transcortical sensory aphasia. Transcortical motor aphasia corresponds to anterior isolation, whereas transcortical sensory aphasia has been called posterior isolation. Luria's (1966, 1970; Luria & Hutton, 1977) frontal dynamic aphasia and transcortical motor aphasia appear to be the same syndrome. The transcortical aphasias are important because they offer the neurolinguist the opportunity to examine the language competence of the isolated peri-Sylvian language zone, and are important to the neurologist because acute transcortical aphasia usually indicates complete or partial sparing of the peri-Sylvian language core. Therefore, the lesion is placed at the periphery of the middle cerebral artery territory, its border zone, or within the territory of the anterior or posterior cerebral arteries (Kertesz, Lesk, & McCabe, 1977; Naeser & Hayward, 1978).

Transcortical Motor Aphasia (TMA)

Introduction

TMA is characterized by a marked reduction in the amount and complexity of spontaneous speech with retained ability to repeat sentences, to name objects presented through a particular sensory modality, and to read aloud. Spontaneous speech is disproportionately reduced in quality and quantity compared to speech evoked by external stimulation of any kind. Comprehension of spoken and written language is relatively preserved, often at the level seen with Broca's aphasia. Writing ability is usually impaired to the same degree as spoken speech. In the acute phase, speech may be severely limited, sometimes to the point of mutism. In patients with mild or recovered forms of TMA, the only remaining deficit may be in word fluency, with inability to produce lists of words belonging to specific letter or semantic categories. The underlying deficit common to moderately and severely affected patients is the inability to prop-ositionalize, to produce a free-flowing sentence, or a short string of sentences that provide answers to specific questions.

Acute lesions of the dominant superior premotor zone commonly result in total muteness lasting several days. The patient rapidly re-gains the ability to mouth words silently or in a dysphonic whisper. At this stage, spontaneous speech is sparse and limited to single-word or short, overlearned phrases; yet, the patient may be able to repeat long complicated sentences. Phonation and quantity of spon-taneous speech then improve considerably over several weeks or months. Phonemic paraphasia and agrammatism are not prominent features. When the lesion involves the lower premotor zone—par-tially affecting the anterior peri-Sylvian language area—mild dys-arthria, phonemic paraphasias, and short-lasting agrammatism may be prominent. There is a less striking discrepancy between spon-taneous speech and repetition. Goldstein (1915, 1948) attributed this form of TMA to subtotal damage with decreased excitibility thresh-old of Broca's area.

At first, patients with TMA may appear to have a severe memory deficit or dementia, because their answers are evasive and vague. This is because they cannot easily produce propositional utterances. In response to general questions that require a connected discourse ("Tell me about your illness."), a common response might be "I don't know." However, when questions do not require more than a single word or a simple sentence answers may be surprisingly informative.

As is true of many large frontal lesions, perseveration is common. They contaminate written, pointing, practic, and spoken responses. This complicates the interpretation of tests of auditory comprehen-sion and apraxia. It is rare for the TMA patient to point to more than two objects in proper sequence. Pointing and naming usually fall off after a number of successful responses because of persev-erations. The patient may be aware of his perseverations but is un-able to avoid them. Recently, Luria and Hutton (1977) made a point of distinguishing between two forms of TMA. In one, verbal persev-erations are prominent; in the other, the absence of perseverations allows for repetition of long, complicated sentences. They call the former perseverative aphasia. In this syndrome, the patient is able to repeat only a word or a brief sentence before perseverations in-terfere with repetition. In the second form, Luria's "dynamic aphasia," there are no perseverations and repetition of complicated sentences is unimpaired, although spontaneous speech is scanty and uninformative.

Neurological findings with lesions in the premotor zone include right hemiparesis involving the leg more than the arm, a right grasp reflex, and rigidity of the right upper extremity. Urinary and bowel incontinence are often present early. With involvement of the anterior and mid corpus callosum, there may be agraphia, apraxia, and tactile anomia of the left upper extremity.

ANATOMY

Lesions responsible for TMA are located in the language-dominant frontal lobe either directly anterior or superior to Broca's area (Goldstein, 1948; Luria, 1970), or within the mid and upper premotor zone in the neighborhood of the supplementary motor cortex (Alexander & Schmitt, 1980; Goldstein, 1948; Jonas, 1981; Környey, 1975; Luria, 1970; Naeser and Hayward, 1978; Rubens, 1975, 1976; von Stockert, 1974), (Figures 1 and 2).

The importance of the left superior premotor region to the speech act has been demonstrated. An extensive literature on the production of aphasia implicates lesions of this region. Lesions situated in the superior premotor zone, far from the classical speech area, routinely produce profound speech and language abnormalities. The literature indicates that aphasia with and without dysphonia often accompanies left frontal parasagittal tumors (Alajouanine, Castaigne, Sabourand, & Contamin, 1959; Arseni & Botez, 1961; Carrieri, 1963; Chusid, de Gutierrez-Mahoney, & Margules-Labergne, 1954; Guidetti, 1957; Magnan, 1880; Maroun, Jacob, & Gowing, 1970; Penfield & Roberts, 1959; Petit–Dutaillis, Guiot, Messing, & Bourdillon, 1954; Sweet, 1951). Persistent dysphonia and mutism have occurred after commissurotomy (Bogen, 1976), possibly on the basis of trauma to the mesial frontal area during surgery.

Surgical excision of the left superior premotor zone is followed by severe, but transient, motor aphasia (Arseni & Botez, 1961; Chavany & Rongerie, 1958; Chusid et al., 1954; Erickson & Woolsey, 1951; Guidetti, 1957; Schwab, 1927). Schwab (1927) commented on the sparing of repetition in aphasia after excision of cortical Area 6 for post-traumatic epilepsy. The diagrams of Conrad (1954), Russell and Espir (1961), and Luria (1970) report many examples of left premotor frontal penetrating missile injuries that cause severe motor aphasia. Luria emphasized sparing of repetition in his patients. Aphasia with cerebrovascular accidents in the territory of the an-

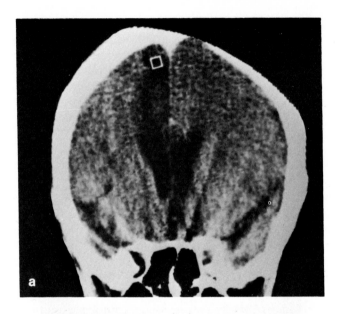

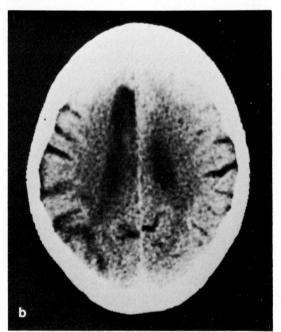

Figure 1. Coronal (la) and 15° from horizontal (lb) CT cuts showing infarction of mesial left frontal lobe with destruction of supplementary motor cortex and anterior corpus callosum in patient with TMA, unilateral apraxia, and agraphia of the left hand.

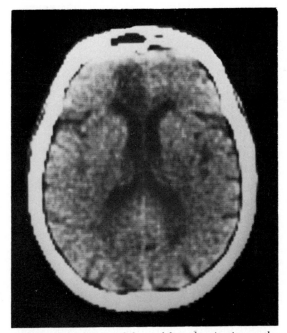

Figure 2. Left mesial frontal low density in another patient with TMA due to infarction in the territory of the left anterior cerebral artery.

terior cerebral artery is well documented (Alexander & Schmidt, 1980; Bonhoeffer, 1914; Critchley, 1930; Damasio & Kassel, 1978; Dimitri & Victoria, 1936; Guidetti, 1957; Hyland, 1933; Jonas, 1981; Környey, 1956, 1975; Liepmann & Maas, 1907; Luria & Tsvetkova, 1968; Masdeu, Schoene, & Funkenstein, 1978; Petit-Dutaillis *et al.*, 1954; Poppen, 1939; Racy, Jannotta, & Lehner, 1979; Rubens, 1975; von Stockert, 1974). With few exceptions, when there were sufficient details of speech and language performance, repetition was disproportionally preserved. Echolalia was not unusual.

Mild and partial forms of this syndrome have been reported, but not referred to as TMA. Milner (1964) reported that left frontal lobectomy results in a reduction of spontaneous speech marked by a tendency to use as few words as possible. Formal tests reveal no obvious aphasia or reduction in verbal intelligence; however, there is a marked reduction of word fluency in tests of the kind described by Thurstone and Thurstone (1949). The deficit does not appear to occur with similar lesions of the right frontal lobe or of the left anterior temporal lobe. This reduction of word fluency with left frontal lobe lesions that spare the language zone has been confirmed both by Benton (1968) and Ramier and Hécaen (1970). The latter (1970) also report minimal but measurable impairment in word fluency with right frontal lobe lesions. They attribute the deficit of word fluency associated with left hemisphere lesions to the combined effects of reduced initiation of action associated with frontal lobe disease in general, and impaired verbal performance associated with left hemisphere damage, in particular.

Sparing of repetition in aphasia associated with lesions just superior to Broca's area is also discussed in the older literature. Marie and Foix (1917) described slowness of speech and idea formation in the presence of normal naming ability and auditory comprehension resulting from missile wounds of the posterior portion of the second frontal gyrus just above Broca's area. Marie's patients were unable to condense ideas into phrases. Kleist (1934) described, using the German term, *Adynamie der Sprache*, speech and language of patients with lesions in Area 9 of Brodmann. These patients were not formally aphasic, but manifested a marked reduction of spontaneous speech, with difficulty in evoking appropriate words and sentences without impaired articulation or repetition.

The pathophysiology of TMA has been much debated. Some have suggested that lack of speech initiative represents nothing more than a part of a general frontal lobe hypokinetic syndrome. However, many patients manifest struggle behavior and considerable frustration after repeated failures. We have observed patients in whom repeated struggle behavior terminated in a catastrophic reaction. The recent literature points to the role of the superior premotor zone in the initiation and inhibition of speech, specifically the left supplementary motor region and its cortical and subcortical connections with cingulate gyrus.

Electrical stimulation of the supplementary motor cortex of either hemisphere in man results in either speech arrest or involuntary repetitive monosyllabic vocalizations (Brickner, 1940; Erickson and Woolsey, 1951; Penfield & Roberts, 1959; Penfield & Welch, 1951). Similar abnormal vocal behavior is known to occur with left frontal parasagittal epileptigenic tumors within or near the supplementary motor cortex (Alajouanine et al., 1959; Arseni & Botez, 1961; Carrieri, 1963; Erickson & Woolsey, 1951; Guidetti, 1957; Petit-Dutaillis et al., 1954; Sweet, 1951). Cerebral blood flow increases bilaterally over frontal parasagittal regions during speech, and, apparently, any repetitial, sequential movement, verbal or nonverbal (Ingvar, Philipson, Torlof, & Ardo, 1975; Larson, Skinhøj, & Lassen, 1978; Lassen, Roland, Larsen, Melamed, & Soh, 1977). It appears that the supplementary motor region plays a major role in mediating the production of sequential, voluntary motor activity of which speech is, by far, the most complex. Botez and Barbeau (1971) believe that the supplementary motor region is the cortical structure that mediates the starting mechanism of speech. The system begins in the periaqueductal gray matter of the mesencephalon and is represented within the ventrolateral nucleus of the thalamus. Cytoarchetecturally, the supplementary motor area appears to represent a paralimbic expansion of limbic cortex (Sanides, 1970). This suggests a link between the limbic system and volitional control of speech.

It is impossible to noticeably alter vocal behavior in nonhuman primates by either bilateral excision or electrical stimulation of facial motor areas. It is only when limbic structures are manipulated that vocal behavior changes (Myers, 1976; Robinson, 1976). Transcortical motor aphasia, therefore, may represent a limbic aphasia in the broadest sense.

Transcortical Sensory Aphasia (TSA)

INTRODUCTION

Transcortical sensory aphasia (TSA) is defined as a syndrome of fluent aphasia with poor comprehension and preserved repetition. In establishing the concept, Lichtheim (1885) stressed the hypothetical rather than the strict anatomical nature of his model of damage to structures outside the language areas, severing them from concepts and memories in the brain. The entity was not accepted at once. Many authors at the turn of the century doubted its existence or ignored it. Henschen's (1920–1922) use of the adjective "so-called" in discussing transcortical sensory aphasia reflects the ambivalence. He distinguished two main groups, one with generalized cerebral atrophy, the other, with lesions of the temporal lobe. Although Henschen emphasized the lesion of the temporal gyri and the underlying white matter, some patients had occipital lobe involvement as well, which was considered incidental. Henschen cited a case of Bernheim with "psychic blindness" in addition to TSA. Many of Henschen's focal cases had inadequate clinical description or poor anatomical documentation. He came to the conclusion that although the term "transcortical aphasia" implies that the source of the disturbance is beyond the cortical areas associated with speech mechanism, the lesions always involve the speech areas. One of the better-documented cases was published by Vix (1910). They examined a posttraumatic patient who also had surgery and found partial word deafness, verbal paraphasias, and automatic repetition. The lesion destroyed the posterior ends of T_1, T_2, T_3. The occipitotemporal area was involved anteriorly (Figure 3).

Dejerine (1914) observed generalized atrophy in cases of TSA and concluded that the syndrome did not have a specific anatomical site. He thought that in cases of atrophy, it is a stage toward complete word deafness and in cases of stroke, a stage in the recovery from Wernicke's aphasia or word deafness. Subsequently, Goldstein (1917, 1948) reviewed the issue and republished some of Liepmann's cases and some of his own. He noted that nearly identical lesions of the posterior superior temporal lobe producing Wernicke's aphasia may result in transcortical sensory aphasia in some patients.

Unlike TMA, the modern literature does not furnish much convincing information about lesion location in TSA. Therefore, we summarize our own experience with computerized tomography (CT) scan localization in this syndrome. We have already published three cases in an isotope localization study (Kertesz *et al.*, 1977). These are included in this subsequent series, with CT scan localization.

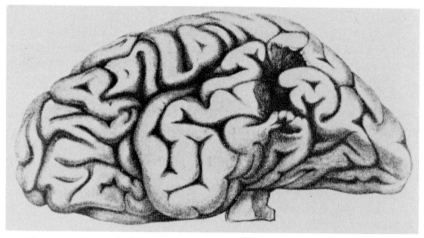

Figure 3. This is the lateral surface of the brain of a case with transcortical sensory aphasia published by Vix. The darkly shaded area of infarction involves the posterior temporal regions and the junction of the occipital and temporal lobes. The brain is viewed from the side and somewhat from below.

THE METHODS OF OUR STUDY

We examined our aphasic population with the Western Aphasia Battery (Kertesz, 1982) and diagnosed 31 patients with TSA, based on a repetition score better than 8 and a comprehension score worse than 7, according to our objective taxonomic criteria. The patients had to be in a fluent category. Their spontaneous speech is often semantic jargon, but this is not an obligatory feature. All the diagnoses were made in the acute state and 22 of these had localizing information, either on computerized tomography or isotope scans or both. Five tumor cases were excluded because of distance effects or gradual growth which lessened the deficit. Two patients with infarcts were excluded because of multiple lesions. The anatomical conclusions are based on the remaining 15 stroke patients (Kertesz, Sheppard, & MacKenzie, 1982).

CT scan lesions were traced on oblique templates by a radiologist who did not know the clinical diagnoses or language scores of the patients; the isotope brain scans (IS) on lateral and posterior templates were made by an isotope specialist in a similarly objective fashion (Figure 4). The methods of overlapping and determining the size of the lesions have been discussed in detail elsewhere (Kertesz,

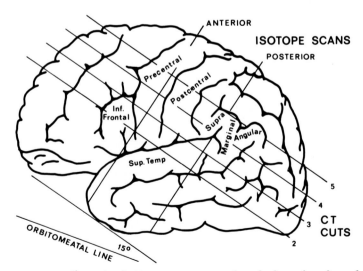

Figure 4. The angle of CT cuts are presented on the lateral surface of the brain template from Sobotta's atlas. Reprinted with permission from *Archives of Neurology* by Kertesz, Sheppard, and MacKenzie (1982).

1979). The levels of the CT templates include the important areas for language and represent the bulk of the lesions (Figure 4). They were drawn after the CT atlas of Gonzales, Grossman, and Palacios (1976).

CLINICAL FEATURES

The characteristic clinical features are summarized in Table 1. Most of the patients had hemianopia, and at least five were noted to have visual object agnosia. A few had well-documented contra-lateral sensory loss and bilateral tactile agnosia (astereognosis). Their speech was fluent and circumlocutory; at times, much of it appeared to be semantic jargon. This distinctive speech disturbance consists of well-articulated and recognizable strings of words, al-though semantically not relevant to the questions asked or to the previous sentence. The sentences were syntactically complete, but word-finding difficulties were often evident. The poor comprehension and preserved repetition were the basis of classification for inclusion into the series as transcortical aphasics.

THE OVERLAP OF THE LESIONS

The lesions were superimposed. The overlap area covers the left parietooccipital region and the occipitotemporal fasciculus but spares the striate cortex. The CT overlap (Figure 5) indicates that the lesions are mainly in the temporo-occipital junction and the oc-cipital lobe. The lateral isotope overlap (Figure 6) illustrates the two areas that are characteristically involved in TSA. Most of the lesions are in the inferior parietotemporo-occipital area in the territory of the posterior cerebral artery or in the posterior cerebral–middle cerebral watershed area. The coronal posterior–anterior view shows the lesions to be medial and inferior, clearly indicating posterior cerebral artery infarcts (Figure 7).

Representative CT (Figure 8) and isotope lesions (Figure 9) are shown from Cases 7 and 12 to illustrate the typical posterior–inferior loca-tion of the lesions, indicating posterior cerebral territory infarcts.

A smaller number of lesions (three) with TSA overlap higher in the parieto-occipital convexity. These lesions are lower and more posterior than those producing the Gerstmann syndrome and alexia

TABLE 1

Clinical Features of Patients with Transcortical Sensory Aphasia

No.	Age	Sex	Visual Loss	Sensory Loss	Paralysis	Speech Output[a]	Recovery of Speech	Location of Lesion[b]	Localization[c]	Comment
1	59	M	Right	Present	Slight	S. Jargon	Died with another stroke	L.T.O.	IS, A	Autopsy confirmation.
2	56	F	Right	Present	—	S. Jargon	Anomic	L.T.O.	IS	Visual agnosia AVM.
3	70	M	Right	Present	—	Empty	Another stroke	L.T.O.	IS	Visual agnosia
4	58	M	Left inferior Quadrant	Slight	—	Empty	Recovered except agraphia	R.P.O.	IS, CT	Left handed, right lesion.
5	74	F	Right	Present	Slight	Paraphasic empty	Unknown	L.P.O.	IS	
6	58	M	Right	Transient	Slight	S. Jargon	Same 6 mo. Died 9 mos.	L.T.O.	IS	Visual agnosia. Balint's syndrome
7	80	F	Right	Mild	—	Empty	Anomic	L.T.O.	IS, CT	Visual agnosia.
8	51	M	Transient	Present	Moderate	S. Jargon	Anomic	L.T.P.	IS, CT	
9	67	M	—	—	—	Empty	Anomic	L.T.P	CT	Initial word deafness.
10	64	M	Right	Present	—	Empty	Anomic	L.T.O.	IS, CT	Some atrophy
11	78	F	—	—	—	Anomic	Unknown	L.T.O.	IS, CT	Frontal lesion superimposed.
12	79	M	Right	—	—	Empty	Unknown	L.P.O.	IS, CT	
13	75	F	Right	Present	—	S. Jargon	Recovered	L.T.O.	CT	Visual agnosia.
14	76	M	Right	Present	Transient	Paraphasic	Improved	L.T.O.	IS, CT	
15	58	M	—	—	—	S. Jargon	Unknown	L.T.P.	IS	

[a] S. Jargon = Semantic Jargon
[b] T. = Temporal   O. = Occipital   P. = Parietal   L. = Left   R. = Right
[c] IS = Isotope Scan   CT = Computerized Tomography   A = Autopsy

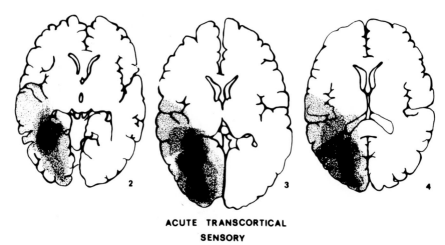

ACUTE TRANSCORTICAL
SENSORY

Figure 5. The overlap of the lesions on CT and isotope scans. The CT cuts, numbered, are referred to in the subsequent figures. Reprinted with permission from *Archives of Neurology*, by Kertesz, Sheppard, and MacKenzie (1982).

and agraphia. A few tumor cases that were not included in the overlap showed similar locations (Figure 10). The temporal lobe is involved in a smaller number of cases.

The lesion size was measured by tracing the lesion outlines with a digitizer program (Kertesz, Harlock, & Coates, 1979). The corre-

LATERAL ISOTOPE OVERLAP

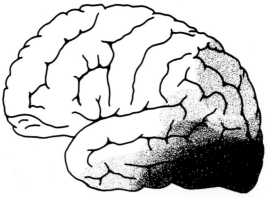

Figure 6. The lateral isotope overlap from the cases on Table 1. Reprinted by permission from *Archives of Neurology*, by Kertesz, Sheppard, and MacKenzie (1982).

POSTERIOR ISOTOPE OVERLAP

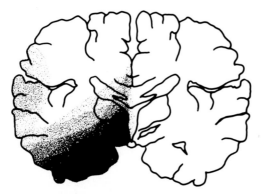

Figure 7. The isotope overlap in the posterior coronal view. Reprinted with permission from *Archives of Neurology*, by Kertesz, Sheppard, and McKenzie (1982).

lations were relatively low between initial severity and lesion size as well as the extent of recovery and lesion size. It appears that the location of the lesion is more important than the size in the development of the syndrome. The test scores at 1 year after stroke as a measure of outcome correlated negatively with lesion size but not enough long-term follow-up cases were available for statistical proof.

DISCUSSION

When transcortical sensory aphasia is seen with focal lesions, their location in the temporo-occipital areas is very consistent. This clear-cut localization escaped attention in the past, as many of the florid cases of fluent echolalic aphasia were seen with Alzheimer's disease (without obvious localizable lesion except diffuse atrophy or trauma where the language disturbance was dismissed as confusion). The post-traumatic instances of TSA are usually very transient and have not been investigated in detail. Alzheimer patients, on the other hand, show a declining course, and when semantic jargon appears with echolalia and poor comprehension, it is not usually considered an aphasia but labeled as the "language of confusion" (Darley, 1964). Even in stroke cases, infarcts of the posterior

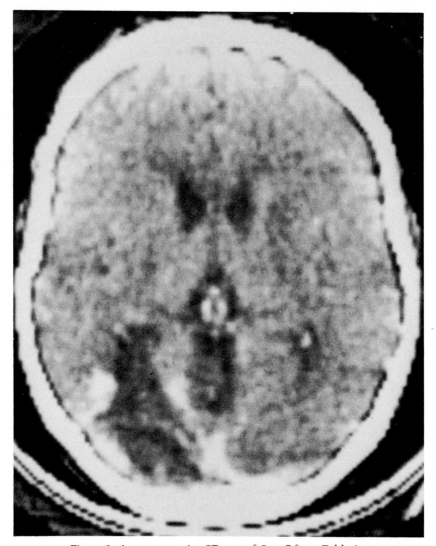

Figure 8. A representative CT scan of Case 7 from Table 1.

cerebral artery often have brain stem signs, diplopia, vertigo, hemianopia, alexia, amnesia, and other disturbances that attract the attention of the examiners obscuring the underlying language disturbance.

The identification of the syndrome depends on the definition of

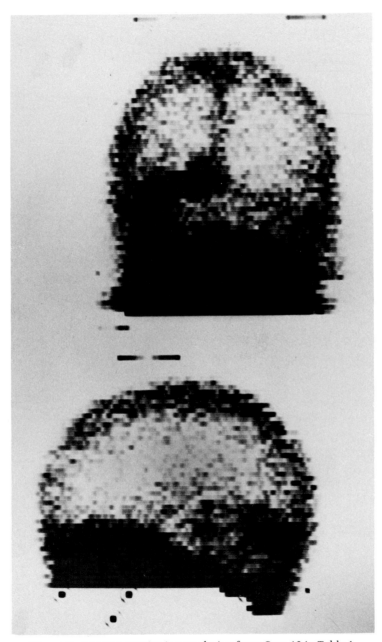

Figure 9. A representative isotope lesion from Case 12 in Table 1.

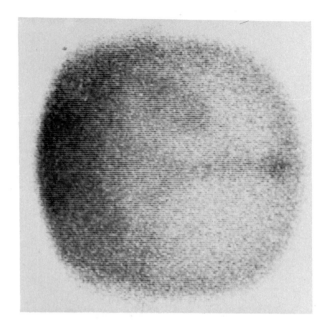

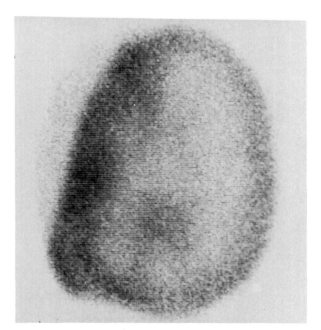

Figure 10. A brain tumor causing transcortical sensory aphasia shows a similar location. The tumor cases were not included in the overlap.

the components and the tests used to measure them. Our standardized test includes repetition as well as other modalities of the usual
aphasia batteries. The difficult levels of these subtests are similar;
therefore, the emphasis placed on preserved repetition to distinguish TSA from Wernicke's aphasia is taxonomically valid. Objective taxonomic criteria based on test scores are much more
preferable than just a clinical judgment that repetition was good
and comprehension poor in a fluent aphasic. The subjective nature
of such a definition leaves the possibility of bias in choosing cases
for localization. Any taxonomic criteria is arbitrary to some extent,
but those based on measurements and scores in a systematic fashion are consistent within an examined population.

Tumor cases were not added to the overlap because of the frequently considerable distance effect and the so-called serial lesion
effect. Just as the smaller serial lesions in animals are shown to be
different from a large lesion occurring at once (Ades & Raab, 1946),
the effect of a slowly growing tumor in behavior may be expected
to be different from a sudden stroke.

Five of our TSA cases were found to be associated with visual
agnosia alone in addition to the more usual bilateral lesions (Chapter 16). The involvement of the splenium of the corpus callosum or
the tapetum (the occipital portion of the subcortical outflow) is considered essential in these cases. It is not surprising that the involvement of the temporoparieto-occipital junction in TSA may be
associated with visual agnosia if the dominant occipital lobe is in
farcted as well. The occipital infarct alone probably would only produce a hemianopia; the subcortical involvement of the callosal fibers
may add alexia or visual agnosia to the clinical picture. Conversely,
the more anterior portion of the lesion without the occipital involvement would result in the syndrome of TSA. In most of our cases
of TSA and visual agnosia, tactile agnosia was also present. Word-
finding difficulty in spontaneous speech, responsive speech, and
sentence completion were much better indicating that amnesia or
word-finding disturbance cannot account alone for the visual and
tactile recognition problem. Even after auditory cues such as the
name of the objects were mentioned, the patients remained dubious
and continued with misnaming or confabulatory behavior.

This unusual language disorder is often characterized by semantic jargon—copious, fluent, irrelevant speech—but distinct from
neologistic jargon in that the substitutions of substantive words—
nouns and verbs especially—are otherwise acceptable lexical items.
And there are no neologisms or any significant number of phonemic

paraphasias. There is a plausible disconnection between the auditory input and the semantic processors that was postulated by Lichtheim (1885). These patients have severely impaired comprehension; yet, phonological and syntactic processing is not affected and repetition is very good. These behavioral features correlated with the relatively well-preserved temporoparietal, periSylvian connections necessary for syntactic and phonological function and repetition, and involvement of the posterior association areas important for comprehension.

Recovery from TSA is usually quite good. These patients improve their comprehension and are considered anomic aphasias subsequently, often by the third month post-stroke. Eventual full recovertly is common. At times, a more permanent syndrome of TSA evolves from acute Wernicke's aphasia. These patients often have more extensive lesions, involving the temporal lobe as a rule, similar to Henschen's cases. The parietal location of the chronic persisting syndrome of TSA was published in our survey of CT localization of aphasia (Kertesz et al., 1979). This difference between the lesion sites of the chronic and acute cases of TSA is a fundamental one that is overlooked in many reviews of localization.

Mixed Transcortical Aphasia

Mixed transcortical aphasia is characterized by near or complete absence of meaningful spontaneous speech and severely impaired comprehension of spoken and written language. Sparse, meaningless, repetitive, stereotypic utterances occur. In the complete picture, there is total absence of propositional speech and little, if any, comprehension. Output consists mainly of echolalic responses to questions and commands and short, stereotyped meaningless utterances. Echolalia is considered by many authors to represent automatic involuntary parrot-like verbal output, always signaling the presence of faulty comprehension (Brain, 1965; Denny–Brown, 1963; Goldstein, 1948). However, some TMA patients with good comprehension are echolalic (Luria, 1970; Rubens, 1976). Researchers have shown, by making use of the echolalic response, that transcortical patients can produce grammatically correct sentences when given incorrect models (Whitaker, 1976). Patients with TMA are more able to recognize and correct semantic errors whereas patients with TSA and mixed transcortical aphasia cannot (Davis, Foldi, Gardner, &

Zurif, 1978). This suggests that the peri-Sylvian language zone, though isolated and unable to perform semantic operations, has the capacity to recognize syntactically incorrect sentences and to change them into their correct form. There are several well-documented reports of this syndrome (Geschwind *et al.*, 1968; Heilman, Tucker, & Valenstein, 1976; Ross, 1980; Whitaker, 1976). The syndrome is associated with multiple focal and/or diffuse pathology affecting widespread areas of anterior and posterior association cortex with relative sparing of the peri-Sylvian language area. Etiology, therefore, includes the dementias (particularly Pick's disease). Dementia is often seen with widespread vascular border zone lesions, carbon monoxide poisoning, and extensive medial frontal–parietal infarction in the territory of the left anterior cerebral artery (Környey, 1975; Ross, 1980). It is rarely seen with a left mainstem middle cerebral artery infarct destroying the periSylvian language zone (Stengel, 1936, 1947).

References

Ades, H. W., & Raab, D. H. (1946). Recovery of motor function after two-stage extirpation of area 4 in monkeys. *Journal of Neurophysiology, 9*, 55–60.

Alajouanine, T., Castaigne, P., Sabourand, O., & Contamin, F. (1959). Palilalie paroxystique et vocalizations itératives au cours de crises épileptiques, etc. *Revue Neurologique, 101*, 685–697.

Alexander, M. P., & Schmitt, M. A. (1980). The aphasia syndrome of stroke in the left anterior cerebral artery territory. *Archives of Neurology. (Chicago), 37*, 97–100.

Arseni, C., & Botez, M. I. (1961). Speech disturbances caused by tumors of the supplementary motor area. *Acta Psychiatrica Scandinavica, 36*, 279–299.

Bastian, H. (1897). Some problems in connexion with aphasia and other speech defects. *Lancet, 1*, 933–942, 1005–1017, 1131–1137, 1187–1194.

Benton, A. L. (1968). Differential behavioral effects in frontal lobe disease. *Neuropsychologia, 6*, 53–60.

Bogen, J. E. (1976). Linguistic performance in the short-term following cerebral commissurotomy. In H. Whitaker & H. A. Whitaker (Eds.), *Studies in neurolinguistics* (Vol. 2). New York: Academic Press.

Botez, M. I., & Barbeau, A. (1971). Role of subcortical structures and particularly the thalamus in the mechanisms of speech and language. *International Journal of Neurology, 8*, 300–320.

Brain, W. R. (1965). *Speech disorders* (2nd ed.). London: Butterworth.

Brickner, R. (1940). A human cortical area producing repetitive phenomena when stimulated. *Journal of Neurophysiology, 3*, 128–130.

Carrieri, G. (1963). Syndrome of disturbance of the left motor supplementary area associated with a parasagittal meningioma. *Rivista di Patologia Nervosa e Mentale, 84*, 29–48.

Chavany, J. A., & Rongerie, J. (1958). L'aphémie post-opératoire transitoire après lobectomie frontale gauche. *Presse Medicale, 66,* 1191–1192.
Chusid, J., de Gutierrez-Mahoney, C., & Margules-Lavergne, M. (1954). Speech disturbances in association with parasagittal frontal lesions. *Journal of Neurosur-
gery, 11,* 193–204.
Conrad, K. (1954). New problems of aphasia. *Brain, 77,* 491–509.
Critchley, M. (1930). Anterior cerebral artery and its syndromes. *Brain, 53,* 120–165.
Damasio, A. R., & Kassel, N. F. (1978). Transcortical motor aphasia in relation to
lesions of the supplementary motor area. *Neurology, 28,* 396.
Darley, F. L. (1964). Diagnosis and Appraisal of Communication Disorders. Engle-
wood Cliffs, N.J.: Prentice Hall.
Davis, L., Foldi, N. S., Gardner, H., Zurif, E. (1978). Repetition in the transcortical
aphasias. *Brain and Language, 6,* 226–238.
Dejerine, J. (1914). *Semiologie des affections du système nerveux.* Paris: Masson.
Denny-Brown, D. (1963). The physiological basis of perception and speech. In L. Hal-
pern (Ed.), *Problems of dynamic neurology.* Jerusalem: Hebrew University Press,
pp. 30–62.
Dimitri, V., & Victoria, M. (1936). Sindrome de la arteria cerebral anterior. *Revista
Neurologica de Buenos Aires, 1,* 81–97.
Erickson, T. C., & Woolsey, C. N. (1951). Observations on the supplementary motor
area of man. *Transactions of the American Neurological Association,* 50–56.
Geschwind, N., Quadfasel, F., & Segarra, J. (1968). Isolation of the speech area. *Neu-
ropsychologia, 6,* 327–340.
Gloning, I., Gloning, K., & Hoff, H. (1963). Aphasia: A clinical syndrome. In L. Halpern
(Ed.), *Problems of dynamic neurology* Jerusalem: Hebrew University Press.
Goldstein, K. (1915). *Die transkortikalen Aphasien.* Jena: Fischer.
Goldstein, K. (1917). *Die transkortikalen Aphasien.* Jena: Fisher.
Goldstein, K. (1948). *Language and language disturbances.* New York: Grune & Strat-
ton.
Gonzalez, C. F., Grossman, C. B., & Palacios, E. (1976). *Computed brain and orbital
tomography—technique and interpretation.* New York: Wiley.
Guidetti, B. (1957). Disturbi della parola associati a lesioni della parte posteriore
dell'area supplementare motoria. *Rivista di Neurologia, 27,* 195–201.
Heilman, K. M., Tucker, D. M., & Valenstein, E. (1976). A case of mixed transcortical
aphasia with intact naming. *Brain, 99,* 415–426.
Henschen, S. E. (1920–1922). *Klinische und anatomische Beitrage zur Pathologie des
Gehirns* (Vols. 5–7). Stockholm: Nordiska Bokhandel'n.
Hyland, H. H. (1933). Thrombosis of intracranial arteries: Report of three cases in-
volving respectively, the anterior cerebral, basilar, and internal carotid arteries.
Archives of Neurology and Psychiatry, 30, 342–356.
Ingvar, D. H., Philipson, L., Torlof, P., & Ardo A. (1975). The average rCBF pattern of
resting consciousness studied with a new colour display system. *Acta Neurol-
ogica Scandinavica, 56, Supplementum* 64, 252–253.
Jonas, S. (1981). The supplementary motor region and speech emission. *Journal of
Communication Disorders, 14,* 349–373.
Kertesz, A. (1979). *Aphasia and associated disorders. Taxonomy, localization and re-
covery.* New York: Grune & Stratton.
Kertesz, A. (1982). *The western aphasia battery.* New York: Grune & Stratton.
Kertesz, A., Harlock, W., & Coates, R. (1979). Computer tomographic localization,
lesion size, and prognosis in aphasia and nonverbal impairment. *Brain and Lan-
guage, 8,* 34–50.

Kertesz, A., Lesk, D., McCabe, P. (1977). Isotope localization of infarcts in aphasia. *Archives of Neurology (Chicago), 34,* 590–601.

Kertesz, A., Sheppard, A., MacKenzie, R. (1982). Localization in transcortical sensory aphasia. *Archives of Neurology (Chicago), 39,* 475–478.

Kleist, K. (1934). *Gehirnpathologie.* Leipzig: Barth.

Környey, E. (1956). Stirnloppen, Balken, und Sprachstörung. *Deutsche Zeitschrift fuer Nervenheilkunde, 175,* 87.

Környey, E. (1975). Aphasie transcorticale et echolalie: Le problème de l'initiative de la parole. *Revue Neurologique, 131,* 347–363.

Larsen, B., Skinhoj, E., & Lassen, N. A. (1978). Variations in regional cortical blood flow in the right and left hemispheres during automatic speech. *Brain, 101,* 193–210.

Lassen, N. A., Roland, P. E., Larsen, B., Melamed, E., & Soh, K. (1977). Mapping of human cerebral functions: A study of the regional cerebral blood flow pattern during rest, its reproducibility and the activation seen during basic sensory and motor functions. *Acta Neurologica Scandinavica, 56, Supplementum 64,* 262–263.

Lichtheim, L. (1885). On aphasia. *Brain, 7,* 433–484.

Liepmann, H., & Maas, O. (1907). Fall von linksseitiger Agraphie und Apraxie bei rechtsseitiger Lahmung. *Journal fuer Psychologie und Neurologie, 10,* 214–227.

Luria, A. (1966). *Human brain and psychological processes.* New York: Macmillan.

Luria, A. (1970). *Traumatic aphasia.* The Hague: Mouton.

Luria, A., & Hutton, J. T. (1977). The modern assessment of the basic forms of aphasia. *Brain and Language, 4,* 129–151.

Luria, A., & Tsvetkova, L. S. (1968). *The mechanisms of "Dynamic aphaia"* Foundations of Language, 4, 296–307.

Magnan, D. R. (1880). On simple aphasia, and aphasia with incoherence. *Brain, 2,* 112–123.

Marie, P., & Foix, C. (1917). Les aphasies de guerre. *Revue Neurologique, 24,* 53–87.

Maroun, F. B., Jacob, J. C., & Gowing, P. (1970). Dysphonia associated with cortical neoplasms. *Journal of Neurosurgery, 32,* 671–676.

Masdeu, J. C., Schoene, W. C., & Funkenstein, H. (1978). Aphasia following infarction of the left supplementary motor area: A clinicopathologic study. *Neurology, 28,* 1220–1223.

Milner, B. (1964). Some effects of frontal lobectomy in man. In J. M. Warren, K. Akert (Eds.), *The frontal granular cortex and behavior.* New York: McGraw-Hill.

Mohr, J. P., Pessin, M. S., Finkelstein, S., Funkenstein, H., Duncan, G., and Davis, K. (1978). Broca's aphasia: Pathological and clinical aspects. *Neurology, 28,* 311–324.

Myers, R. E. (1976). Comparative neurology of vocalization and speech: Proof of a dichotomy. In S. R. Harnad, H. Steklis, & J. Lancaster (Eds.), *Origins and evolution of language and speech.* New York: New York Academy of Sciences.

Naeser, M. A., & Hayward, R. W. (1978). Lesion localization in aphasia with cranial computed tomography and the Boston Diagnostic Aphasia Exam. *Neurology, 28,* 545–551.

Niessl von Mayendorf, E. (1911). *Die aphasischen Symptome und ihre kortikale Lokalization.* Leipzig: Barth.

Penfield, W., & Roberts, I. (1959). *Speech and brain mechanisms.* Princeton, N.J.: Princeton University Press.

Penfield, W., & Welch, K. (1951). The supplementary motor area of the cerebral cortex: A clinical and experimental study. *AMA Archives of Neurology and Psychiatry, 66,* 289–317.

Petit-Dutaillis, D., Guiot, G., Messing, R., Bourdillon, C. (1954). A propos d'une aphémie par atteintée de la zone matrice supplémentaire de Penfield. *Revue Neurologique, 90,* 95–106.

Poppen, V. L. (1939). Ligation of the left anterior cerebral artery. *Archives of Neurology and Psychiatry, 41,* 495–503.

Racy, A., Jannotta, F., & Lehner, L. (1979). Aphasia resulting from occlusion of the left anterior cerebral artery: Report of a case with an old infarct in the left Rolandic region. *Archives of Neurology (Chicago), 36,* 221–224.

Ramier, A. M., & Hécaen, H. (1970). Role respectif des atteintes frontales et de la latéralisation lesionnelle dans les deficits de la "fluence verbale." *Revue Neurologique, 123,* 17–22.

Robinson, B. W. (1976). Limbic influences on human speech. In S. R. Harnad, H. Senlis, & J. Lancaster (Eds.), *Origins and evolution of language and speech.* New York: New York Academy of Sciences.

Ross, E. D. (1980). Left medial parietal lobe and receptive language functions: Mixed transcortical aphasia after left anterior cerebral artery infarction. *Neurology, 30,* 144–151.

Rubens, A. B. (1975). Aphasia with infarction in the territory of the anterior cerebral artery. *Cortex, 11,* 239–250.

Rubens, A. B. (1976). Transcortical motor aphasia. In H. Whitaker & H. A. Whitaker (Eds.), *Studies in neurolinguistics* (Vol. 1). New York: Academic Press, pp. 293–306.

Russell, W. R., & Espir, M. L. (1961). *Traumatic aphasia: A study of aphasia in war wounds of the brain.* London & New York: Oxford University Press.

Sanides, F. (1970). Functional architecture of motor and sensory cortices in primates in the light of a new concept of neocortex evolution. In C. R. Noback & W. Montagna (Eds.), *The primate brain* New York: Appleton, pp. 137–208.

Schwab, O. (1927). Uber Stutzreaktionen (Magnus) beim Menschen. (Zugleich ein Beitrag zur Auffassung der sogenannten Gelenksreflexe.) *Zeitschrift fuer die Gesamte Neurologie und Psychiatrie, 108,* 585–593.

Stengel, E. (1936). Zur Lehre von den transkorticalen Aphasien. *Zeitschrift fuer die Gesamte Neurologie und Psychiatrie, 154,* 778–782.

Stengel, E. (1947). A clinical and psychological study of echo-reactions. *Journal of Mental Science, 93,* 598–612.

Sweet, W. (1951). Discussion of Erickson and Woolsey. *Transactions of the American Neurological Association, 76,* 55.

Thurstone, I. L., Thurstone, T. (1949). *Examiner manual Aphasie. for the SRA primary mental abilities* (Rev. ed.). Chicago: Illinois Scientific Research Association.

Vix, E. (1910). Anatomischer Befund. bei transkortikaler sensorisher Aphasie. *Archiv fuer Psychiatrie und Nervenkrankheiten, 47,* 200–213.

von Stockert, T. R. (1974). Ein neues Konzept zum Verstandnis der cerebralen Sprachztorungen. *Nervenarzt, 45,* 94–97.

Wernicke, C. (1874). *Der aphasische Symptomenkomplex.* Breslau: Cohn & Weigart.

Wernicke, C. (1886). Einige Neuere Arbeiten uber Aphasie. *Fortschritte der Medizin, 4,* 377–463.

Wernicke, C. (1908). The symptom-complex of aphasia. In A. Church (Ed.), *Modern clinical medical disease of the nervous system.* New York: Appleton.

Whitaker, H. (1976). A case of the isolation of the language function. In H. Whitaker & H. A. Whitaker (Eds.), *Studies in neurolinguistics* (Vol. 1). New York: Academic Press.

11

Thalamic Lesions and Syndromes

J. P. Mohr

Introduction

For many years, no specific role in speech and language was attributed to the thalamus (Brain, 1965; Nielsen, 1962). In some classifications for aphasia, the alleged lack of a thalamic role even played a part in the formulation of the theories of aphasia (Geschwind, 1965).

Special emphasis in the present review is placed on the details of the published clinical material to point up the role of the thalamus in language disorders. The clinical syndrome formulated from this material may add to many current opinions that a thalamic lesion causes a disturbance fitting the traditional definition of aphasia. However, the syndrome does not fit neatly into current classification of aphasia.

The case material of thalamic lesions includes tumors, infarcts, stereotaxic operations, and hemorrhage. Despite these several etiologies, the number of published cases is small.

LOCALIZATION
IN NEUROPSYCHOLOGY

269

Thalamic Tumors

Few cases of thalamic tumors have been reported; even fewer with aphasia have been described in detail. Even in the rare examples with aphasia, it takes little effort to see how such cases could have been set aside as a poor source of syndrome analysis, since the distortion of adjacent structures produced by tumor easily might be the explanation for any language disturbances that occur.

Smythe and Stern (1938) are credited with the first mention of aphasia. They noted it in three of their six cases as thalamic tumor, all of which involved the left thalamus. It is not clear from the case descriptions whether the aphasia occurred early or late in the course, nor how the severity of the aphasia related to disturbances in sensation, motor function, or consciousness. McKissock and Paine (1958), in noting aphasia with thalamic tumors, postulated that the disturbances in behavior and language were due to increased intracranial pressure. Cheek and Taveras (1966), who also described aphasia with thalamic tumors, postulated that the language disturbance was "more specific" for the thalamic lesion.

Unfortunately, none of the cases of thalamic tumors found in the literature contributes much to the characterization of a clinical syndrome.

Thalamic Infarction

This material holds the greatest hope of providing a series of cases with a discrete lesion occurring in a previously healthy brain. However, in the types of infarcts encountered, no such syndrome has yet emerged.

BILATERAL INFARCTS

Mills and Swanson (1978) described the only known case where bilateral infarction was confined to the medial thalamus. Aphasia was not described; however, detailed analysis of language was hindered by the presence of apathy and a hypersomnolent state. Similar infarction occurs from occlusion of the top of the basilar artery (Caplan, 1980) but no specific aphasic disturbances have been reported.

LACUNAR INFARCTS

Two syndromes of focal thalamic infarction have been described. These are pure sensory stroke (Fisher, 1965, 1978), and sensorimotor stroke (Mohr, Kase, Meckler, & Fisher, 1977). In each instance, the lacunes were due to occlusion of one or more branches of the thalamoperforant arteries (tiny vessels penetrating the midbrain to supply the thalamus). The reported cases with autopsy studies have shown the infarcts in the ventral posterior nucleus. Both syndromes feature contralateral disturbance in sensation, one also having contralateral hemiparesis. However, neither syndrome has been reported with dysphasia.

POSTERIOR CEREBRAL ARTERY TERRITORY INFARCTS

There is no dearth of cases of unilateral infarction involving the posterior cerebral artery territory, but all, without exception, have been due to infarction involving the cortical territory of the posterior cerebral artery supply. The thalamic component of the infarct is an unusual event, encountered only with the larger lesions. Infarction confined to the thalamus has not yet been isolated in a case of posterior cerebral artery occlusion. But even in the few cases with thalamic involvement, the syndrome seems no different from those in which the thalamus is spared.

In bilateral posterior cerebral artery territory infarction, a state described as "agitated delirium" (Caplan, 1980; Horenstein, Chamberlain, & Conomy, 1962; Medina, Chokroverty, & Rubino, 1976; Medina, Rubino, & Ross, 1974)—lasting days to weeks—has been encountered. Infarction has been extensive enough to involve fusiform, lingual, and hippocampal gyri. Involvement of the thalamus could occur in such cases, but has not been described.

Thalamotomy

During its heyday, stereotaxic surgery of the thalamus was the treatment of choice for parkinsonism. After medical therapy largely replaced thalamotomy, the operation failed to find much application for other purposes. Since most of the interest in aphasia and the thalamus developed after thalamotomy had already faded, there now seems little likelihood that much further data will be developed concerning this potentially important subject; therefore, the observations scattered through the available literature assume special significance.

The surgical lesions were usually produced by means of radio-frequency or cryothermal injury. The size was usually 35–100mm^3 (Sem-Jacobsen, 1965), roughly equivalent to that of a lacunar infarct. For an individual case—usually—one lesion was produced. Bilateral lesions were rarely employed. The preferred location of the lesion for control of parkinsonism was the ventral lateral (VL) nucleus of the thalamus because of the importance of this nucleus as an extrapyramidal motor pathway. Except for special investigations involving transient stimulations, such as the careful studies by Ojemann and colleagues, effects outside VL were unwelcome errors in stereotaxic placement or the results of too large a lesion. Because the CT scan had not been invented during the period when thalamotomy was in fashion, only the rare autopsy exists to document the actual lesion size in these cases. There are virtually no data on the incidence of operative-induced hemorrhage that could have enlarged the surgical lesion.

THALAMOTOMY AND TRANSIENT DYSPHASIA

In early reports, the subject of dysphasia following thalamotomy was not mentioned (Spiegel, Wycis, Szekely, Adams, Flanagan, & Baird, 1963) or was described only as arrest of speech (Guiot, Hertzog, Rondot, & Molina, 1961). In other reports, the occurrence of a dysphasia or disturbed mental state was noted, although few details were given (Allen, Turner, & Gadea-Ciria, 1966; Bravo, Parera, & Seiquer, 1966; Gillingham, Watson, Donaldson, & Naughton, 1960; Hermann, Turner, Gillingham, & Gaze, 1966; Laitinen, 1966; Lin & Cooper, 1960; Riechert, 1964; Watkins & Oppenheimer, 1962). However, the early incidence data suggest dysphasia was a common occurrence: Fully 13 of 18 dysphasics were described in the series studied by Mundinger and Riechert (1964).

Despite the few authors who denied a correlation between lesion side and dysphasia (Krayenbühl, Wyss, & Yasargil, 1961; Waltz, Riklan, Stellar, & Cooper, 1966), most found dysphasia was produced by a lesion involving the left side (Allen *et al.*, 1966; Bell, 1968; Krayenbuhl, Siegfried, Kohenof, & Yasargil, 1965; Riechert, 1964; Selby, 1969; Shapiro, Sadowsky, Henderson, & Van Buren, 1973).

Laitinen (1966) noted a "real dysphasia in connection with right hemiparesis" in one case among 224 thalamotomies, but no mention was made as to the side or exact site of the lesion. Bravo *et al.* (1966) described 650 cases: 15 had a "mental or behavioral deficit," 11 transient, 4 permanent, but the deficit was described only as "disorientation, lethargy and apathy," and no details were given concerning laterality or exact lesion location. Riechert (1964) noted a 2% incidence in "speech disturbances of the motor aphasia type, or of subcortical aphasia type . . ."

Gillingham *et al.* (1960) described their experience with 60 cases, 19 of which underwent left thalamotomy (see Figure 1); the others had a lesion placed in the pallidum or in the right side. In two cases (Case 7, Case 10), moderately severe dysphasia developed from the surgery, lasting 4 and 6 weeks, respectively. In both cases, the lesion placed was in the pallidum, and the authors were convinced the capsule was also affected. In two other cases (Case 34, Case 51), left thalamotomy was followed by disordered behavior described in one as "florid psychotic reaction" that persisted 3 weeks. In another, "a severe confusional state" that persisted 4 weeks, "settling down to a somewhat fluctuating degree of confusion." A later publication from the same service (Hermann *et al.*, 1966) reported a more detailed study of the problems, noting dysphasia, dysarthria, and changes in voice volume as complications from thalamotomy (see

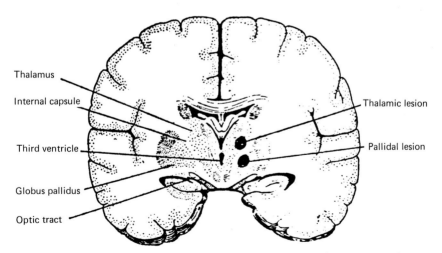

Figure 1. Coronal view of the brain showing the location of the stereotaxic lesions placed in the thalamuc and globus pallidus by Gillingham, Watson, Donaldson, and Naughton (1960).

Figure 2). In this later study, an additional 118 cases were reported. Left-sided operations were performed on 37 cases, among whom six developed dysphasia. No details of the dysphasia were reported, but the authors noted that these cases suffered a somewhat larger lesion (296mm³, *SD* 52mm³) than did those without dysphasia (218mm³, *SD* 75mm³). When the scattergrams of lesion location were compared in the two groups, no difference was evident between the dysphasic and normal cases.

DESCRIPTIONS OF DYSPHASIA

In later studies, some detailed descriptions of dysphasia appeared. A diminished "verbal memory" was noted in cases tested 4–6 days postoperatively by Krayenbühl *et al.* (1965) but only for left, not right-sided, operations. A transient dysphasia that subsided after 10–14 days was noted in 42% of left thalamotomies by Selby (1969). Jurko and Andy (1964) noted no problems in the vocabulary subtests but found a slight reduction in verbal IQ among 25 thalamotomies tested pre- and postoperatively. Shapiro *et al.* (1973) found a diminished verbal IQ in left thalamotomy cases tested at 2 weeks. In this group, the disturbance improved but was still present on retests at 17 months.

The most detailed clinical description of the deficits, up to that

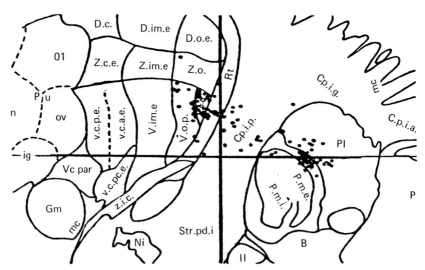

Figure 2. Scattergram of stereotaxic lesions in the thalamus produced by Hermann, Turner, Gillingham, and Gaze (1966).

time, was presented by Bell (1968). None of his 22 cases of right thalamotomy showed dysphasia, but 10 of 31 (29%) experienced dysphasia following left thalamotomy. The spectrum of severity ranged from a mild difficulty in word finding and object naming to incomprehensible speech. Disturbances of expression exceeded those of comprehension. Repetition of speech was normal, but "rapid fatigability was prominent in the more severe disorders."

In the three cases with a mild deficit, Bell noted laconic, hesitant speech with periods of silence and word-finding difficulties. Paraphasias and faulty grammar were superimposed on these disturbances in the four cases with dysphasia of moderate severity. The three cases of severe dysphasia had "additional disabilities" not further elaborated. Two experienced disturbances of consciousness that appeared to have limited the quality of observations on their language disturbance. The third case developed the dysphasia after a thalamic hemorrhage complicated the clinical state. Unfortunately, the clinical details were not described.

TRANSIENT DYSPHASIA

In all the reports describing the course of the disorder, the dysphasia appeared either immediately postoperative, or worsened for several days (Bell, 1968; Selby, 1969; Shapiro et al., 1973), then improved steadily. In six of Bell's cases, the disturbance subsided within a few weeks, whereas in four it persisted as long as 25 and 32 months. However, in some cases, no significant change was noted at followup as late as 4 or more months (Christensen, Juul-Jensen, Malmros, & Harmsen, 1970; Jurko & Andy, 1964; Shut, 1970).

LESION FOCUS AND DYSPHASIA

According to earlier workers (Riklan, Levita, Zimmerman, & Cooper, 1969; Sem-Jacobsen, 1965), the needling of the thalamus alone was insufficient to produce the dysphasia. A focal lesion was required.

In living cases before the advent of CT scanning, the site of the lesion was inferred to be in VL. Few postmortem studies exist on the subject; of these, the clinical details are not as complete as might be desired. Sameral, Wright, Sergay, and Tyler (1976) reported a case with the lesion confined to VL. Hermann et al. (1966) had cases with the lesion in the globus pallidus sparing the thalamus. The case of thalamic lesion described by Ojemann, Fedio, and Van Buren (1968) was "mildly dysnomic" for the 17 days from operation until death.

Lesions in sites other than VL thalamus have produced some disturbance in speech and language function, but apparently only rarely. Spiegel and Wycis (1962) described only 1 of 90 with aphasia from a lesion of the dorsomedial thalamus compared with 3 of 16 from a lesion of VL. Brown, Riklan, Waltz, Jackson, and Cooper (1971) found a language disturbance in only 1 case among 11 from a pulvinar lesion. In this case, the disturbance developed during the operation. Repetition was

> good even for complex phrases. Speech was less intelligible with perseveration, mumbling and occasional pallilalic responses. Jargon phrases were noted. Thus, asked his profession he replied, . . . "I worked as a rigger. Oh, well, a rigger is pull water, rigs up and that is what he is . . . well he rigs business." Series speech was good. Reading was possible.

In careful stimulation studies involving VL and the pulvinar (Figure 3) carried out by Ojemann et al. (1968; Ojemann and Ward, 1971), stimulation of the lateral or superior portions of VL failed to alter naming. However, altered object naming occurred in some but not all cases from stimulation in the anterior portion and in the posterior inferior medial portion. This latter region abutted the pulvinar, stimulation of which produced similar alterations in naming in all cases studied.

Ojemann and colleagues used the terms anomia, perseveration, and anarthria to categorize the errors. By anomia, they meant "inability to name the object correctly, but with demonstrated ability to speak, such as would be indicated by being able to say 'that is a. . . .'" Anomic errors occurred as omissions and as misnames. In stimulation of the pulvinar, the omissions and misnamings occurred with approximately equal frequency.

Perseveration was defined as "the repetition of part or all of a correct object name." Perseveration affected fewer cases, but also occurred whether VL or the pulvinar was stimulated.

Stimulaton of subsections of VL that produced errors appears to have been in the same regions noted by Hermann et al. (1966). In the pulvinar, stimulations that yielded errors occurred in the anterior and superior portion most reliably (Ojemann et al., 1968). These data contrast with those of Brown et al. (1971) who noted only 1 among 11 cases in which a left pulvinar lesion produced change in language fuction. However, in none of Brown's cases was the exact site of the lesion within the pulvinar described and a permanent lesion, not stimulation, was the source of the data.

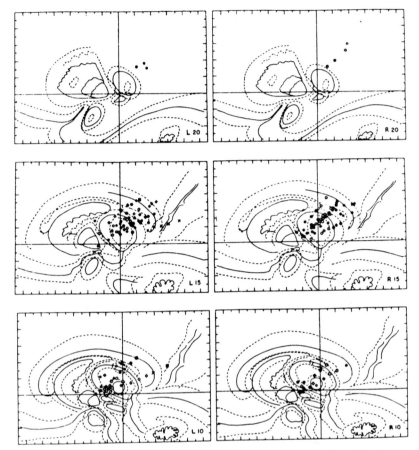

Figure 3. Sagittal sections of the left (L) and right (R) sides of the brain stimulated by Ojemann, Fedio, and Van Buren (1968). The stimulation occurred mostly in the centrum medianum and nucleus lateralis dorsalis of the thalamus. Responses included no errors (O); anomia (black ball); motor speech disruption (black box); anarthria (black triangle); sensory speech disruption (open diamond); visual speech disruption (x).

Thalamic Hemorrhage

Cases of thalamic hemorrhage are not common, but they far out-number all other causes of focal unilateral thalamic injury suitable for the study of dysphasia. Hemorrhage in any brain location ac-counts for only 18% of strokes, and the thalamus is the site involved in a mere 13% of cases of hemorrhage (Mohr, Caplan, Melski, Duncan, Kistler, Pessin, Goldstein, & Bleich, 1978). By simple arithmetic, 13% of hemorrhages, given 18% of strokes due to hemorrhage leaves but 2% of all cases of stroke attributable to thalamic hemorrhage, half of which occur in the hemisphere dominant for speech and language. In the majority of this small number of cases, the thalamic hemorrhage develops so quickly to a large size that the patient is either untestable or only for a very brief time before coma supervenes. In the unpublished data from the ongoing Pilot National Stroke Data Bank Project, for example, only seven hematomas confined to the left thalamus occurred among 909 prospectively analyzed cases of stroke at four cooperating institutions. None of the seven presented with aphasia.

Given all these constraints, it is, perhaps, no surprise that the number of reported cases is small. This scanty literature is presented here in considerable detail as it represents almost all of the cases described to date, and because it conveys a flavor of the clinical presentation of importance in the analysis of the syndrome.

PERSONAL CASES

Mohr, Watters, and Duncan (1975) described a 72-year-old, right-handed, hypertensive physician's widow engaged in conversation when she suddenly put her hand to her head and said, "Oh, my, I've never felt like this before," and then, according to a witness, "began talking way out, muttering, never finishing a sentence." Within moments, she became somnolent and weak on the right side.

At the hospital emergency ward 1 hour later, she was described as sleepy, following simple commands to open her eyes, her mouth, and move her left arm. She spoke understandable words, although most of her speech was considered unintelligible jargon. CT scan on the day after admission showed a left thalamic hemorrhage extending laterally and inferiorly from the thalamic region toward the left insula (see Figure 4).

The following day, she appeared asleep, yet readily participated in testing, even though she frequently kept her eyes closed when speaking. She proved testable only for a few seconds at a time, due to an unpreventable lapse into a state of fading vocal volume, logorrheic paraphasia, then silence. A sharp word or prod produced prompt remission to the more alert state for a few seconds when she conversed accurately, only to relapse to the original logorrheic state followed by silence.

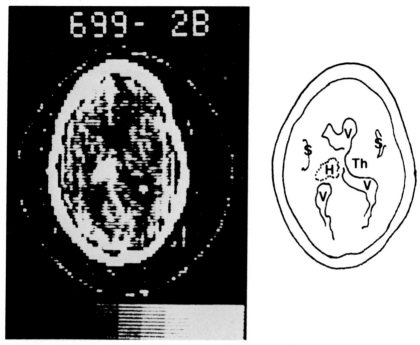

Figure 4. CT scan view of the hematoma affecting the left thalamus in personal case 1 (Mohr, Watters, & Duncan, 1975).

During the many brief testable periods, she performed so well on a wide range of language tests that none present suspected any disturbance in language during these periods. These satisfactory performances included repeating aloud of long, familiar and unfamiliar words and syllable groups (e.g., "Massachusetts," "settsachumass," "Philadelphia," "Moscow," "Popocatepetl," "xytaceuatl," "consiwis," "opicancanoe"). She named short words dictated in spelled form and spelled aloud dictated words; named states of the Union whose initials were dictated (e.g., "NH"); named objects characteristic of body parts or actions (e.g., "What do you wear on your head?" "What does a policeman blow?"; named animals producing a characteristic sound (e.g., "moo"); named the usual color characteristically associated with objects whose names were dictated ("grass"); read aloud large headlines ("Scandalous epidemic of tooth decay is sweeping America"); and named individual items presented visually in the form of a montage line drawing of five objects.

By contrast, in the logorrheic state, she uttered so many unwonted neologistic paraphasias as to cause examiners in that phase of testing to wonder if she would ever again speak normally.

The cycles of examiner-produced remission and ready relapse were too brief for sustained testing, and within 1 hour the patient refused to continue.

Re-examination 7 days later showed improvement but the same characteristic performance, in addition to a perseverative component not previously noted. When re-examined 2 months after hemorrhage, her language and behavior deficits had completely cleared. She had no recall for her entire hospitalization.

Case 2 A 74-year-old, right-handed, hypertensive man was admitted the day he was found incontinent and unresponsive on the floor next to his bed. A CT scan (see Figure 5) on the day of admission showed a large hemorrhage involving the left caudate and anterior thalamus which extended into the mid-putamen. He was lethargic, agitated, and disoriented. Speech was fluent but language content was an incoherent mixture of his native Italian and American English. The most

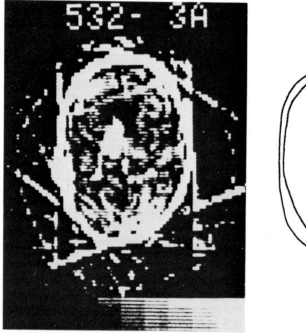 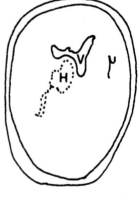

Figure 5. CT scan view of the hematoma affecting the left thalamus in personal case 2 (Mohr, Watters, & Duncan, 1975).

obvious disturbance was fading speech volume and a rapidly appearing logorrheic paraphasia followed by silence, unless vigorously prompted by the examiner.

He replied to questioning with normal prosody, intonation, and emphasis, but demonstrated a remarkable degree of echolalia. He repeated long and unfamiliar sets of syllables including "Massachusetts", "settsachumass", "Mississippi", "Salerno," "Popocatepetl", "xytaceuatl". Replies were interspersed with occasional appropriate social phrases. However, many verbal responses were so paraphasic to be virtually unintelligible. The tendency for perseverative utterances was very strong and frequently a spontaneous series of responses occurred, such as counting in Italian. These perseverations always could be interrupted by the examiner.

He was worse on re-examination the next day. He casually uttered the grossest of errors but seemed satisfied with his responses. Most striking was his behavior when not rigidly controlled by the examiner: Upon initially being engaged in conversation, he was smoothly conversational but rapidly became logorrheic and poorly controlled until interrupted.

OTHER PERSONALLY REVIEWED CASES

Eleven cases of thalamic hemorrhage were found among 16,000 autopsies performed over 15 years in a survey done by the author and colleagues at the Massachusetts General Hospital in 1975. Of these 11, all but 4 were either comatose or insufficiently examined. One of the cases was reported by Ciemins (1970), and is summarized later in the literature survey. The others are described in as full detail as records permit.

Case 3 A 57-year-old, right-handed, hypertensive man suffered an autopsy-documented left thalamic hemorrhage, which involved the medial dorsal, lateral posterior and ventral posterior nuclei, including the pulvinar to its posterior tip.

Examination by Dr. Robert Layzer showed

nominal aphasia only partial—names tie, button, shirt, pen; misses belt, buckle, shoe. Dysarthria also present. Jargon in burst intermixed with true speech. Often substitutes one wrong letter in a word. Oriented as to place, time, gave 4:30 [2:30 correct], month as "seven" date as 22 [correct]. Seems to understand spoken voice correctly. Performs simple commands correctly. Quiet, unspontaneous. The right face, arm, and leg were weak, but moved somewhat, and the right plantar response was extensor. Visual field examination showed probable right hemianopia.

Neurologic consultation by Dr. P. R. Dodge the next day

agreed with those recorded. Language disturbance makes history taking
difficult but . . . Follows simple commands, e.g. "open mouth," "close eyes,"
but doesn't carry out those requiring two steps or two simultaneous actions. Speech is flowing but frequently words have no meaning in fact aren't
words. This is typical jargon though performance is variable. States function of watch but can't name it—"stooch." After giving him alternatives,
he selects the correct name, only to forget it a minute later.

By the fourth hospital day, his improvement showed "gradual
clearing of dysphasia and hemiparesis." At discharge on the forty-
second day, he "does test phrases well and can subtract seven from
100 quite well."

Case 4 A 46-year-old, right-handed, hypertensive man developed a
left thalamic hemorrhage 1.5 × 2 cm in size, affecting the anterior
nucleus including the ventrolateral and centromedian nuclei and adjacent anterior limb of the internal capsule, as confirmed by an autopsy subsequently.

He presented with right-sided weakness and "he had slurred
speech." On examination two days later, he showed "no apraxia,
aphasia. Claims to be right handed." He was found "alert, cooper-
ative, oriented ×3. Calculation: 6 × 7 = 42, 10 × 2 = 20, 100 − 7
= 93. Memory $\frac{3}{3}$ retention. Can spell. Reading adequate. Identifies
detailed parts of five objects. Attention span adequate for a very ill
man." He was found to have a right hemiparesis, arm exceeding leg,
with a right extensor plantar response, no sensory or visual field
abnormalities, "mild dysarthria without aphasia." No worsening
occurred and the patient was discharged slightly improved 46 days
later.

LITERATURE CASES

Penfield and Roberts (1959) made passing reference to a "severe
aphasia" with considerable misnaming, perseveration, and una-
wareness of the occurrence of errors in a case of a "small hemorrhagic lesion" in the pulvinar of the thalamus in the hemisphere
dominant for speech and language.

Bugiani, Conforto, and Sacco (1969) described a 74-year-old
hypertensive male whose autopsy showed hemorrhage throughout
the entire left thalamus. It was considered to have occurred in two

separate episodes, the first confined to the anterior thalamus; the second was massive and fatal.

The speech disturbance in the first episode featured lowered voice volume and normal articulation. The language disturbance showed syntactic errors, paraphasias, verbal stereotypes occurring in spontaneous speech, and poor comprehension. However, repetition of words was intact.

Ciemins (1970) reported a 53-year-old male with a 2.5 × 1 × 1.2 cm area of hemorrhage in the left thalamus extending from the anterior nuclei to the posterior commissure, a smaller, 4 × 2.2 mm cystic lesion in the right thalamus, a 6 × 7 × 4 mm hemorrhagic infarct in the left occipital cortex, and a 1.5 × 2.5 × 3 mm vacuolated lesion in Area 40 of the left parietal lobe. The hemorrhage involved all the left thalamic nuclei and was confined to the thalamus. It did not invade the internal capsule nor did it enter into the ventricular system.

The illness began as sudden "confusion," posterior head pain and somnolence. Examination 5 days after admission showed reduced spontaneous speech. Language responses featured incomplete, fragmentary, but syntactically correct, sentences; ability to name up to four objects after which perseveration would set in; perseverative writing; difficulty in carrying out complex commands; and inability to carry out even simple written commands. The patient had no disturbance in repetition of spoken words.

Ciemins' (1970) second case was from the Massachusetts General Hospital series. The patient was a 58-year-old hypertensive female, whose autopsy 3 years after the ictus showed a 1.6 cm cavity in the left thalamus involving the lateral aspect of the ventral posterior and lateral posterior nuclei, including the medial third of the pulvinar. She was described only as "aphasic" during admission, and, on later evaluations over the next three years, as having "mild aphasia," "slight expressive aphasia," and "feeble speech." She had right arm numbness and weakness initially.

Sager, Mares, and Nestianu (1965) reported two striking cases. Both were presumed to be hemorrhages. Neither showed other lesions. One was a 62-year-old man with hemorrhagic softening in the posterior part of the thalamus. He was described as showing a "definite receptive dysphasia, alexia, acalculia, and amnestic aphasia." No other details were given. The second was a right-handed, 55-year-old man with a "hemorrhagic softening" in the left lateral posterior nucleus of the thalamus and in the pulvinar. He "displayed alexia and receptive dysphasia."

Sameral, Wright, Sergay, and Tyler (1976) described a case documented by CT scan with a hemorrhage involving the posterior left thalamus. The main deficits were "absent spontaneous speech, anomia perseverations, trailing off of words, decreased vocal volume, and neologisms in the presence of intact repetition and comprehension testing." Moderate improvement had occurred when he was examined 3 and 6 months later.

Cappa and Vignolo (1979) described *transcortical* features of aphasia, that is, repeating aloud was perserved, in three cases with left thalamic hemorrhage. All three showed dysnomias on confrontation naming, poor reading, and writing, but adequate repeating aloud. Case 1, a 62-year-old woman with a small left thalamic hemorrhage documented by CT scan, showed severe reduction in spontaneous speech, adequate naming of common objects, and apparently intact comprehension on initial examination. Extreme expressive inertia despite prompting by the examiner was a major finding. "The patient tended to stop talking after each utterance, and continuous prompting by the examiner was necessary."

Case 2 was a 76-year-old man, examined 4 days after onset. "Oral expression was markedly reduced, with frequent perseverations and echolalic repetitions." By 3 months, only a slight improvement had occurred.

The last case, a 65-year-old woman, on admission was "fluent with several paraphasias and comprehension was impaired." Tested in detail on Day 13, her oral descriptions were "scanty with marked inertia" and a mild tendency to perseveration. Prompting by the examiner was necessary after nearly every sentence.

Reynolds, Turner, Harris, and Ojemann (1979) described five cases with "dysphasia." Their first case was a man, aged 61, with a CT-documented small hematoma involving the posterolateral left thalamus who presented with "a fluent aphasia, anomia, frequent perseverations, and neologisms." He could repeat verbal input. One year later, he denied any language difficulties. Their second case, a 40-year-old man with a CT-documented large, left thalamic hematoma shown later to be due to a vascular tumor presented acutely with "dysphasia, supranuclear paralysis of upward gaze, and sensory and motor deficits of the right side." His speech contained language errors characterized as "perseverations and non-sense syllables." A third case, a man, aged 23, with a left thalamic cryptic arteriovenous malformation acutely developed "a paucity of spontaneous speech with fading vocal volume. In addition, anomia, perseveration, and neologisms were present. . . . Language comprehension appeared intact. On a standard object-naming test, there was a 31% error rate with marked perseveration. These perseverations often were words or phrases completely unrelated to the test material." A month later, he had improved considerably. Case 4 was a 37-year-old man with a large, left thalamic mass, with "no spontaneous speech, garbled words and occasional meaningful words." The final case was a 51-year-old woman whose abnormality is described only as "aphasia."

Walshe, Davis, and Fisher (1977) described 10 cases of left thalamic hemorrhage with CT scan documentation. Four were said to be aphasic, described as ranging from a few paraphasic errors to a complete receptive and expressive disorder. Most disorders improved with time.

Alexander and LoVerme (1980) reviewed 15 cases—13 had CT scans—all showing a deep hematoma varying from small to large size. Judging from the CT scan location and by description in their Table 1, eight appear to have been of thalamic location. The cases all were studied by the Boston Diagnostic Aphasia Examination or by the Porch Index of Communicative Ability. None of the cases were reported in raw data form as they were individually examined at

TABLE 1

Language Behavior in 8 Cases of Deep Hemorrhage Involving the Region of the Thalamus (Alexander & LoVerme, 1980).

	Case							
	1	2	3	4	7	8	9	13
Fluency	0[a]	0	0	0	0	0	0	1
Articulation	1[a]	0	1	0	1	1	1	1
Comprehension	0	0	0	0	0	1	2[a]	2
Repetition	0	0	0	0	0	0	1	1
Naming	1	2	1	1	2	2	2	3[a]
Paraphasias	1	0	2	0	1	2	2	2
Reading	0	0	2	1	1	1	0	2
Writing	1	0	2	1	3	2	3	1
Constructions	1	0	1	1	3	1	1	2
Calculations	0	0	0	0	3	3	·	3
Praxis	0	0	0	0	1	—	1	0
Memory	2	2	0	2	3	0	2	2
Perseveration	0	0	0	0	2	2	3	3
Affect	1	0	1	1	2	1	1	3
Attention	1	0	1	0	3	1	1	1

[a]0 = normal, 1 = mild, 2 = moderate, 3 = severe.

different times by different examiners. The earliest examination was 2 days in one case, the remainder at 3 weeks (four cases), 5 weeks (three cases), and a final case examined first at 8 months.

Six cases showed extended jargon, described as "paraphasic speech that runs beyond the level of a simple phonemic or semantic alteration," but the authors did not report the site of the hemorrhage (putaminal versus thalamic).

Syndrome Formulation

REVIEW OF TERMS USED

The thread of a distinctive but unusual condition seems to run throughout the scanty literature. There has been a remarkable array of descriptive terms. Apart from aphasia, these terms include inattention (Smythe & Stern, 1938), dementia (Schulman, 1957), decreased concentration (Schulman, 1957), florid psychotic reaction (Gillingham et al., 1960), severe confusional state (Gillingham et al., 1960), disorientation (Bravo et al., 1966), and apathy (Mills & Swanson, 1978). Speech has been described as feeble (Ciemins, 1970), irrelevant (Smythe & Stern, 1938), rapid fatigability, laconic, hesitant (Bell, 1968), unintelligible, garbled (Van Buren & Borke, 1969), perseveration, mumbling, occasional palilalia, jargon (Brown et al., 1971), and paraphasic (Alexander & LoVerme, 1980).

Terms used to describe the aphasia itself have ranged among real (Laitinen, 1966), total (Smythe & Stern, 1938), mixed (Bugiani et al., 1969), complete receptive and expressive (Walshe et al., 1977), slight expressive (Ciemins, 1970), motor aphasia type (Riechert, 1964), definite receptive (Sager et al., 1965), fluent (Reynolds et al., 1979), mildly dysnomic (Ojemann et al., 1968), anomic (Sager et al., 1965; Sameral et al., 1976), subcortical aphasia type (Riechert 1964), transcortical (Cappa & Vignolo, 1979), and diminished verbal memory (Krayenbühl et al., 1965). The assessment of severity varied from mild (Ciemins, 1970), moderately severe (Gillingham et al., 1960), and severe (Bell, 1968) to residual (Van Buren & Borke, 1969).

No single eponym or distinctive term has risen from the many as yet. The very variety suggests some unusual features not easily classified according to traditional formulations.

ATTEMPTS TO CLASSIFY BY TRADITIONAL CRITERIA

The features of the syndrome of motor or Broca's aphasia do not characterize cases with thalamic lesions, even though the terms, "expressive" or "motor aphasia," have been used in some reports. None of the published cases have demonstrated the dysprosody, effortful speech, and agrammatism characteristic of motor aphasia as currently understood (Mohr, Pessin, Finkelstein, Funkenstein, Duncan, & Davis, 1978).

Nor can the syndrome be classified as a conduction aphasia. Although few cases appear to have been tested to settle the point, it is remarkable that there is little or no reported disturbance in repeating aloud. This point stands out in sharp contrast to the occurrence of a wide array of other disturbances in language. Repeating aloud is not completely normal, however, since many cases with thalamic lesions make errors when tested with complex materials. But at the level of word complexity where repeating aloud is accomplished without errors, gross disturbances are encountered in tests of comprehension and naming to such a degree that impaired repeating aloud cannot be considered a feature of the syndrome of thalamic aphasia.

The lack of impaired repeating aloud is of particular importance, considering the anatomy of the lesions involved. In naturally occurring lesions, chief among them hemorrhage, the presence of the mass in the thalamus could easily be postulated to achieve its main language effects by pressure on the adjacent isthmus of the temporal lobe. As the resultant syndrome of the temporal isthmus (Nielsen, 1962) is considered to be identical with Wernicke aphasia, a disturbance in repeating aloud should be a central element. It is currently assumed—an assumption that may not be entirely warranted by facts from other cases—that impaired repeating aloud reflects a disturbance to the arcuate fasciculus (Benson, Sheremata, Bouchard, Segarra, Price, & Geschwind, 1973). The presence of this fasciculus in the temporal isthmus should insure that it is injured by a thalamic mass. This injury should produce impaired repeating aloud. By this argument, the intact repeating aloud in thalamic lesions should mean that the language disturbances arise from the thalamic lesion itself.

These arguments against the applicability of classification of these cases as Broca's aphasia or conduction aphasia leave Wernicke aphasia, transcortical aphasia and subcortical aphasia to be considered. The disturbances encountered include dysnomia, paraphasia, and disturbance in comprehension, terms that should allow one or more of these syndrome names to apply in cases of thalamic lesion.

Aphasic Delirium

Before too casual an application is made of one of these traditional syndrome names, some of the associated features of the behavior of thalamic cases need to be taken into consideration.

Many authors have been impressed that these cases show a gross disturbance in alertness, and a remarkable inconstancy in response rate, content, and accuracy. Whether seen as an obstacle to the analysis of the aphasia, the striking features of the behavior have prompted the use of such terms (quoted individually in the reports previously cited) as disorientation, lethargy, apathy, severe confusional state, fluctuating degrees of confusion, extreme expressive inertia, incomplete and fragmentary speech, mumbling, less intelligible speech, rapid fatigability, trailing off of words, periods of silence, patient tended to stop talking after each utterance, continuous prompting by the examiner was necessary, perseveration, jargon in bursts intermixed with true speech, perseveration often of words or phrases completely unrelated to the test material, and paraphasic speech that runs beyond the level of simple phonemic or semantic alteration.

These observations, made in all types of thalamic lesions, including thalamotomy, all strike a central theme of a fluctuation in performance akin to a delirium. At the least affected end of the clinical spectrum, the patient passes for normal; at the most severe, there is virtually no normal language behavior. And these two ends of the spectrum are encountered in the same patient from minute to minute, making an overall quantitative assessment of language difficult, at times, even impossible.

It is this delirial fluctuation in alertness—and with it the unwonted paraphasias—that are the most characteristic features of the acute syndrome of a thalamic lesion, not just the occurrence or the types of errors in language use. Indeed, the language disturbance appears to this observer to be but one of the elements in the disorder, the severity of which mirrors but is not independent of the disorder in alertness.

As in other forms of delirium, the condition is rarely persistent. The whole syndrome usually fades within days—weeks at most. In addition, as in other forms of delirium, at the end of this time, the patients are totally amnestic for the entire period and have recovered normal performance on all language tasks. This latter result also suggests that the language disorder is but part of a bigger syndrome and not a separate phenomenon.

In a further effort to reinforce this observation, it is useful at this point to cite behavioral observations made on other forms of delirium. These citations should help separate the aphasic delirium of thalamic lesions from other syndromes.

FEATURES OF METABOLIC DELIRIUM

Unfortunately, the literature on metabolic delirium contains discouragingly few detailed descriptions of the behavior in individual cases. Most of the texts are descriptions of the examiner's conclusions rather than of the behavior itself. As a result, few descriptions are complete enough to be certain how closely the cases of differing etiology resemble one another. The available literature suggests only that the syndromes of differing etiology are more alike than different in their language content.

The terms used for the behavior in delirium are most often drawn from accounts of delerium tremens. They include "pressure of speech with repeated stereotypic exclamations or incoherent flight of ideas . . . not uncommonly the clinical picture shows rapid changes from phases of overactivity to periods of apathy and aspontaneity. . . . Speech is usually slurred and with paraphasic errors. In severe examples it may be incoherent and fragmented" (Lishman, 1978, pp. 13, 709); "resembles . . . hypnagogic or hypnopompic phenomena. . . . conversation becomes limited, with a tendency to short monosyllablic phrases. Thought becomes disordered and fragmented with perseveration . . . drowsiness follows in many patients, while others are restless . . . thinking may be so disconnected as to produce incoherent speech" (Heller & Kornfeld, 1975, p. 45).

These quotes typify the type of descriptions available for delirium from alcohol withdrawal, sleep deprivation, hallucinogens, and postcardiac surgery states; in all, some degree of thalamic derangement may play a role in the genesis of the symptoms.

There are many features shared between these cases and those of

tical functioning; more particularly, right–left disorientation, writing difficulty (*agraphia*) and a calculation defect (*acalculia*)
(Gerstmann, 1927, 1930). He regarded these deficits as related to a
dissolution of both the morphologic knowledge of the hand and of
its highly skilled use in writing and calculation. Although other
symptoms were noted in his material, Gerstmann considered that
four of the signs—finger agnosia, right–left disorientation, agraphia,
and acalculia—formed a distinct constellation. From his pathologic
data, he showed that all patients who demonstrated all four symptoms had lesions in the dominant parietal lobe, more specifically,
in the region of the angular gyrus and adjacent occipital lobe. Because of the strong correlation of the symptom cluster with focal
pathology, Gerstmann considered that the four components formed
a genuine symptom cluster; others soon assigned his name as an
eponym.

The localizing significance of purely behavioral signs such as
aphasia and alexia had been well accepted in clinical practice since
the late nineteenth century. Therefore, neurologists quickly accepted Gerstmann's findings as being another behavioral syndrome
that could assist them in localizing lesions in the cerebral cortex.
Neurologists examining patients at the bedside are usually limited
by time in their evaluation of behavior and, therefore, typically make
primarily qualitative judgments as to the presence or absence of
particular deficits. This is certainly true in the case of the Gerstmann syndrome as each sign is complicated and even a qualitative
assessment of performance is often difficult.

There has been considerable study as well as rather vigorous debate about the Gerstmann syndrome in the past 20 years. In this
chapter, we review and comment on the syndrome and its symptoms; we discuss its anatomical and neuropsychological implications and, hopefully without undue bias, analyze the controversy
that the syndrome has engendered.

Description of the Syndrome

The Gerstmann syndrome, as used in clinical neurology, is a constellation of four distinct behavioral features: finger agnosia, right–
left disorientation, agraphia, and acalculia. Each symptom represents a specific disturbance in higher cortical functioning. Although
the individual deficits are specific, each is complex and may be elic-

ited by a variety of testing methods. Because of the basic clinical nature of the syndrome, the testing must be applicable for bedside and office examination. We discuss each symptom in detail, but it must be kept in mind that the syndrome can be considered definitely to be present only if all four elements can be shown to be present.

FINGER AGNOSIA

The pivotal sign in the Gerstmann syndrome is finger agnosia (Gerstmann, 1924). *Finger agnosia* does not mean, as the name implies, that the patient does not recognize fingers as fingers and therefore misidentifies them as, let us say, toes, arms, or toothbrushes; but rather, in Gerstmann's own words, that the patient has a "disability for recognizing, naming, selecting, differentiating and indicating the individual fingers of either hand, the patient's own as well as those of other persons" (Gerstmann, 1940:398). Gerstmann was the first to stress the significance of this unusual sign, and in Critchley's words his "shrewd and original communication . . . virtually started a new chapter in the story of parietal symptomatology" (Critchley, 1953:203).

In Gerstmann's original patient, and in many patients subsequently reported, the finger recognition problem was pervasive, being present regardless of the method tested. From the definition, however, it is obvious that the faculty of finger recognition is far from a unitary function. Naming, pointing to named fingers, and moving a finger on one hand that corresponds to one that an examiner has moved on his own opposite hand are all quite different functions, each requiring different neuropsychologic mechanisms for successful completion. In some patients, one aspect of finger agnosia may be more prominent than others. At one point in the history of finger gnosis, these separate functions were differentially labeled; "finger aphasia" for the inability to name fingers, "finger apraxia" for the inability to individually move fingers, and so forth (Schilder, 1931). Although such labels emphasize the various aspects of finger agnosia, this proliferation of terms is neither necessary nor practical. One observation that has been made by all clinicians testing finger recognition is that it is the middle three fingers that are most frequently misidentified.

In general, when testing for finger agnosia at the bedside, several methods of examination should be utilized; these are outlined here.

unilateral variety using nonverbal tests only has been described in the opposite-hand unilateral hemispheric lesions (Gainotti & Tiacci, 1973). Why a generalized dysfunction of finger sense should be found after a focal lesion in the left parietal lobe has been a matter of much speculation. It is thought by some authors that finger agnosia is a restricted aspect of autotopagnosia or failure to appreciate ones topographical body scheme; but finger agnosia usually occurs in isolation from a generalized autotopagnosia. Many theories have attempted to explain the function of finger gnosis but none has adequately explained the phenomenon. Why a left-sided lesion should cause bilateral loss of finger sense is also uncertain. It is well recognized that a left-sided lesion can cause bilateral ideomotor apraxia; therefore, it appears that the left hemisphere is dominant for both sensory knowledge and complex motor performance of both hands (Geschwind, 1975).

RIGHT–LEFT DISORIENTATION

Right–left disorientation is a term used to describe a patient's inability to differentiate right from left either on himself or on another. The definition implies that the right–left problem represents a generalized difficulty in applying a spatial concept of lateral orientation to the body rather than merely a linguistic defect in which the labels right and left are misapplied. As with finger agnosia, right–left disorientation is complex and both verbal and nonverbal testing methods are commonly employed in identifying the defect.

In testing for right–left disorientation, tasks of graded difficulty should be given. Because each question has only two possible answers (i.e., right or left), enough trials must be given to overcome chance factors.

1. Verbal tasks
    a. Naming side indicated by examiner
        1. on patient
        2. on examiner facing patient
        3. on examiner in unusual orientation (e.g., seated sideways with legs crossed; ask patient to identify one foot or knee).
    b. Ask patient to point to body parts on one side of the body named by examiner, (e.g., "point to my right ear"):
        1. on patient
        2. on examiner facing patient
        3. on examiner in unusual positions.

    c. Crossed commands. Ask patient to point with specific hand to specific part (e.g., "point to left ear with right hand").
      1. on patient
      2. on examiner facing patient
      3. on examiner in different postures.
2. Nonverbal tests (Head, 1926). With the patient seated opposite the examiner; instruct patient to point to the exact part on his own body that the examiner has pointed to on his (e.g., examiner points to his own right eye and the patient then points to his own right eye). The examiner can also cross his arms or legs and move one part and ask patient to move the similar part.

This series of tests can be administered in a few minutes and can provide the examiner with a comprehensive assessment of the patient's right–left orientation. In mild cases of right–left disorientation, the patient fails only the complex crossed commands. With moderate impairment, the patient consistently fails on tasks with the examiner facing him; with a marked deficit, the patient shows right–left confusion on himself.

Several important factors must be appreciated when interpreting failure on these right–left tasks. One factor is that there are many people in the normal population (including educated people) that have significant difficulties with right–left orientation. Interestingly, this is twice as common in females (17.5%) as in males (8.8%) (Wolf, 1973). A second factor is aphasia. It has been shown repeatedly that aphasic patients usually perform quite poorly on the verbal right–left tasks (Benton, 1979; Dennis, 1976; Sauguet et al., 1971). Accordingly, it is wise to be very cautious in diagnosing right–left disorientation in an aphasic patient unless significant errors are made on nonverbal tasks as well. A third factor is denial. Some patients with denial or unilateral neglect have difficulty with right–left tasks on the basis of a neglected side alone (usually left) (Nielsen, 1938).

Being cognizant of the influencing factors outlined here, it is possible to further analyze the neuropsychologic mechanism involved in right–left discrimination. The major requirement is the development of an autotopographical concept of the body and its inherent right–left symmetry. It is precisely this symmetry that causes confusion; it is a rare patient whose body schema disorientation includes an inability to distinguish nonsymmetrical regions, that is, top from bottom or front from back (Stengel & Vienna, 1944).

During development, the individual initially forms a basic spatial concept of the body and its symmetry. Having done so, he or she is then able to accomplish the more complex operation of reversing and reorienting this right–left symmetry (Benton, 1968). With this higher level of conceptualization of laterality, the individual can correctly identify the right and left of others regardless of their orientation—facing him, walking in the opposite direction, or hanging upside down. It is this spatial conceptualization of right–left that is the essence of right–left orientation. This function, best tested by the nonverbal imitation tasks, can be disturbed by lesions in either right or left hemisphere (Sauguet et al., 1971).

Concomitant with the development of right–left sense, as discussed previously, is the application of verbal labels to the sides of the body. On occasion, errors in right–left orientation are due to the misapplication of the linguistic labels, "right" and "left." This mislabeling can occur by three mechanisms: (1) from aphasia (anomia particularly); (2) because basic spatial disorientation does not allow the individual to appreciate the correct side to label (discussed in this chapter; and (3) a disconnection of the temporoparietal language system that contains the labels from the parieto-occipital tactile–visual system from which the spatial concept of right–left arises. The first and third mechanisms would be seen only in left hemisphere lesions.

AGRAPHIA

Agraphia is a disorder in the expression of written language that occurs as a result of brain damage (Hécaen & Albert, 1978). As with other complex higher cortical functions, agraphia can be caused by the disruption of a variety of neuropsychologic functions. The patient who is aphasic in speech, for example, almost inevitably is agraphic[1] and produces writing errors that are distinctly aphasic in nature. Some patients who do not demonstrate aphasic speech, however, can exhibit an agraphia that is characterized by misspellings, omissions or intrusions of letters or words, letter or word substitution (paragraphias), syntax errors, and, on occasion, completely nonsensical writing (jargon agraphia). Such cases are classified as *aphasic agraphia*.

There are other examples of agraphia in which the patients are unable to properly align letters and words on the page and may even

---

[1]Exceptions to this rule are, at best, extremely rare.

have difficulty producing recognizable letters. This disorder, often called *spatial agraphia*, appears to be part of a more generalized constructional impairment. Patients with spatial agraphia, unlike many of those with aphasic agraphia, also have a pronounced defect in copying written language.

A third major type of agraphia distinguished by some authors is an *apraxic agraphia*. Not all authors, however, accept this as a separate category. As usually described, the syndrome has the following characteristics: no primary sensory, motor, constructional, or language deficit; yet, the patient is unable to correctly form letters spontaneously or from dictation. The agraphia is due to the loss of the sensory–motor engrams (stored patterns of letters and words) necessary for writing. It is this type of agraphia that is generally felt to be present in patients with the Gerstmann syndrome, however, performance varies (Critchley, 1953; Hécaen & Albert, 1978). In general, most perform more adequately when copying than when writing either spontaneously or from dictation. Spatial problems as well as misspellings due to letter order errors and letter omissions have been described (Kinsbourne & Warrington, 1964). In some patients, a combination of writing errors is demonstrated.

In testing for agraphia, it is important to give the patient material of graded complexity; some patients fail at a very basic level of letter formation whereas others demonstrate their agraphia only in the form of syntax errors in sentence length material.

1. Writing to dictation—ask the patient to write letters, numbers, then words, and finally, sentences.
2. Spontaneous writing—have the patient write his name and address, numbers 1–10, the first 10 letters of the alphabet, then the names of objects and finally some sentences. (e.g., about the weather, their job, how they would change an automobile tire, etc.)
3. Copying—numbers, letters, words, and sentences.
4. Anagrams or typewriter—if available. Some patients with severe apraxic or spatial agraphia can succeed in composing messages with a typewriter or anagram letters (Valenstein & Heilman, 1979).

Writing is a high-level, complex, cognitive process and a series of steps—each a distinct neuropsychologic function—is required for its successful execution (Luria, 1964, 1966). The individual functions are carried out in separate brain regions and, because of this, a focal cerebral lesion can disturb the writing process in a selective fashion, depending upon the location and extent of the damage.

In the hearing population, written language is predicated upon the auditory–verbal language system. Luria (1966) has demonstrated this by developmental studies. He asked children to write stories but prevented them from vocalizing by having them clench their tongues between their teeth. When thus restricted, the children's writing became grossly agraphic. The written language system in many people appears not to escape fully this reliance on verbal language; therefore, it is likely that in many instances the first step in writing is the mental production of a spoken message. The second step would require the transformation of this verbal phonemic system into a visual–spatial symbolic system. In Western languages, this involves a direct translation into a grapheme or letter-sound system, which is not always fully phonetic. These letters and their combinations become the basic visual–spatial building blocks of the written language system.

Serial ordering is an additional function which obviously is critical in both the phoneme selection of spoken language and the grapheme choice in written language. The actual act of writing requires a third step—the reproduction on paper of the graphemic symbol system. This final step requires a transformation of the visual–spatial symbol into a kinesthetic motor pattern that guides the hand and fingers through the writing motions.

Any lesion producing an aphasia in spoken speech will cause a concomitant agraphia. Left hemisphere posterior temporal lesions and lesions in the peri-Sylvian area posteriorly (supramarginal gyrus) (see Figure 1) will produce a fluent form of aphasia and an aphasic agraphia. If the lesion is more posterior in the parietal lobe (angular gyrus region), spoken language often is spared yet the visual–spatial symbol is deranged; the patient can neither interpret nor reproduce the symbols. This lesion produces an alexia as well as an agraphia (a syndrome discussed in greater detail elsewhere in this volume).

Some authors hypothesize that if a lesion is so placed as to damage the kinesthetic–motor patterns for writing—yet leaves undisturbed both the verbal language system and the visual–spatial symbolic representation system—a pure agraphia would be produced. This type of agraphia would be an apraxic agraphia, the variety usually described with the Gerstmann syndrome.

The existence of pure agraphia has been debated since Exner (1881) first postulated that an isolated agraphia would be produced

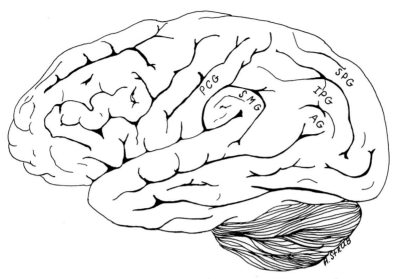

Figure 1. Left hemisphere of human brain. Post central gyrus (PCG) (areas 3, 1, 2-Brodmann); supramarginal gyrus (SMG) (area 40-Brodmann); angular (AG) gyrus (Area 39—Brodmann); superior and inferior parietal gyri (SPG and IPG)—superior parietal lobule (Areas 5 and 7—Brodmann).

by a lesion in the posterior portion of the second frontal gyrus. He contended that a lesion anterior to the hand region of the motor strip could produce a writing disturbance similar to the aphasia described by Broca (a lesion in the third frontal gyrus). The existence of isolated agraphia with frontal lesions continues to be controversal. Hécaen and Consoli (1973) have described some patients with mild, relatively pure agraphias from frontal lesions but these have been principally in the third frontal convolution rather than the second. Furthermore, these patients were all lefthanders and this may represent a special case.

Lesions in the superior, anterior, and mid parietal area, however, have been reported to produce a pure agraphia (superior and inferior parietal gyrus—Areas 5 and 7 (Basso, Taborelli, & Vignolo, 1978; Russell & Espir, 1961). (See Figure 1.)

It is in this parietal cortex that kinesthetic images for the hand movements necessary for writing are thought to be integrated with the visual–spatial percept of the letters stored in the inferior parietal and parietal–occipital area (angular gyrus and surrounds). Lesions in this area produce, according to some authors, an apraxic agraphia, the type mostly commonly described in patients with the

Gerstmann syndrome. A lesion in this area seems either to destroy the kinesthetic engrams of the graphemes or prevent their integration with the verbal and visual language systems. As patients with Gerstmann syndrome usually can copy much more adequately than they write spontaneously, it is doubtful that there is complete destruction of the sensory–motor engrams.

Several additional aspects of pure agraphia should be mentioned although these have little relevance to the agraphia seen in the Gerstmann syndrome. Patients with severe constructional impairment, particularly with right or bilateral parietal lesions, often will have a severe spatial agraphia; their writing may either be extremely distorted, or, at times, be reduced to an illegible scrawl. This defect will produce an agraphia that is, in a sense, pure, as there is no aphasia but the agraphia is more correctly only part of a more generalized constructional defect.

Several individual cases of pure agraphia have been reported. Rosati, DeBastiani, and Pinna (1979) have described a single case of aphasic agraphia in a right-handed individual with a deep left temporal lesion. This patient had a mild comprehension deficit but demonstrated a severe agraphic disturbance. Assal, Chapuis, and Zander (1970) also reported a patient with a pure agraphia with a left hemisphere insult but of unspecified localization. Also, a rare form of isolated agraphia of the left hand has been described in a right-handed patient with a lesion in the anterior corpus callosum (N. Geschwind & E. Kaplan, 1962).

Left-handed patients demonstrate some interesting agraphic syndromes after hemispheric lesions. In general, they may have an agraphia that persists after a widespread aphasic disturbance clears. More specifically, an isolated apraxic agraphia has been described in several left-handed patients with right hemisphere lesions (Heilman, Coyle, Gonyea, & Geschwind, 1973; Valenstein & Heilman, 1979). One of the patients had no aphasia and seemed to have suffered destruction of sensory–motor engrams because he could produce normal written messages on a typewriter.

Chédru and Geschwind (1972) have noted a very high incidence of isolated spatial and aphasic agraphia in patients during acute confusional or delirious states. They comment that writing is a more difficult, less-practiced task that is very delicate and fragile. They raise the possibility that because many patients with pure agraphia have brain tumors, the agraphia they demonstrate may be secondary to the generalized effects of increased intracranial pressure and not the locus of the tumor. This mechanism may well explain many cases of pure agraphia, but it does not account for those seen secondary to stable vascular lesions, stable syndromes after missile wounds, or in the left-handed patient after recovery from a more significant aphasic disturbance.

ACALCULIA

Calculation is a very interesting, complex, cognitive ability. It is built on a set of very rudimentary, innate capacities and has developed to a high level through the use of various symbol systems. There are almost certainly innate functions necessary for the development of the ability to calculate, for example, an innate sense of number, the basic concepts of more and less, and an appreciation of the relationship of parts to the whole. On the other hand, much of the process of calculation is, like language, a culturally learned skill. A number of factors are necessary: first, a symbolic numbering system with some type of ordering as to magnitude; second, a decimal or place value or similar notation; third, a basic set of rules and concepts governing the manipulation of these symbols (e.g., adding, subtracting) and a set of signs to indicate the operations (e.g., $+$, $-$, $\times$). The act of calculation itself refers to this manipulation process.

In the Gerstmann syndrome, a defect in calculating ability or *acalculia* constitutes the fourth and final element. As with the other features of the syndrome, acalculia is a multifaceted abstract and very complex disturbance. Calculation and acalculia have been quite extensively studied and discussed (Grewel, 1952, 1969; Hécaen, Angelergues, & Houllier, 1961; Henschen, 1920) with three main categories of disturbance identified (Hécaen *et al.*, 1961).

The first category is a *spatial acalculia* in which visual spatial impairment prevents the patient from properly organizing figures on the page when carrying out complex written problems. Alignment errors abound and orthographic features are distorted. Although this type of error principally disturbs the performance of complex written problems, complicated oral arithmetic problems requiring mental visualization may also be affected.

The second category of disturbance is a loss of the appreciation of basic arithmetic processes: carrying, borrowing, stepwise computation in complex multiplication, and so forth. This disorder has been labeled *anarithmetria* by Hécaen *et al.* (1961) and represents the purest form of acalculia.

The third form of acalculia is based on an inability to use the symbolic notation for both numbers and computational signs. This can be aphasic in nature (the patient produces incorrect number substitutions or paraphasias when solving oral calculations). Also, it can take the form of a number-and-sign alexia and agraphia in which the patient is unable to understand and use these written symbols. In one such case, studied by Benson and Denckla (1969), the patient produced both incorrect verbal and written answers to simple problems yet consistently could point to the correct answer from a number display. As is probably true of other cases, actual computational skills are intact although errors in phoneme or grapheme choice prevent the patient from demonstrating his competence.

In severe cases of acalculia, in addition to the deficits discussed, patients also may demonstrate a loss of memory for rote arithmetic tables and some may even lose their basic number concepts.

The acalculia in the Gerstmann syndrome has not received extensive study and there does not seem to be any agreement as to the type of calculation abnormality exhibited by the patients. Gerstmann (1940) felt it was a basic defect in arithmetic operations (anarithmetria) that, in severe cases, would manifest itself as a failure to understand number sequence and decimal value. Hécaen and Albert (1978) agree. Critchley (1953), on the other hand, considered it to be primarily a parietal or spatial acalculia which was evident most prominently on written calculation. Kinsbourne and Warrington (1962) observed a combination of errors: computational, spatial, and symbolic. They felt that automatic rote problems were least affected.

Since the exact nature of the acalculia in the Gerstmann syndrome is not well formulated, the evaluation of calculating ability should be comprehensive.

1. Counting—Have the patient count up to 30 (errors do not often show up in simple one-digit numbers).
2. Assessing number concept—ask the patient which two numbers or stacks of coins is larger, and so on. Unfortunately, this type of testing requires verbal instructions and may show errors based on failure to comprehend complex relational, grammatical forms.
3. Translation of number concept into verbal and written symbol:
   a. Ask patient to tell and write down the number of objects shown to him (e.g., fingers, coins, etc.)
   b. Ask patient to read numbers and hold up the number of fingers indicated.

4. Oral calculations—start with rote sums and proceed to subtraction, multiplication, division, and then to complex calculations (e.g., 38 + 56). If incorrect answers are given, see if the patient can write or point to correct answer in a display or list of numbers.
5. Written calculations—use the same hierarchy suggested in Number 4. Vary signs and difficulty. Dictate problems for the patient to write and provide written examples.

Lesions in almost any region of the cortex can produce a disturbance in calculation; therefore, localization based on the presence of acalculia alone is impossible. There are, however, certain aspects of calculation errors that indicate damage in more defined areas of the cortex. Spatial acalculia is almost always associated with a parietal lesion, with right parietal lesions being more likely to produce a severe defect than left. Aphasic, agraphic, or alexic calculation problems are seen with lesions of the speech-dominant hemisphere. Anarithmetria usually is seen in bilateral disease but also can be seen with left parietal involvement. In the Gerstmann syndrome, the type of acalculia is uncertain so it is difficult to attach any specific localization significance to that specific symptom in isolation.

DISCUSSION OF THE SYNDROME

It is these four behavioral signs that constitute the classic Gerstmann syndrome. The diagnosis should not be made unless all four elements are present; to speak of a partial Gerstmann syndrome only serves to muddy already turbid waters. One problem that arises when assessing any behavioral sign is the specification of the quality or severity of failure necessary before a patient is considered to be suffering from a deficit in the corresponding function. Operational definitions have been devised that include quantitative cutoff scores on extensive test batteries. On the other hand, the presence of the four behavioral signs can often be satisfactorily ascertained at the bedside. If an adequate sample of behavior is obtained using the various modes of testing outlined, the diagnosis can be made, in most instances, without great difficulty.

In a medical syndrome, ideally, the principal symptoms or signs of the syndrome should be present in isolation or at least stand out clearly against any other behavioral or neurologic signs. In the

Gerstmann syndrome, this luxury is seldom if ever enjoyed. In cases of the full Gerstmann syndrome, it is very common to find other accompanying signs; some, particularly constructional impairment, nearly always present; others, alexia, color agnosia, and right hemianopia, are found less frequently. Anomic aphasia is very commonly present but can be quite mild; and, as we have noted, aphasia may be totally absent. Despite the fact that associated symptoms are present to varying degrees, this does not detract from the localizing significance of the full syndrome as we discuss in the following section.

Localization

In the many cases of the Gerstmann syndrome described in the literature, the overwhelming majority of patients have had a lesion involving the left parietal lobe (Table 1). Not unexpectedly, a patient with bilateral parietal or diffuse brain disease also can show the full syndrome. Rarely have cases been reported with right hemisphere lesions and these have either been in left-handed patients or in patients whose right parietal lesion was a large tumor with widespread dysfunction from raised intracranial pressure. In general, a right-handed patient presenting with a full Gerstmann syndrome is very likely to have a left parietal lesion. In the study by Heimburger, Demyer, and Reitan (1964), 95% of the patients with the full syndrome had a left parietal lesion.

The syndrome has its greatest utility when other, more strongly, localizing signs are not present. The presence of significant aphasia in a right-handed patient, for example, very quickly and certainly identifies a left hemisphere lesion regardless of the presence or absence of finger agnosia. But the demonstration of the Gerstmann signs in a nonaphasic patient can be of great clinical value. The syndrome can be present in a progressive lesion such as a tumor or noted only as a more significant deficit is regressing. This latter group is no less interesting scientifically yet is of less obvious clinical usefulness.

Of theoretical interest has been the attempt to localize the lesion more discretely within the left parietal lobe. Although of no great additional clinical importance, such an exercise may help us to further understand the complex functioning of the parietal lobe. We disagree with Critchley (1953) that any attempt at more discrete lo-

TABLE 1

Cases of Full Gerstmann Reported in Literature

Author	Case Number	Hemisphere	Location and Type of Lesion
Gerstmann (1924)	1	L	Angular gyrus—vascular
Herrmann and Pötzl (1926)	2	R	Angular gyrus—second occipital gyrus (ambidextrous patient)
Gerstmann (1927, 1930)	1	L	Parieto-occipital—tumor
	2	L	Parieto-occipital—vascular
Lange (1930)		L	Parieto-occipital—temporal
Lange (1933)		L	Parietal
Mussio-Fournier and Rawak (1934)		L	Hemisphere—tumor
Muncie (1935)	1	L	Parieto-occipital—Tumor
	2		Bilateral
Nielsen (1938)	1	L	Hemisphere—posterior, metastatic tumors
Olsen and Ruby (1941)		L	Parietal—vascular
Stengel and Vienna (1944)			Bilateral—vascular
Arbuse (1947)		L	Parieto-occipital—tumor
Critchley (1953)	35118	L	Parietal tumor
	C. S.	L	Parietal tumor
	J. W.	L	Hemisphere vascular
	32579	L	Parietal tumor
	22019	L	Parietal vascular
	25140	L	Hemisphere vascular
	L. B.–J.	L	Temporoparietal—tumor
	A. P.		Bilateral—vascular
	23452		Bilateral parietal—vascular
	F. E. W.		Bilateral atrophy
	24033		Bilateral parieto-occipital vascular
	12621	L	Bilateral—vascular
	36459	L	Angular gyrus—tumor
	35427	L	Hemisphere—tumor

(continued)

TABLE 1 (*continued*)

Author	Case Number	Hemisphere	Location and Type of Lesion
Russell and Espir (1961)	68	L	Anterior superior parietal—missle
Kinsbourne and Warrington (1962)	1		Bilateral atrophy
	2		Bilateral atrophy
	3		Bilateral atrophy
	4		Bilateral atrophy
	5	L & R	Multiple sclerosis
	6	L	Degeneration
	7	L	Posterior parietal—tumor
	8	L	Parieto-occipital—tumor (left-handed)
	9	R	Parieto-temporal—vascular (left-handed)
Heimburger *et al.* (1964)	23 cases Statistical study showing		
	78%	L	Posterior
	13%		Bilateral
	9%	R	Hemisphere (large tumor, no comment as to handedness)
Poeck and Orgass (1966)	4 cases		All left hemisphere or bilateral
Benson and Denckla (1969)	1	L	Posterior parietal—vascular
	2	L	Posterior parietal—tumor
Kinsbourne and Rosenfield (1974)	1	L	Posterior parietotemporal vascular
Strub and Geschwind (1974)	1		Bilateral atrophy
Hrbek (1977)	1	L	Upper-mid parietal—tumor
	2	L	Parietal—tumor
	3	L	Hemisphere—tumor
	4	L	Parietotemporal—hemorrhage
	5	L	Pareital—vascular
	6	L	Inferior parietal—vascular
	7	L	Anterior—mid parietal
	8	L	Parietotemporal—trauma
	9	L	Parietal—not well-localized encephalitis

10	L	Inferior parietal—vascular
11		Bilateral atrophy
12	L	Temporal—tumor (transient symptoms)
13	L	Temporal hemorrhage
14	L	Frontotemporal—tumor
15	L	Frontotemporal—tumor
17		Diffuse embolization
Kertesz (1979) 1	L	Parietal—vascular
2	L	Parietal—vascular
3	L	Parietal—aneurysm
4	L	Parietal—hemorrhage
5		Unspecified—trauma
6	L	Parietal—tumor
7	L	Parietal—tumor
8	L	Parietal—tumor
9		Bilateral—tumor
Rosati et al. (1979) 1	L	Parietotemporo-occipital—tumor
Roeltgen et al. (1983) 1	L	Parietal—infarct

Total	L	Hemisphere	68
		Bilateral	20
	R	Hemisphere	4
	Either L or Bilateral		4 (Poeck & Orgass, 1969)
			96

calization is "a vain and unpromising task." Some of the pathologic material may allow a certain degree of regional localization within the left parietal lobe and can supply indication for further research.

Gerstmann (1930, 1940) felt that the lesion involved the angular gyrus (Figure 1) and contiguous second occipital convolution. Heimburger *et al.* (1964) agreed that the angular gyrus was involved, but not in all cases. They also described some cases in which a lesion restricted to this gyrus did not produce the syndrome. Judging from their data, damage to the angular gyrus is neither essential nor sufficient for the appearance of the syndrome. It should be noted that all their patients with the four Gerstmann signs had large lesions which invariably produced a picture of widespread neurologic dysfunction. Specific localization data for their cases are not reported but their conclusions are well founded.

In a missile wound case reported by Russell and Espir (1961), a severe, nonaphasic Gerstmann syndrome was described with a lesion in the mid and superior left parietal lobe, somewhat superior to, but including, the angular gyrus (Case 68). Hrbek (1977), in an extensive discussion of the syndrome with a description of 17 personally collected cases, argues that the necessary lesion is on the border between supramarginal gyrus and superior parietal lobule. Roeltgen, Sevush, and Heilman (1983) have reported a case of a pure Gerstmann syndrome (all four components and no evidence of aphasia or constructional impairment) in which the lesion in the superior angular gyrus that extended into the supramarginal gyrus and minimally into the inferior parietal gyrus (inferior portion of the superior parietal lobule).

From a review of the reported cases, it appears that the most likely lesion to produce the Gerstmann syndrome is posteriorly placed in the parietal lobe, in the angular gyrus as suggested originally by Gerstmann, but extending into the superior parietal lobule (superior and inferior parietal gyrus) rather than into occipital lobe. Such a lesion seems to produce the syndrome in its least contaminated form. This high lesion, such as the one described by Russell and Espir (1961, Case 68), Kertesz (1979, cases 1 and 7), and Roeltgen, Sevush, and Heilman (1983) is well away from the classic language zone and therefore produces neither aphasia nor alexia. Constructional impairment is present in all but the case of Roeltgen, Sevush and Heilman (1983) and seems almost inexorably associated with the classic four components of the syndrome. It is clear that many patients will show evidence of aphasia because the language zone is quite close and frequently involved.

It is true, and not too surprising, that most lesions of the left parietal lobe will not produce the Gerstmann syndrome but will show other interesting and important neurologic and behavioral signs. This is a separate issue entirely and in no way negates the utility and certainly not the existence of the syndrome.

Discussion

PATHOPHYSIOLOGY AND NEUROPSYCHOLOGY
OF THE SYNDROME

From an analysis of the symptomatology and a description of pathologic data, it is evident that the Gerstmann syndrome represents a complex multifaceted disturbance of dominant parietal function. The basis of the neuropsychologic deficits have been debated and various attempts have been made to establish a single unifying mechanism to explain all findings. Gerstmann attempted to show that a basic disturbance in body schema could explain the entire syndrome. The principal features of finger agnosia and right–left disorientation are aspects of a spatial knowledge of the body, particularly the hand. However, to associate calculation ontogenetically with counting on the fingers and writing with a physiologic differentiation of the fingers may be stretching the concept of body scheme beyond its definition.

Stengel and Vienna (1944) believed that the defect in constructional ability was the basic disturbance. Constructional impairment is admittedly commonly seen with the syndrome and Stengel's case could certainly be explained on the basis of constructional impairment alone. There are, however, many other cases that clearly would not support this hypothesis.

Poeck and Orgass (1966) propose that the Gerstmann syndrome merely reflects a more generalized language disturbance or aphasia. Aphasia often is present because of the propinquity of the language zone to the angular gyrus and superior parietal lobule. An aphasic will demonstrate agraphia and may show difficulty on verbal testing of finger identification, right–left, and calculation. The syndrome produced is often an artifactual Gerstmann syndrome but not as it is commonly understood. We disagree with Poeck and Orgass and also Russell (1963) that to separate the Gerstmann symptoms from an aphasic disorder is an artificial exercise. Agraphia and acalculia are certainly language-related but the concepts of body schema embodied in finger agnosia and right–left sense are very likely distinctly spatial and may not be related to language except through the verbal method of testing.

Kinsbourne and Warrington (1964) suggest that the Gerstmann syndrome is basically a disorder of spatiotemporal sequencing. The correct ordering of fingers on the hand, letters in the word, numbers in the continuum and sides of the body are directly related to spatial and temporal ordering. This is an appealing hypothesis as ordering is a common feature; yet, it may merely reflect a basic analytic function ascribed to the entire left hemisphere. Thus, a common underlying feature may be present but may, in fact, actually be too general a function to be classified as a unifying mechanism.

In our view, there is, at present, no single underlying neuropsychologic defect that can explain the four cardinal symptoms seen in the Gerstmann syndrome. The parietal lobe is a complex and very highly developed region of cortex in which visual, tactile, and auditory–sensory information is processed and stored (Luria, 1966). It is in the parietal lobe that cross-modal associations are probably formed between the sense modalities. Complex kinesthetic patterns also are developed and stored in the parietal lobe; these, in turn, guide highly skilled and complex motor activity. It is obvious that the parietal lobe has many diverse functions and that any lesion will (in all likelihood) disrupt several separate yet interlocking cortical systems. Depending on the exact location and extent of the lesion and the peculiarities of the individual brain in which the lesion occurs, a variety of symptoms and symptom clusters may be seen. In some patients, a specific left parietal lesion will produce a clinical picture of the Gerstmann syndrome. Careful analysis of the individual symptoms and localization data gives us a realistic understanding of the pathophysiology of the symptom complex and allows us to postulate the region of the dominant parietal most likely to be involved (Hrbek, 1977). It seems that a lesion involving the symbolic system of the angular gyrus and kinesthetic system of the superior parietal lobule can produce, in relatively isolated fashion, the four signs of the Gerstmann syndrome accompanied by constructional impairment.

CRITICISM OF THE SYNDROME

In recent years, the Gerstmann syndrome has been assailed on several fronts. To some, it is an enigma (Critchley, 1966); to others, a fiction (Benton, 1961, 1977; Heimburger et al., 1964; Poeck & Orgass, 1966). Since the syndrome has engendered so much controversy in the recent literature, we feel that the principal arguments should be aired to make the reader aware of the issues surrounding the controversy.

Some investigators have argued that the syndrome is intrinsically a part of a broader aphasic disorder (Poeck & Orgass, 1966). In support of this view, Critchley (1966, 1970) speaks of latent or pre-aphasia as a possible explanation of many of the symptoms. We discussed this issue earlier in the chapter and summarize here.

It is true that many individuals with significant aphasia will—because of their aphasia—be unable adequately to perform the more complex tasks described by Gerstmann. The Gerstmann syndrome may be seen in patients with only mild aphasia, in which the Gerstmann components are severe and cannot, therefore, be accounted for by the aphasia. In such a case, it would be unjustified to consider the syndrome as resulting from aphasia. There are, of course, cases of the syndrome in which no aphasia has been demonstrated, evidence that substantially negates the argument that the syndrome is actually part of an aphasic disorder. The question of a latent or preaphasia in this context is somewhat cryptic. Whereas it is true that many functions tested in the Gerstmann components have drawn to a greater or lesser extent on verbal language during development, it seems illogical to call on language errors to explain this syndrome in a clinically nonaphasic patient.

A second issue revolves around a basic misunderstanding about the concept of a syndrome as used in clinical medicine. It has been stated that the correlation among the Gerstmann components is weak and that individual components are more strongly correlated with other deficits (Benton, 1961). Benton (1961) and others state that it is, therefore, not a syndrome at all. We believe, however, that this analysis is based on a fundamental misunderstanding of what traditionally is meant by a syndrome.

The essence of a medical syndrome is that a collection of signs or symptoms, when all present, indicate the presence of a specific disease. The correlation between elements in a syndrome can be low, high, or in-between. Thus, the combination of hoarseness, nystagmus, a Horner's syndrome, pain loss on one side of the face and on the opposite side of the body would lead to the diagnosis of an infarction in the lateral medulla, most commonly as a result of an occlusion in the posterior inferior cerebellar artery or in the vertebral artery from which it springs. It is obvious that, if one were to study a great number of patients, one would find a very low correlation between hoarseness and nystagmus, or between a Horner's syndrome and either of these.

Indeed, a syndrome is most useful as a diagnostic tool precisely when the elements usually are not found together. When they are found together, this strongly points to some special pathological process. Furthermore, the lateral medullary syndrome is composed of elements not based on a disturbance of some common physiological foundation but on proximity of anatomical systems. Other syndromes, in particular, those based on some underlying pathologic disturbance, do have symptoms which have a common pathophysiology, that is, the components of Addison's syndrome or of congestive heart failure. The anatomic studies have shown that the Gerstmann syndrome does predict—with high accuracy—damage to the left parietal lobe and, because of this, the Gerstmann syndrome qualifies as a true clinical syndrome.

A final and very important criticism of the Gerstmann syndrome is that the four elements of the syndrome are not seen in isolation from other neurologic and behavioral findings. Many authors, including Gerstmann himself, have noted that their patients demonstrate associated symptoms. The major point of the criticism is that Gerstmann arbitrarily chose the four elements from personal bias, and might just as easily have chosen another cluster of left parietal symptoms. Certainly, this is a valid point. It is clear, however, that Gerstmann chose his four components very well since, in fact, they do predict left parietal disease with high accuracy. Future research can discover whether there is some other constellation that is even more strongly predictive. There are many interesting behavioral deficits associated with dominant parietal lesions and clinical neurologists (as well as psychologists) should be aware of them. One would hope that, through increased study of cases, a variety of focal behavioral syndromes can be identified. Because of the many functions performed by the dominant parietal lobe, it is obvious that a number of typical syndromes have evolved and will continue to do so. The syndrome of alexia with agraphia with or without anomic aphasia is one well-established example. Unfortunately, much time has been spent in the last 20 years seeking to discredit or support the Gerstmann syndrome rather than establishing the validity of other behavioral syndromes associated with parietal disease.

In conclusion, we can say that Gerstmann made a definite contribution to the study of higher cognitive functioning and that his syndrome is still of clinical value. We would, however, strongly agree with Benton (1961) that many investigators, in their adherence to the four classic symptoms, have often prejudiced their clinical observations and not given adequate attention to other behavioral signs of parietal disease. At this point, it seems far better to end the condemnation or praise of the syndrome and let time place it in its proper perspective in the field of neurobehavior.

References

Arbuse, D. I. (1947). The Gerstmann Syndrome. Case report and review of the literature. *Journal of Nervous and Mental Disease, 105,* 359–371.

Assal, G., Chapuis, G., & Zander, E. (1970). Isolated writing disorders in a patient with stenosis of the left internal carotid artery. *Cortex, 6,* 241–248.

Badal, J. (1888). Contribution à l'étude des cécités psychiques; alexie, agraphe, hémianope inférieure, trouble du sens de l'espace. *Archives Ophtalmologie (Paris), 8,* 97–117.

Basso, A., Taborelli, A., & Vignolo, A. (1978). Dissociated disorders of speaking and writing in aphasia. *Journal of Neurology, Neurosurgery and Psychiatry, 41,* 556–563.

Benson, D. F., & Denckla, M. B. (1969). Verbal paraphasia as a source of calculation disturbance. *Archives of Neurology (Chicago), 21,* 96–102.

Benton, A. L. (1961). The fiction of the "Gerstmann syndrome." *Journal of Neurology, Neurosurgery and Psychiatry, 24,* 176–181.

Benton, A. L., (1968). Right-left discrimination. *Pediatric Clinics of North America, 15,* 747–758.

Benton, A. L. (1977). Reflections on the Gerstmann Syndrome. *Brain and Language, 4,* 45–62.

Benton, A. L. (1979). Body schema disturbances: Finger agnosia and right-left disorientation. In K. M. Heilman & E. Valenstein (Eds.), *Clinical neuropsychology.* London & New York: Oxford University Press, pp. 141–158.

Chédru, F., & Geschwind, N. (1972). Writing disturbances in acute confusional states. *Neuropsychologia, 10,* 343–353.

Critchley, M. (1953). *The parietal lobes.* London: Arnold.

Critchley, M. (1966). The enigma of Gerstmann's syndrome. *Brain, 89,* 183–198.

Critchley, M. (1970). *Aphasiology and other aspects of language.* London: Arnold.

Dennis, M. (1976). Dissociated naming and locating of body parts after left anterior temporal lobe resection: An experimental case study. *Brain and Language, 3,* 147–163.

Exner, S. (1881). *Untersuchungen über die Lokalisation der Funktionen in der Grosshirnrinde des Menschen.* Vienna: W. Braumuller.

Gainotti, G., & Tiacci, C. (1973). The unilateral forms of finger agnosia. *Confinia Neurologia, 35,* 271–284.

Gerstmann, J. (1924). Fingeragnosie: Eine umschriebene Störung der Orientierung am eigenen Körper. *Wiener Klinische Wochenschrift, 37,* 1010–1012.

Gerstmann, J. (1927). Fingeragnosie und isolierte Agraphie, ein neues Syndrom. *Zeitschrift fuer die Gesamte Neurologie und Psychiatrie, 108,* 381–402.

Gerstmann, J. (1930). Zur Symptomatologie der Hirnläsionen im Uebergangsgbeit der unteren Parietal und mittleren Occipitalwindung. *Nervenarzt, 3,* 691–695.

Gerstmann, J. (1940). Syndrome of finger agnosia, disorientation for right and left, agraphia and acalculia. *Archives of Neurology and Psychiatry, 44,* 398–408.

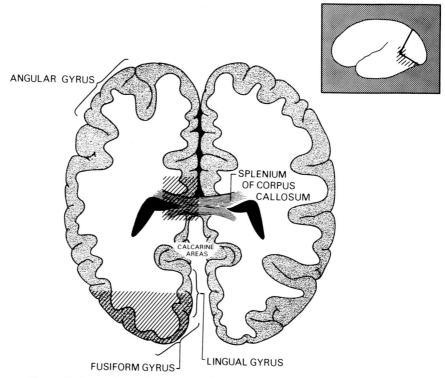

Figure 3. Approximate location of the lesion in cases of splenio-occipital alexia without agraphia or hemianopsia. Note that the lesion spares the left calcarine cortex but undercuts it.

malformations (Ajax *et al.*, 1977), carbon monoxide poisoning (Adler, 1944; Goldstein, Joynt, & Goldblatt, 1971), and trauma (Heilman, 1971). Lühdorf and Paulson (1977) have questioned whether hemianopsia was truly absent in some of these cases.

Color agnosia is one of the most fascinating and least understood concomitants of alexia without agraphia (Benson & Geschwind, 1969; Geschwind & Fusillo, 1966). It is reported to be present in 70% of all cases (I. Gloning *et al.*, 1968). Although many studies have been reported (Damasio, McKee, & Damasio, 1979; Oxbury, Oxbury, & Humphrey, 1969; Stachowiak & Poeck, 1976; Zihl & von Cramon, 1980), the exact nature of the causative lesion remains unknown. In considering this problem, it is important to remember that there are two aspects of color agnosia: color anomia (inability to name colors on visual confrontation) and inability to point to the correct color when the name is given. The former is frequently tested; the latter is not. (See Chapter 17 on achromatopsia.)

Preservation of color naming (i.e., absence of color anomia) is often seen in patients whose occipital lesions are largely ventral to the calcarine regions (Ajax et al., 1977; Greenblatt, 1973; Johansson & Fahlgren, 1979; F. M. Vincent, Sadowsky, Saunders, & Reeves, 1977). This finding suggests that color naming can be mediated by the dorsal outflow tracts of the calcarine regions (cuneus and transverse fasciculus of the cuneus). Even when the patient has a complete right hemianopsia, preservation of the dorsal fibers of the splenium may be sufficient to allow preserved color naming by transfer of visual color information from the intact right calcarine cortex (Cumming et al., 1970). Thus, the clinical absence of color anomia in alexia without agraphia implies either that a splenio-occipital lesion has spared the dorsal outflow tracts of the calcarine cortices or that the lesion is not splenio-occipital (see subangular alexia, this chapter).

HEMIALEXIA

Hemialexia refers to the loss of reading ability in one visual half field. The existence of the syndrome is predictable from Dejerine's original model, in which a lesion of the splenial fibers of the corpus callosum disconnects the right visual cortex from the left hemisphere's language apparatus (Figure 4). Thus, the model also predicts that hemialexia will appear only in the dominant (left) visual field, with preservation of reading on the dominant side.

Clinical evidence for the reality of the syndrome was first reported by Trescher and Ford in 1937 and confirmed by Maspes in 1948. Their patients had posterior callosal sections for surgical approaches to colloid cysts and a tumor. The tests of "reading" were limited to single letters. In 1962, Gazzaniga, Bogen, and Sperry reported left hemialexia for words after complete callosal section for seizure disorders. Subsequent studies have shown that hemialexia for words will result from lesions limited to the posterior corpus callosum (splenium) (Gazzaniga & Freedman, 1973).

Further studies have also shown that hemialexia does not occur in callosal-sectioned patients when the splenium is not involved (Gazzaniga, Risse, Springer, Clark, & Wilson, 1975; Goldstein & Joynt, 1969; Gordon, Bogen, & Sperry, 1971). In fact, normal reading of single words may be demonstrated tachistoscopically even when

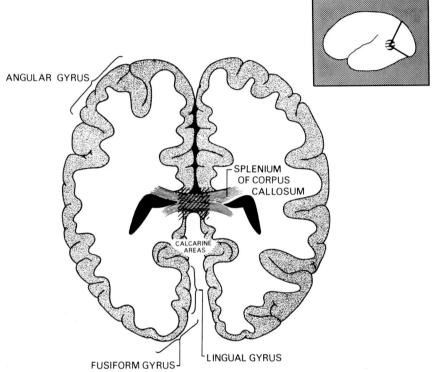

Figure 4. Approximate location of the lesion in hemialexia. The splenial fibers may actually be interrupted somewhat more to either side of the midline.

the splenium is only partially cut (Greenblatt *et al.*, 1980). Analysis of these cases of partial splenial section indicates that the ventral splenial fibers are critical for interhemispheric transfer of written information (Greenblatt *et al.*, 1980). Recent studies in callosal-sectioned patients by Zaidel (1978) indicated that the type of alexia in the right hemisphere patients is similar to that seen in Wernicke's aphasia.

Although the vast majority of hemialexia cases have been related to surgical lesions, there is one report of a transient case in a patient who had a ruptured vascular malformation of the medial anterior occipital lobe, just under the splenium (Wechsler, 1972). When similar tachistoscopic testing is performed on patients who have agenesis of the corpus callosum, there are some deficiencies in reading of single words, especially among those whose agenesis is complete rather than partial (Ettlinger, Blakemore, Milner, & Wilson, 1972, 1974).

Occipital Alexia

It follows from Dejerine's original explanation of pure alexia that removal of the dominant occipital lobe should produce the syndrome if the angular gyrus is spared. The reality of this prediction was established in 1952 by the report of Hécaen *et al.*, who described the alexic sequelae of occipital lobectomies in seven patients. Two broad generalizations have been elicited from their report: (1) Post-occipital lobectomy alexias are usually transient; but (2) even when there is significant functional recovery of reading, patients often find sustained reading to be difficult or even downright disagreeable (Geschwind, 1965). In other words, reading is no longer an automatic and efficient process. Despite the importance of their observations, the lengthy paper of Hécaen *et al.* is subject to the same criticisms that apply to the scattered case reports that preceded it (Foerster, 1929; German & Fox, 1934; Penfield & Evans, 1934; C. Vincent, David, & Puech, 1930). The lesions themselves were of varying types, sizes, and shapes. More importantly, the surgical resections varied considerably in location and size. Theoretically, it might be logical to talk about three kinds of occipital lobectomies: complete lobectomies, partial lateral lobectomies, and partial medial lobectomies. In practice, however, the first two types can be dealt with together, because lateral lobectomies are often done for decompression of lesions that are invading the whole occipital lobe.

The above generalizations, derived from the report of Hécaen *et al.*, actually apply best to the alexias after complete or lateral occipital lobectomies for infiltrating lesions (Figure 5). These patients usually have right (dominant) hemianopsia, so one can conclude that the splenial fibers coming from the intact right hemisphere are affected either by edema related to the surgery or by direct infiltration by the lesion. Because many of these patients have malignant tumors, long-term followup is precluded by deterioration and death (Hamanaka & Ikemura, 1968; Thiébaut, Philippides, Helle, & Ruch, 1954).

In contrast to this situation, alexias after medial occipital lobectomies often have a better prognosis (Greenblatt, Mattis, Swerdlow, & Ancede, 1979). In fact, these cases are actually medial occipital lobe retractions, usually done for excision of medial occipital (falx or medial tentorial) meningiomas or other medially located, extra-axial masses (Figure 6). In other words, the surgical maneuver requires relatively little tissue removal. Most of the occipital lobe is simply retracted to allow access to the tumor. These patients have

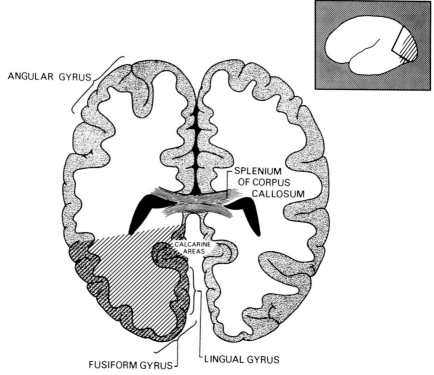

Figure 5. Approximate location of the lesion in lateral or holo-occipital alexia resulting from large occipital lobectomies that spare the angular gyrus. If the surgical or pathological lesion invades the splenium, then the anatomical situation is the same as in splenio-occipital alexia without agraphia (Figure 2).

better long-term prognoses, both for reading and for life itself. However, they may require 1 year or more to recover reasonably efficient reading.

The existence of this syndrome of pure alexia after medial occipital lobectomy carries with it some interesting anatomical implications. Like almost all occipital lobectomy patients, these people have right (dominant) hemianopsias, but their spleniums have not been invaded. In the immediate postoperative period, one could (and probably should) attribute their alexias to edema in the white matter, affecting the splenial fibers. However, if that were the only explanation, they should recover reading in a matter of weeks, not months or years. Moreover, this would be especially true if there were *direct* splenial fibers from right visual association cortex to

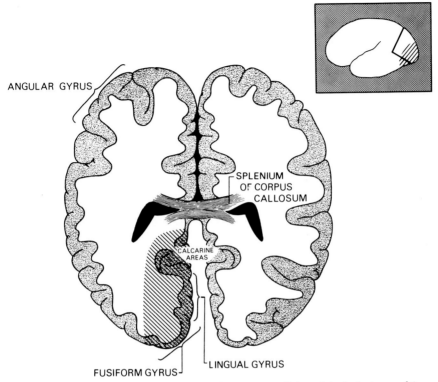

Figure 6. Approximate location of the lesion in medial occipital alexia resulting from surgical approaches to medial occipital lesions. Note the relative sparing of the lateral occipital cortex. If the surgical or pathological lesion invades the splenium, then the anatomical situation is the same as in splenio-occipital alexia without agraphia (Figure 2).

the left angular gyrus. That is, if such fibers do exist, they would be well on the periphery of the lobectomy and retraction. One would then expect the alexia to recover rapidly and thoroughly. Since it does not, the likelihood is that the angulopedal pathway from the right visual association areas has an obligatory connection with homologous areas on the left, in accordance with Flechsig's rule (Flechsig, 1901). Only through this connection can lexic signals from the right hemisphere reach the left angular gyrus.

The preceding anatomical conclusions allow clarification of some of the difficulties in understanding the post-occipital lobectomy alexias. In the complete or lateral lobectomy syndrome, most of the ventral occipital association cortex is removed or invaded by tumor. Even if the splenial fibers from the right are preserved, they find no occipital association cortex with which to connect on the left. Recovery of reading is never fully efficient. On the other hand, in the medial lobectomy syndrome, the entire field of left lateral occipital cortex remains unscathed. Therefore, the splenial fibers from the right can connect to a substantial amount of left occipital association cortex and thence to the angular gyrus. From this, one further conclusion can be reached. It is unlikely that the left lingual gyrus is absolutely critical for reading, as it is usually invaded by medial occipital retraction.

Although it was stated above that alexias resulting from lateral or complete occipital lobectomies can usually be considered together, this is not always the case. Ventrolateral, noninfiltrating tumors have been found in association with pure alexia (C. Vincent *et al.*, 1930; F. M. Vincent & Reeves, 1980). In addition, infarctions limited to the left ventrolateral occipital regions also have been reported in pure alexia (Johansson & Fahlgren, 1979). It is presumed that these infarctions have occurred in the distribution of the lateral branch of the posterior cerebral artery. In these ventrolateral cases, whether caused by tumor or infarction, contralateral hemianopsia has been a variable feature and color anomia has been absent. Although the lesions in these cases may be largely confined to the left occipital lobe, they are subangular in terms of the disconnection mechanism that is responsible for their associated alexias.

SUBANGULAR ALEXIA

Given the central importance of the angular gyrus for reading, any lesion (or combination of lesions) that disconnects the angular gyrus from its visual lexic input should cause alexia without agraphia. Dejerine, and others since his time (Benson & Geschwind, 1969; Goldstein, *et al.*, 1971), have predicted that a lesion undercutting the afferent white matter connections to the angular gyrus would cause pure alexia (Figure 7). Such a case was reported by Greenblatt in 1976. The patient was a right-handed woman who had an unruptured arteriovenous malformation just deep to the left posterior insula. It was excised through a cortical incision at the temporooccipital junction, although the incision may have extended slightly upward into parietal cortex. In the immediate postoperative period, the patient had a severe alexia without agraphia. This finding began

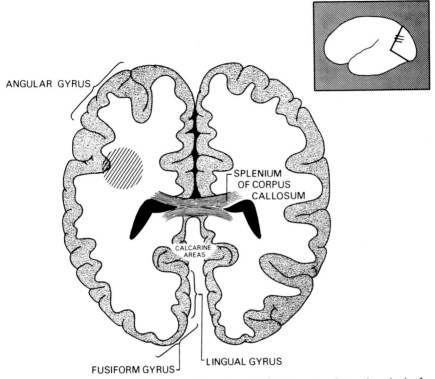

ANGULAR GYRUS

SPLENIUM
OF CORPUS
CALLOSUM

CALCARINE
AREAS

FUSIFORM GYRUS

LINGUAL GYRUS

Figure 7. Approximate location of the subcortical lesion in subangular alexia. In most cases, the actual lesion is larger; the illustration shows the critical part of those lesions, that undercut the angular gyrus on its afferent side. As shown, the lesion would not produce an accompanying hemianopsia. It would do so if it extended further inferiorly into the optic radiations.

to clear in a few days, but some reading disability persisted for a few months. The anatomical localization of this surgical lesion was described by Greenblatt as "subangular."

Since Greenblatt's report, three other cases of pure alexia have been ascribed to this subangular mechanism (Orgogozo, Pere, & Strube, 1979; Pirozzolo, Kerr, Obrzut, Morley, Haxby, & Lundgren, 1981). The report of Pirozzolo et al. (1981) is particularly interesting, because their patient also had mixed transcortical aphasia. This additional finding implies that the white matter lesion associated with subangular alexia is probably in the posterior subcortical watershed distribution of the left hemisphere's vascular supply.

Several other reports in the literature can also be interpreted as having had subangular lesions, though their authors did not specifically explain them by that mechanism (Assal & Hadj-Djilani, 1976; Beauvois, Saillant, Meininger, & Lhermitte, 1978; Brust, 1980; Denckla & Bowen, 1973; Fincham, Nibbelink, & Aschenbrener, 1975; Hoff & Pötzl, 1937; Sroka, Solsi, & Bornstein, 1973; Staller, Buchanan, Singer, Lappin, & Webb, 1978; Turgman et al., 1979; F. M. Vincent et al., 1977). The cases of lateral occipital infarction discussed by Johansson and Fahlgren (1979) also can be added to this list, noting that the kinds of pathology in these cases have been quite variable. In addition to the vascular malformations (Greenblatt, 1976; Sroka et al., 1973) and infarctions (Orgogozo et al., 1979; Pirozzolo et al., 1981) already mentioned, there have been intracerebral hematomas (Assal & Hadj-Djilani, 1976; Beauvois et al., 1978), mtastatic tumors (Fincham et al., 1975; Turgman et al., 1979), head injury (Staller et al., 1978), malignant glioma (Hoff & Pötzl, 1937), and meningioma (F. M. Vincent et al., 1977).

In their report of a case of multiple metastases of malignant melanoma, Fincham et al. (1975) concluded that they could not explain their patient's pure alexia in terms of Dejerine's hypothesis. However, their published anatomical figures show subcortical demyelination and edema under the left occipitoparietal junction.

Visual field deficits are variable in subangular alexia. It is common to have no deficit at all (Assal & Hadj-Djilani, 1976; Greenblatt, 1976; Hoff & Pötzl, 1937; Pirozzolo et al., 1981; F. M. Vincent et al., 1977). Another common pattern is right upper quadrantopsia (Johansson & Fahlgren, 1979; Orgogozo et al., 1979; Staller et al., 1978). Complete right homonymous hemianopsia has been reported (Turgman et al., 1979), but in some cases, this early finding evolves into a right upper quadrantopsia (Sroka et al., 1973). This variability is consistent with the location of the lesions in the lateral left occipitotemporal region. The frequent finding of right upper quadrantopsia (and absence of reports of residual right lower quadrantopsia) emphasizes the location of the lesion inferior to the angular gyrus. If the lesion actually were in the parietal lobe, the visual defect would be in the contralateral inferior quadrant.

In splenio-occipital alexia without hemianopsia, it has been postulated that preservation of color naming is related to the preservation of dorsal outflow tracts from the left calcarine cortex to the cuneus (Greenblatt, 1973). Since these areas are dorsomedial to the lesions responsible for subangular alexia, it makes sense that color anomia is usually mild or absent in subangular alexia.

Angulotemporal Alexias

The alexias associated with lesions of the dominant angular gyrus are generally accompanied by varying degrees of aphasia. Beyond this incontrovertible statement, nothing else is very clear. As usual, the major difficulties concern two different aspects of the problem, the clinical and the anatomical. At the clinical level, the most fundamental problem relates to the severity of the accompanying aphasia (Kertesz, 1979). Anatomically, of course, the important questions have to do with the boundaries of the lesion. In an earlier section of this chapter, the angular gyrus was described as the "central common pathway" for reading. The factors of its critical centrality in the reading process and its relatively small size have combined to make precise analysis of its role in reading very difficult to sort out.

Alexia with Agraphia

Clinically, alexia with agraphia is almost always accompanied by some degree of posterior aphasia, at least to the extent of a mild anomia. Benson and Geschwind (1969) implied that cases with relatively mild aphasic disturbances are not uncommon, but Newcombe and Ratcliff (1979) found they are quite rare. In any case, they are real. When relatively pure cases of alexia with agraphia are found, the location of the lesion invariably involves the left angular gyrus (Albert, 1979; Benson, 1979; Benson & Geschwind, 1969; Kertesz, 1979; Wechsler et al., 1972) (Figure 8). There have been no major attempts to try to correlate particular regions of the angular gyrus with specific varieties of the clinical syndrome. However, Nielsen (1939) made some steps in this direction. He did so by analyzing the boundaries of the lesion that may be associated with alexia with agraphia.

At the clinical level, Nielsen (1939) made the seemingly straightforward distinction between *recognition* of a word and *comprehension* of a word. He assumed that recognition is a necessary prerequisite for comprehension. Using this distinction and its attendant assumption, he studied 3 cases of left temporal lobectomy with known margins of excision. He also analyzed 17 anatomically similar cases from the literature. Nielsen stated that the angular

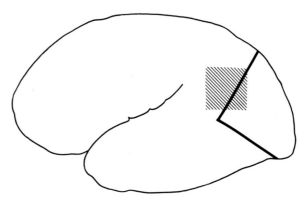

Figure 8. Diagrammatic representation of the cortical lesion in alexia with agraphia. The angular gyrus is destroyed without significant extension into adjacent parietotemporal cortex, except inferiorly.

gyrus suffices to recognize words but not generally to comprehend them. Although the sophistication of clinical neurolinguistics has increased enormously since Nielsen, his anatomical conclusions have not been superseded.

The angular gyrus is bounded anteriorly by the supramarginal gyrus (the other major component of the inferior parietal lobule), superiorly (medially) by the superior parietal gyrus, posteriorly by the occipital lobe, and inferiorly by the first (superior) and second (middle) temporal gyri. Nielsen (1939) concluded that the boundaries of the lesion associated with alexia and agraphia are coterminal with those of the angular gyrus, except inferiorly, where the angular gyrus meets the posterior aspect of the first temporal convolution. This cortical region includes Wernicke's area.

As summarized by Nielsen (1939), Henschen had postulated that the angular gyrus alone could not comprehend words without involving Wernicke's area in the process. As a general rule, Nielsen concurred in this statement. However, Henschen himself described a case in which the angular gyrus appeared to have carried out this function in the absence of Wernicke's area.

Nielsen (1939) described similar cases, and therefore concluded that, *"The area concerned with comprehension of the visual word* extends from Wernicke's area into the angular gyrus. This area is bounded superiorly by Brodmann's area 40, posteriorly by area 39 with which it merges, inferiorly by 21 and anteriorly by 42." Nonetheless, it is also true that, "In a few cases comprehension of the written word can be accomplished without the presence of the posterior portion of the superior temporal convolution if the angular gyrus is intact." This latter statement is also supported by several case reports in the more recent literature (Heilman, Rothi, Campanella, & Wolfson, 1979; Hier & Mohr, 1977; Michel, 1979). In some cases, localization was known only from radioisotope studies (Heilman et al., 1979) that are difficult to interpret, but two cases have been localized in life by CT (Hier & Mohr, 1977; Michel, 1979).

One more intriguing possibility remains. It follows from the preceding discussion that alexia for comprehension might result from a lesion that simply disconnects the angular gyrus from Wernicke's area. Nielsen (1939) summarized a single case report by Heubner that appeared to be a real example of this phenomenon. Interestingly, Heubner's patient had mixed transcortical aphasia but no agraphia. The angulotemporal disconnection in this case was shown by the patient's preserved ability to read aloud (implying normal word recognition), albeit without comprehension. This important finding differentiates Heubner's case from the more recent report of Pirozzolo et al. (1981), whose seemingly similar, subangular patient could not read aloud. The occurrence of transcortical alexia in association with a temporal lesion due to trauma has been documented recently by Bub and Kertesz (1982). This patient could read aloud complex words as well as nonwords without comprehending what she was reading (transcortical alexia) as long as the words were orthographically regular. Orthographically irregular words like "ache" were misread: "atje" (surface dyslexia).

ALEXIA WITH AGRAPHIA AND APHASIA

Alexia, as an accompanying phenomenon in the context of Wernicke's aphasia (Figure 9), is discussed in Chapter 8 of this volume. Suffice it to say here that isolated alexia without aphasia is not seen with strictly temporal lesions. Nielsen (1939) summarized one case by Leva (Nielsen's Case 7) that approximated this situation, but there was some disturbance of auditory comprehension.

Postangular Alexia

Theoretically, it might be argued that the alexias resulting from lesions of the temporal lobe (or at the angulotemporal junction) are actually postangular, because they involve pathways which are ef-

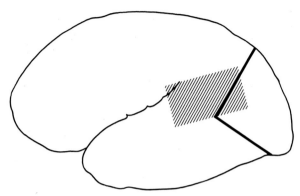

Figure 9. Diagrammatic representation of the cortical lesion in alexia with agraphia and aphasia. The lesion extends anteriorly and inferiorly beyond the angular gyrus.

ferent from the angular gyrus. We have seen, however, that the anatomical and functional interrelationships of the angular gyrus and adjacent temporal regions are so intimate as to defy anatomical classification at this time. For practical purposes, therefore, my use of the term "postangular alexia" is essentially synonymous with Benson's use of the terms "frontal alexia" (1979) and "anterior alexia" (1977).

As Benson (1977) pointed out, it has been known for a long time that some alexic elements often accompany Broca's aphasia (Figure 10). Because of theoretical problems, however, it has been difficult for many authorities to accept the existence of alexia in the context of an anterior aphasic lesion. Nonetheless, the phenomenon is real. Given the nonfluent nature of their concomitant auditory language disorder, it is not surprising that Broca's aphasics have trouble reading aloud, but they have more trouble reading single letters than whole words. The important point is that these patients have "true" alexias, because they have varying degrees of comprehension difficulties, and they make characteristic semantic and phonological errors. The distinction of impaired letter versus word reading, which has been known since Wernicke, has been further elaborated by the recent interest in deep dyslexia (Marshall & Newcombe, 1973). Deep dyslexics read whole words but they cannot read through phonological analysis. It has been found on a preliminary analysis that there is a higher incidence of deep dyslexia among Broca's aphasics (Kertesz, 1982).

Until recently, the only localizing information for postangular alexia was based largely on clinical examination (Benson, 1977).

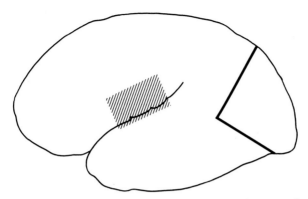

Figure 10. Diagrammatic representation of the cortical
lesion in preangular alexia. The lesion probably involves
Broca's area and significant amounts of adjacent cortex.

Among all of Benson's 61 patients, alexia was the only clinical feature suggestive of a lesion outside the frontal lobe. In 1982 Kirshner
and Webb reported the presence of postangular alexia in 2 Broca's
patients and in 2 patients with global aphasia. A CT scan in 1 Broca's
patient showed a large left frontal infarct sparing the temporal lobe,
and a CT in a global patient showed a large left frontotemporal and
parietal lesion.

Since the lesion responsible for Broca's aphasia often is extensive,
it is difficult to know exactly which part of the lesion is responsible
for the reading abnormality. In some recent studies (Kertesz, 1979;
Mohr, Pessin, Finkelstein, Funkenstein, Duncan, & Davis, 1978) it
has been shown that the posterior margins of lesions causing Broca's aphasia may extend well into the opercular and even peri-Sylvian regions. This leads to the speculation that postangular alexia
may be due to disconnection of the angular area from the more frontal region by lesions deep in the white matter under the parieto-
frontal cortex. This idea is supported by the observation that reading
comprehension is not generally disturbed in aphemia, a condition
whose causative lesion is usually said to be more tightly restricted
to the frontal lobe (Brown, 1972; Ruff & Arbit, 1981).

Ideographic Alexia

Most Western alphabets are essentially phonetic symbol systems.
However, some writing systems are more directly pictographic
(ideographic), notably Chinese. Japanese writing is a combination

of both, the *kana* portion being phonetic and the *kanji* (ideographic) part being derived from Chinese. Because of this unusual mixture in their written language, the analysis of Japanese alexics holds special interest for the investigation of the anatomical correlates of the acquired alexias. Among the small number of Japanese cases that have been adequately reported, it appears that *kana* and *kanji* are equally impaired in the preangular alexias (Hirose *et al.*, 1977; Kurachi, Yamaguchi, Inasaka, & Torii, 1979), but there is a dissociation when the lesion is angulotemporal (Yamadori, 1975) or more diffusely peri-Sylvian (Sasanuma, 1975). With the angular and peri-Sylvian lesions, the patients lose their ability to read the phonetic alphabet (*kana*) much more than they lose the ideographic (*kanji*).

The two preangular patients (with alexia for *kana* and *kanji*) had posterior cerebral artery infarctions resulting in classical splenio-occipital alexia with contralateral hemianopsias (Hirose *et al.*, 1977; Kurachi *et al.*, 1979). Therefore, lexic information had to enter the nondominant hemispheres initially. If the *kanji* were being selectively processed by the nondominant hemispheres, then these patients should have been able to read in that ideographic script.

Further evidence along the same lines is provided by a recent study of three Japanese hemialexics (Sugishita, Iwata, Toyokura, Yoshioka, & Yamada, 1978). During the first year after their splenial sections, these patients had equal difficulties with *kana* and *kanji*. It was only later that the investigators began to find some differential improvement of *kanji* reading in the left visual fields. This very late and quite relative recovery of *kanji* does not allow one to decide whether the improvement was mediated by processes in the right or left hemispheres, or both. Since there have not been any reports of right brain lesions resulting in selective *kanji* alexia, it seems unlikely that the nondominant hemisphere plays any major interpretive role in the normal reading of *kanji* script.

Among three Japanese patients who had presumed or proven angular gyrus lesions, two had no visual field defects (Yamadori, 1975). Therefore, lexic information was available to both hemispheres. Although reading was impaired in both alphabet systems, the *kana* (phonetic) suffered more in the absence of the dominant angular gyrus. The preceding information concerning Japanese reading in the preangular alexias makes it unlikely that the nondominant hemisphere is responsible for the greater preservation of *kanji* in angulotemporal alexia. Therefore, one is forced to conclude either that the *kanji* is selectively processed elsewhere in the dominant hemisphere, or, more likely, that it is processed more diffusely on the dominant side. This conclusion is somewhat at variance with that of Benson (1979), who interprets the contemporary literature to mean that *kana* is processed more anteriorly than *kanji* in the language apparatus of the dominant hemisphere. In support of Benson is the suggested evidence that deep dyslexics (who cannot read phonologically, like *kana* impairment) have frontoparietal lesions (Marin, 1980) and are often associated with Broca's aphasia (Kertesz, 1982).

Musical Alexia

The ability to read, write, and perform music is similar to the reading of other language systems in that it requires extensive training and practice to reach a reasonable level of efficiency. However, the multiplicity of the various interdigitated skills is so complex that attempts to localize the amusias have been largely unrewarding (Wertheim, 1977). *Musical alexia*, the acquired inability to read music, is one of the amusias. In proficient musicians who suffer focal brain insults, musical alexias may accompany alexia for ordinary language, but isolated alexia for music has not been reported in the absence of other linguistic or musical disabilities (Benton, 1977).

In general, there is a tantalizing tendency for specific musical disabilities to be similar to individual patients' other language disorders (e.g., musical alexia with alexia for words [Brust, 1980; Levin & Rose, 1979]) but the clinical syndromes are complicated by the complexities of musical interpretation and performance.

Thalamic Alexia

The problem of thalamic participation in language and its disorders is discussed in Chapter 11 of the present volume. For the purposes of this chapter, the present state of affairs in this highly unsettled area is summarized by these statements: (1) When disorders of auditory language are found in patients with known thalamic lesions, alexia and/or agraphia are often part of the clinical picture. However, the severity of the reading disability is usually proportional to the degree of aphasia (Benson, 1979; Darley, Brown, & Swenson, 1975). (2) Although thalamic and other diencephalic lesions have been anatomically well defined in patients who had alexia with or without agraphia (Barat, Mazaux, Bioulac, Giroire, Vital, & Arné, 1981; Van Buren, 1979), there has never been a clear case report of an alexic patient without aphasia with only a thalamic lesion.

Acquired Alexias in Childhood

Despite the potential importance of this subject, very little is known about it. This dearth of information is particularly striking in view of the huge debate that has been engendered by questions of lateralization and localization in developmental dyslexia (Benton & Pearl, 1978).

Localization of acquired auditory disorders in childhood has also received some attention (Ludlow, 1980). Perhaps the problem is related to the difficulty of defining the end of the period of childhood in relationship to the acquisition of efficient, adult literacy. This should not be insurmountable. In contemporary Western society, large numbers of normal children achieve functional literacy in the last few years of their first decade. Even so, in the recent literature, there is but one report of acquired alexia in childhood that includes localizing information.

Skoglund (1979) described a normally intelligent, 11-year-old boy who developed mitochondrial myopathy associated with left hemianopsia and alexia without agraphia. His initial CT was normal, but 9 months later, there were bilateral parietooccipital lucencies. The smaller, left-sided lucency was located just where one might expect to see the lesion of subangular alexia. The patient's reading improved with steroid therapy. Because of the bilateral nature of the lesions and the concomitant hemianopsia, one cannot use this case to draw valid conclusions about lateralization of alexogenic lesions at this child's age. However, it does show that focal hemispheric lesions in children may be associated with specific alexia syndromes.

References

Adler, A. (1944). Disintegration and restoration of optic recognition in visual agnosia. *Archives of Neurology and Psychiatry, 51,* 243–259.

Ajax, E. T. (1967). Dyslexia without agraphia. *Archives of Neurology (Chicago), 17,* 645–652.

Ajax, E. T., Schenkenberg, T., & Kosteljanetz, M. (1977). Alexia without agraphia and the inferior splenium. *Neurology, 27,* 685–688.

Alajouanine, P. T. (1960). *Les grandes activités du lobe occipital.* Paris: Masson.

Albert, M. L. (1979). Alexia. In K. M. Heilman, E. Valenstein (Eds.), *Clinical neuropsychology.* London & New York: Oxford, pp. 59–91.

Assal, G., & Hadj-Djilani, M. (1976). Une nouvelle observation d'aléxie pure sans hémianopsie. *Cortex, 12,* 169–174.

Barat, M., Mazaux, J. M., Bioulac, B., Giroire, J. M., Vital, C., & Arné, L. (1981). Troubles du langage de type aphasique et lésions putamino-caudées. *Revue Neurologique, 137,* 343–356.

Beauvois, M., Saillant, B., Meininger, V., & Lhermitte, F. (1978). Bilateral tactile aphasia: A tacto-verbal dysfunction. *Brain, 101,* 381–401.

Benson, D. F. (1977). The third alexia. *Archives of Neurology (Chicago), 34,* 327–331.

Benson, D. F. (1979). *Aphasia, alexia, and agraphia.* Edinburgh & London: Churchill-Livingstone.

Benson, D. F. (1981). Alexia and the neuroanatomical basis of reading. In F. J. Pirozzolo & M. C. Wittrock (Eds.); *Neuropsychological and cognitive processes in reading.* New York: Academic Press, pp. 69–92.

Benson, D. F., & Geschwind, N. (1969). The alexias. In P. Vinken & G. Bruyn (Eds.), *Handbook of clinical neurology* (Vol. 4). Amsterdam: North-Holland, pp. 112–140.

Benson, D. F., & Tomlinson, E. B. (1971). Hemiplegic syndrome of the posterior cerebral artery. *Stroke, 2,* 559–564.

Benton, A. L. (1977). The amusias. In M. Critchley & R. Henson (Eds.), *Music and the brain.* Springfield, Ill.: Thomas, pp. 378–397.

Benton, A. L., & Pearl, D. (Eds.) (1978). *Dyslexia. An appraisal of current knowledge.* London & New York: Oxford University Press.

Boucher, M., Kopp, N., Tommasi, M., & Schott, B. (1976). Observation anatomo-clinique d'un cas d'alexie sans agraphie. *Revue Neurologique, 132,* 656–659.

Boucher, M., Michel, F., Tommasi, M., & Schott, B. (1975). Alexie sans agraphie. In F. Michel & B. Schott (Eds.), *Les syndromes de disconnexion calleuse chez l'homme.* Lyon: Hôpital Neurologique, pp. 371–379.

Brown, J. W. (1972). *Aphasia, apraxia and agnosia.* Springfield, Ill.: Thomas.

Brust, J. C. M. (1980). Music and language. Musical alexia and agraphia. *Brain, 103,* 367–392.

Bub, D., & Kertesz, A. (1982). *Lexical processing in a transcortical alexic.* Presented to the International Neuropsychological Society, Pittsburgh, February.

Caplan, L. R., & Hedley-Whyte, T. (1974). Cuing and memory dysfunction in alexia without agraphia. *Brain, 97,* 251–262.

Cohen, D. N., Salanga, V. D., Hully, W., Steinberg, M. C., & Hardy, R. W. (1976). Alexia without agraphia. *Neurology, 26,* 455–459.

Cumming, W. J. K., Hurwitz, L. J., & Perl, N. T. (1970). A study of a patient who had alexia without agraphia. *Journal of Neurology, Neurosurgery and Psychiatry, 33,* 34–39.

Damasio, A. R., McKee, J., Damasio, H. (1979). Determinants of performance in color anomia. *Brain and Language, 7,* 74–85.

Darley, F. L., Brown, J. R., & Swenson, W. M. (1975). Language changes after neurosurgery for Parkinsonism. *Brain and Language, 2,* 65–69.

Dejerine, J. (1891). Sur un cas de cécité verbale avec agraphie, suivi d'autopsie. *Comptes Rendus des Séances de la Société de Biologie et de Ses Filiales, 3,* 197–201.

Dejerine, J. (1892). Contribution à l'étude anatomo-pathologique et clinique des différentes variétés de cécité verbale. *Comptes Rendus des Séances de la Société de Biologie et de Ses Filiales, 4,* 61–90.

Dejerine, J., & Vialet, N. (1893). Contribution à l'étude de la localisation anatomique de la cécité verbale pure. *Comptes Rendus des Séances de la Société de Biologie et de Ses Filiales, 11,* 790–793.

Denckla, M. B., & Bowen, F. P. (1973). Dyslexia after left occipitotemporal lobectomy: A case report. *Cortex, 9,* 321–328.

Dennis, M., Lovett, M., & Wiegel-Crump, C. A. (1981). Written language acquisition after left or right hemidecortication in infancy. *Brain and Language, 12,* 54–91.

Erkulvrawatr, S. (1978). Alexia and left homonymous hemianopsia in a non-right hander. *Annals of Neurology, 3,* 549–552.

Ettlinger, G., Blakemore, C. B., Milner, A. D., & Wilson, J. (1972). Agenesis of the corpus callosum: A further behavioural investigation. *Brain, 97,* 225–234.

Ettlinger, G., Blakemore, C. B., Milner, A. D., & Wilson, J. (1974). Agenesis of the corpus callosum: A further behavioural investigation. *Brain, 97,* 225–234.

Fincham, F. W., Nibbelink, D. W., & Aschenbrener, C. A. (1975). Alexia with left homonymous hemianopsia without agraphia. *Neurology, 25,* 1164–1168.

Flechsig, P. (1901). Developmental (myelogenetic) localisation in the cerebral cortex in the human subject. *Lancet, 2,* 1027–1029.

Foerster, O. (1929). Beiträge zur pathophysiologie der sehbahn und der sehsphäre. *Journal für Psychologie und Neurologie, 39,* 463–485.

Foix, C., & Hillemand, P. (1925). Role vraisemblable du splénium dans la pathogénie de l'aléxie pure par lésion de la cérébrale postérieure. *Bulletins et Memoires de la Société Médicale des Hôpitaux de Paris, 49,* 393–395.

Gazzaniga, M. S., Bogen, J. E., & Sperry, R. W. (1962). Some functional effects of sectioning the cerebral commissures in man. *Proceedings of the National Academy of Sciences of the U.S.A., 48,* 1765–1769.

Gazzaniga, M. S., & Freedman, H. (1973). Observations on visual processes after posterior callosal section. *Neurology, 23,* 1126–1130.

Gazzaniga, M. S., Risse, G. L., Springer, S. P., Clark, E., & Wilson, D. H. (1975). Psychologic and neurologic consequences of partial and complete cerebral commissurotomy. *Neurology, 25,* 10–15.

German, W. J., & Fox, J. C. (1934). Observations following unilateral lobectomies. *Research Publications—Association for Research in Nervous and Mental Disease, 13,* 378–434.

Geschwind, N. (1962). The anatomy of acquired disorders of reading. In J. Money (Ed.), *Reading disability.* Baltimore: Johns Hopkins Press, pp. 115–129.

Geschwind, N. (1965). Disconnexion syndromes in animals and man. Part I. *Brain, 88,* 237–294.

Geschwind, N., & Fusillo, M. (1966). Color-naming defects in association with alexia. *Archives of Neurology (Chicago), 15,* 137–146.

Gloning, I., Gloning, K., & Hoff, H. (1968). *Neuropsychological symptoms and syndromes in lesions of the occipital lobe and the adjacent areas.* Paris: Gauthier-Villars.

Gloning, I., Gloning, K., & Jellinger, K. (1966). *Tschabitscher:* Zur dominanzfrage beim syndrom: Reine wortblindheit-farbagnosie. *Neuropsychologia, 4,* 27–40.

Gloning, I., Gloning, K., Seitelberger, F., & Tschabitscher, H. (1955). Ein fall von reiner wortblindheit mit obduktionsbefund. *Wiener Zeitschrift für Nervenheilkunde und Deren Grenzgebiete, 12,* 194–215.

Gloning, K. (1977). Handedness and aphasia. *Neuropsychologia, 15,* 355–358.

Goldstein, M. N., & Joynt, R. J. (1969). Long-term follow-up of a callosal-sectioned patient. *Archives of Neurology (Chicago), 20,* 96–102.

Goldstein, M. N., Joynt, R. J., & Goldblatt, D. (1971). Word blindness with intact central visual fields. *Neurology, 9,* 873–876.

Gordon, H. W., Bogen, J. E., & Sperry, R. W. (1971). Absence of deconnexion syndrome in two patients with partial section of the neocommissures. *Brain, 94,* 327–336.

Greenblatt, S. H. (1973). Alexia without agraphia or hemianopsia. *Brain, 96,* 307–316.

Greenblatt, S. H. (1976). Subangular alexia without agraphia or hemianopsia. *Brain and Language, 3,* 229–245.

Greenblatt, S. H. (1977). Neurosurgery and the anatomy of reading: A practical review. *Neurosurgery, 1,* 6–15.

Greenblatt, S. H., Mattis, S., Swerdlow, J. L., & Ancede, A. (1979). *The alexic syndromes of dominant (left) occipital lobectomy.* Paper presented to the International Neuropsychological Society, New York.

Greenblatt, S. H., Saunders, R. L., Culver, C. M., & Bogdanowicz, W. (1980). Normal interhemispheric visual transfer with incomplete section of the splenium. *Archives of Neurology (Chicago), 37,* 567–571.

Halsey, J. H., Blauenstein, U. W., Wilson, E. M., & Wills, E. L. (1980). rCBF activation in a patient with right homonymous hemianopia and alexia without agraphia. *Brain and Language, 9,* 137–140.

Hamanaka, T., & Ikemura, Y. (1968). On the neuropsychology of pure alexia—a case of pure alexia with an occipital lobectomy. *Psychiatria et Neurologia Japonica, 70,* 689–700 (in Japanese).

Hécaen, H., & Albert, M. L. (1978). *Human neuropsychology.* New York: Wiley.

Hécaen, H., de Ajuriaguerra, J., & David, M. (1952). Les deficits fonctionnels aprés lobectomie occipitale. *Montasschrift fuer Psychiatrie und Neurologie, 123,* 239–291.

Hécaen, H., & Sauguet, J. (1971). Cerebral dominance in left-handed subjects. *Cortex, 7,* 19–48.

Heilman, K. M., Rothi, L., Campanella, D., & Wolfson, S. (1979). Wernicke's and global aphasia without alexia. *Archives of Neurology, (Chicago), 36,* 129–133.

Heilman, K. M., Safran, A., & Geschwind, N. (1971). Closed head trauma and aphasia. *Journal of Neurology, Neurosurgery, and Psychiatry, 34,* 265–269.

Hier, D. B., & Mohr, J. P. (1977). Incongruous oral and written naming. *Brain and Language, 4,* 115–126.

Hirose, G., Kin, T., & Murakami, E. (1977). Alexia without agraphia associated with right occipital lesion. *Journal of Neurology, Neurosurgery, and Psychiatry, 40,* 225–227.

Hoff, H., & Pötzl, O. (1973). Reine wortblindheit bei hirntumor. *Nervenarzt, 10,* 385–394.

Johansson, T., & Fahlgren, H. (1979). Alexia without agraphia: Lateral and medial infarction of left occipital lobe. *Neurology, 29,* 390–393.

Kertesz, A. (1979). *Aphasia and associated disorders.* New York: Grune & Stratton.

Kertesz, A. (1982). *Varieties of reading disorders.* Presented at the Winter Conference on Brain Research, Steamboat Springs, Colorado, January.

Kinsbourne, M., & Warrington, E. K. (1962). A variety of reading disability associated with right hemisphere lesions. *Journal of Neurology, Neurosurgery, and Psychiatry, 25,* 339–344.

Kirshner, H. S., & Webb, W. G. (1982). Word and letter reading and the mechanism of the third alexia. *Archives of Neurology, 39,* 84–87.

Kurachi, M., Yamaguchi, N., Inasaka, T., & Torii, H. (1979). Recovery from alexia without agraphia: Report of an autopsy. *Cortex, 15,* 297–312.

LaBerge, D., & Samuels, S. J. (1974). Toward a theory of automatic information processing in reading. *Cognitive Psychology, 6,* 293–323.

Landis, T., Regard, M., & Serrat, A. (1980). Iconic reading in a case of alexia without agraphia caused by a tumor: A tachistoscopic study. *Brain and Language, 11,* 45–53.

Levin, H. S., & Rose, J. E. (1979). Alexia without agraphia in a musician after transcallosal removal of a left intraventricular meningioma. *Neurosurgery, 4,* 168–174.

Levitt, L. P., Gastinger, J., McClintic, W., & Lin, F. (1978). Alexia without agraphia due to aneurysm. *Pennsylvania Medicine, 81,* 86–87.

Ludlow, C. (1980). Children's language disorders: Recent research advances. *Annals of Neurology, 7,* 497–507.

Lühdorf, K., & Paulson, O. B. (1977). Does alexia without agraphia always include hemianopsia? *Acta Neurologica Scandinavica, 55,* 323–329.

Mani, S. S., Fine, E. J., & Mayberry, Z. (1981). Alexia without agraphia: Localization of the lesions by computerized tomography. *Computerized Tomography, 5,* 95–97.

Marin, O. S. M. (1980). CAT scans of five deep dyslexic patients. In M. Coltheart, K. Patterson, & J. C. Marshall (Eds.), *Deep dyslexia.* London: Routledge & Kegan Paul.

Marshall, J., & Newcombe, F. (1973). Patterns of paralexia: A psycholinguistic approach. *Journal of Psycholinguistic Research, 2,* 175–200.

Maspes, P. E. (1948). Le syndrome expérimental chez l'homme de la section du splénium du corps calleux. Aléxie visuelle pure hémianopsique. *Revue Neurologique, 80,* 100–113.

Matsui, T. , & Hirano, A. (1978). *An atlas of the human brain for computerized tomography.* Tokyo: Igaku-Shoin.

Michel, F. (1979). Preservation du langage écrit malgré un déficit majeur du langage oral. *Lyon Medical, 241,* 141–149.

Michel, F., Schott, B., Boucher, M., & Kopp, N. (1979). Aléxie sans agraphie chez un malade ayant un hémisphère gauche déafférenté. *Revue Neurologique, 135,* 347–364.

Mohr, J. P., Pessin, M. S., Finkelstein, S., Funkenstein, H. H., Duncan, G. W., & Davis, K. R. (1978). Broca aphasia: Pathologic and clinical. *Neurology, 28,* 311–324.

Neville, H. J., Snyder, E., Knight, R., & Galambos, R. (1979). Event related potentials in language and non-language tasks in patients with alexia without agraphia. In D. Lehmann & E. Callaway (Eds.), *Human evoked potentials.* New York: Plenum, pp. 269–283.

Newcombe, F., & Marshall, J. C. (1973). Stages in recovery from dyslexia following a left cerebral abscess. *Cortex, 9,* 329–332.

Newcombe, F., & Ratcliff, G. (1979). Long-term psychological consequences of cerebral lesions. In M. S. Gazzaniga (Ed.), *Handbook of behavioral neurology* (Vol. 2). New York: Plenum, pp. 495–540.

Nielsen, J. M. (1939). The unsolved problems in aphasia. II. Alexia resulting from a temporal lesion. *Bulletin of the Los Angeles Neurological Societies, 4,* 168–183.

Orgogozo, J. M., Pere, J. J., & Strube, E. (1979). Alexie sans agraphie, "agnosie" des couleurs et atteinte de l'hémichamp visuel droit: Un syndrome de l'artère, cérébrale postérieure. *Semaine des Hôpitaux, 55,* 1389–1394.

Oxbury, J. M., Oxbury, S. M., & Humphrey, N. K. (1969). Varieties of colour anomia. *Brain, 92,* 847–860.

Papadakis, N. (1974). Subdural hematoma complicated by homonymous hemianopia alexia. *Surgical Neurology, 2,* 131–132.

Penfield, W., & Evans, J. (1934). Functional defects produced by cerebral lobectomies. *Research Publications—Association for Research in Nervous and Mental Disease, 13,* 352–377.

Péron, N., & Goutner, V. (1944). Alexie pure sans hémianopsie. *Revue Neurologique, 76,* 81–82.

Pirozzolo, F. J., Kerr, K. L., Obrzut, J. E., Morley, G. K., Haxby, J. V., & Lundgren, S. (1981). Neurolinguistic analysis of the language abilities of a patient with a "double disconnection syndrome": A case of subangular alexia in the presence of mixed transcortical aphasia. *Journal of Neurology, Neurosurgery and Psychiatry, 44,* 152–155.

Ruff, R. L., & Arbit, E. (1981). Aphemia resulting from a left frontal hematoma. *Neurology, 31,* 353–356.

Sasanuma, S. (1975). Kana and Kanji processing in Japanese aphasics. *Brain and Language, 2,* 369–383.

Sasanuma, S., & Fujimura, O. (1971). Selective impairment of phonetic and non-phonetic transcription of words in Japanese aphasia patients: Kana vs. Kanji in visual recognition and writing. *Cortex, 7,* 1–18.

Skoglund, R. R. (1979). Reversible alexia, mitochondrial myopathy, and lactic acidemia. *Neurology, 29,* 717–720.

Sroka, H., Solsi, P., & Bornstein, B. (1973). Alexia without agraphia with complete recovery. *Confinia Neurologica, 35,* 167–176.

Stachowiak, F.-J., & Poeck, K. (1976). Functional disconnection in pure alexia and color naming deficit demonstrated by facilitation methods. *Brain and Language, 3,* 135–143.

Staller, J., Buchanan, D., Singer, M., Lappin, J., & Webb, W. (1978). Alexia without agraphia: An experimental case study. *Brain and Language, 5,* 378–387.

Stephens, R. B., & Stilwell, D. L. (1969). *Arteries and veins of the human brain.* Springfield, Ill.: Thomas.

Sugishita, M., Iwata, M., Toyokura, Y., Yoshioka, M., & Yamada, R. (1978). Reading of ideograms and phonograms in Japanese patients after partial commissurotomy. *Neuropsychologia, 16,* 417–426.

Thiébaut, F., Philippidès, D., Helle, J., & Ruch, M. R. (1954). Aléxie occipitale. *Revue d'Oto-Neuro-Ophtalmologie, 3,* 153–157.

Trescher, J. H., & Ford, F. R. (1937). Colloid cyst of the third ventricle. *Archives of Neurology and Psychiatry, 37,* 959–973.

Turgman, J., Goldhammer, Y., & Braham, J. (1979). Alexia, without agraphia, due to brain tumor: A reversible syndrome. *Annals of Neurology, 6,* 265–268.

Van Buren, J. M. (1979). Anatomical study of a posterior cerebral lesion producing dyslexia. *Neurosurgery, 5,* 1–10.

Vincent, C., David, M., & Puech, P. (1930). Sur l'alexie. Production de phénomène à la suite de l'extirpation de la corne occipitale du ventricule latéral gauche. *Revue Neurologique, 1,* 262–272.

Vincent, F. M., & Reeves, A. G. (1980). Alexia without agraphia: A reversible syndrome. *Annals of Neurology, 8,* 206.

Vincent, F. M., Sadowsky, C. H., Saunders, R. L., & Reeves, A. G. (1977). Alexia without agraphia, hemianopia, or color-naming defect: A disconnection syndrome. *Neurology, 27*, 689–691.

Warrington, E., & Zangwill, O. L. (1957). A study of dyslexia. *Journal of Neurology, Neurosurgery and Psychiatry, 20*, 208–215.

Wechsler, A. F. (1972). Transient left hemialexia. *Neurology, 22*, 628–633.

Wechsler, A. F., Weinstein, E. A., & Antin, S. P. (1972). Alexia without agraphia. A clinical and radiographical study of three unusual cases. *Bulletin of the Los Angeles Neurological Societies, 37*, 1–11.

Wertheim, N. (1977). Is there an anatomical localisation for musical faculties? In M. Critchley & R. A. Henson (Eds.), *Music and the brain.* Springfield, Ill.: Thomas, pp. 282–297.

Yamadori, A. (1975). Ideogram reading in alexia. *Brain, 98*, 231–238.

Zaidel, E. (1975). A technique for presenting lateralized visual input with prolonged exposure. *Vision Research, 15*, 283–289.

Zaidel, E. (1978). Lexical organization in the right hemisphere. In P. A. Buser & A. Rougeul-Buser (Eds.), *Cerebral correlates of conscious experience.* Amsterdam: North-Holland, pp. 177–197.

Zihl, J., & von Cramon, D. (1980). Colour anomia restricted to the left visual hemifield after splenial disconnexion. *Journal of Neurology, Neurosurgery and Psychiatry, 43*, 719–724.

14

Modality-Specific Disorders of Written Language

Luigi A. Vignolo

Clinical practice offers examples of verbal behavior disturbances that are strictly confined to one single receptive or expressive modality, and, as such, cannot be easily explained by the sizeable lesions of the cortical language areas that usually entail a multimodality disorder of language. They are the so-called "pure" or "modality-specific" disorders of verbal behavior, the mechanisms of which are still a matter for dispute and research.

In this chapter, we confine ourselves to the clinical–anatomical correlation in patients with modality-specific disorders of written language, that is, pure alexia and agraphia. Correlations are established mainly on the basis of the CT scan findings.

Materials and General Method

The clinico-neuroradiological correlations described here were carried out in adult patients who harbored cerebro-vascular lesions (generally infarcts of the brain, rarely intracerebral hemorrhages). Only those patients whose lesions were stable, demonstrated by a CT scan performed at least 3 weeks post-stroke, were studied.

The *neurological disorder* was evaluated by a number of quantitative tests, including a detailed examination of language. A special battery for patients with reading disorders is described in the Appendix.

The *site and extent of the lesion* was assessed by an Electronic Musical Instruments (EMI) scanner 1000 CT. A routine CT scan exam yields eight 13 mm horizontal sections from the base of the skull to the vertex. These are then projected onto the screen of a Diagnostic Display Console (DDC) and photographed, using a Polaroid. In these photographic reproductions of the sections, the vascular lesions show up as areas of abnormal hypo- or hyperdensity within the brain. The contour of the lesion was identified on each section. If it was thought to be necessary for better comparison, the contour of the lesion was then transferred onto a lateral diagram of the damaged cerebral hemisphere. The procedure is described in detail by Mazzocchi and Vignolo (1978). Basically, it is necessary to carry out two simple operations. First, the angle of the CT sections, with respect to the orbito-meatal line (OML), is established by taking the bone structures of the base of the skull as points of reference. The contour of the lesion is traced on each section and is then transferred onto a standard lateral diagram.

Alexia without Agraphia

Five patients with this syndrome are described in detail. Two (Cases 1 and 2) showed the classical picture of isolated alexia, whereas in the remaining three cases a selective reading slowness was in the foreground (see Boccardi & Vignolo, 1983).

Case 1. A 63-year-old right-handed retired bus driver, 6 years of schooling, with a history of myocardial infarction 14 years before and current high blood pressure, suddenly developed right-sided hemianopia and reading difficulty. A transient mild anomia and right-sided pyramidal syndrome were observed a few days later.

At the standard language examination 1 month post-stroke, he showed a severe defect of both reading comprehension and reading aloud, in contrast with sufficiently preserved writing on dictation and spontaneous writing (writing a letter). A few anomias were present in writing as well as in oral expression; color naming was as good as picture naming. The Token Test score was normal (29/36).

On repeat examination 6 months post-stroke, there still was a dense right homonymous hemianopia, severe alexia without agraphia with inability to read what he had written, and a moderate naming defect on confrontation. Essentially, this picture remained the same except for a progressive reduction of the anomias. The special test battery for reading, carried out 20 months post-stroke, yielded the following results with the patient falling well below cut-off score in the tests: (a) phonological tests (score: 47, 37, and 61, respectively): he merely looked at the first graphemes and then chose by guessing. Reading block letters seemed to be somewhat easier than reading small handwritten letters. By contrast, he obtained an almost perfect score on the perceptual test. (b) reading aloud. (c) reading of texts (score: 64, 0, and 1, respectively): he seemed unable to read words of more than seven letters and, apart from this, he took more than 5 minutes to painfully try to read one single line. (d) ordering of letters of alphabet: he obtained a very low score of 4.5. Although single letters were well recognized, putting them into the right alphabetic sequence was virtually impossible. By contrast, he obtained the maximum score on ordering numerals.

The fact that the visual discrimination of perceptually similar logatomes was normal, and the identification of phonemic variations of logatomes very poor, suggests that the reading disorder did not depend upon the inability to carry out subtle perceptual discriminations in the visual modality; on the other hand, the relatively good spontaneous writing and writing to dictation testified that the repertoire of graphemes was unimpaired. This was confirmed by the high effectiveness of all facilitations (score: 32, 25, and 30, respectively).

The CT scan showed (Figure 1) an ischemic lesion involving a large area in the left occipital lobe. Although the splenium was not damaged, the left occipital lesion extended anteriorly, interrupting the callosal afferents from the right occipital lobe.

Case 2. A 54-year-old right-handed engineer, 8 years of schooling, high blood pressure, came to our observation 7 months after a stroke. He showed a mild right hemiparesis and hemianesthesia, dense right homonymous hemianopia, and total inability to read aloud, understand, and copy words and phrases, with preserved writing to command and to dictation. A few anomias and verbal paraphasias were present both in his speech and his spontaneous writ-

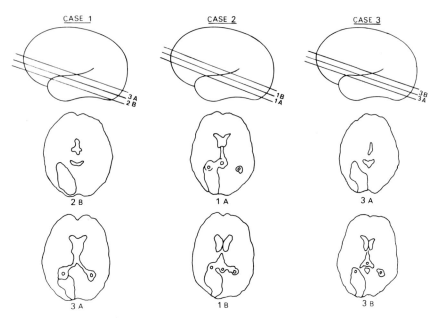

Figure 1. CT scan lesions in patients with alexia without agraphia (cases 1 to 3).

ing. He complained of poor color vision and had difficulty performing the Token Test, although his auditory comprehension was excellent in everyday life and when examined in other standard ways. Both the patient and his relatives volunteered the information that his memory for recent events was somewhat impaired (e.g., he sometimes asked the same questions about things that had happened to him the day before, events his relatives felt he should remember quite well).

In summary, alexia without agraphia was, by far, the most striking aspect of the clinical picture in this patient, although some aphasic, agnosic, and memory defects were also present.

The CT scan performed 7 months post-onset showed (Figure 1) a large infarct of the left occipital lobe extending anteriorly so as to damage the callosal fibers coming from the intact splenium, and inferiorly, to the basal surface of the posterior medial temporal lobe so as to encroach upon the hippocampus.

In patients whose disorder consisted essentially in abnormally slow reading, a careful inquiry of the difficulties and compensation mechanisms associated with such slowness sometimes yielded interesting results, as in Case 3.

Case 3. A 53-year-old right-handed, highly educated, hypertensive patient who had had two transient ischemic attacks in the verte-brobasilar territory was struck in the middle of the night by an intense, transient left temporal headache. The next morning, he realized that he was unable to read any more, whereas writing to dictation was unimpaired and oral language disorders were limited to occasional word substitutions ("yesterday" instead of "today"). A dense right homonymous hemianopia was found. This patient was examined 8 months post-stroke. He had spontaneously developed several compensation mechanisms, interwoven in highly complex behavior. He followed the line with his index finger, moving it to reproduce a given letter kinesthetically whenever necessary, in order to decipher it. He said he was unable to see or pay attention to more than five letters at the same time. He managed, mentally, to assemble "chunks" of the letter sequences by recognizing meaningful di- or tri-grams, such as common prepositions or articles (e.g., *per, da, li*) or di-grams from car plates (e.g., MI = Milano, NA = Napoli); he would then put these di-tri-grams together to get the form of the entire word. To complete the sentence, he filled the gaps by relying heavily on contextual cues; he usually guessed the last word of the sentence—a procedure which sometimes led to the right word and sometimes to semantic paralexias. These mechanisms went on almost simultaneously; the patient read with a tense attitude and a sense of urgency. Continuing daily practice, carried out for 8 months, succeeded in reducing the reading time by one-fourth. In spite of this, the overall results were still unsatisfactory from the point of view of speed. This patient's intelligence, motivation, high educational level, and ingenuity in trying to compensate for the disability—in addition to spontaneous recovery—would have made the reading problem quite minor had he had a less demanding job. As a corporation lawyer, however, he was severely hampered in a number of essential routine reading operations such as rapidly browsing through a series of documents to find one particular point of interest, checking a brief written report at a glance, or even looking up a word in the dictionary.

At the standard aphasia examination, slowness and hesitancies were observed. At the special test battery for reading, the patient fell below cut-off score on both the perceptual and the phonological sections as well as on reading aloud from entire written passages or texts. Slowness, rather than wrong responses, was the cause of the poor scores on these tests. For example, total time for text reading ranged from 300 to 360 sec—more than twice the normal threshold. Occasional errors occurred during the spontaneous somesthetic rewriting of single letters (e.g., *P* was traced as *R*, and then read as such). Facilitations, of course, were highly effective; indeed, the patient had discovered some of them himself long before the examination.

In conclusion, the pure alexia in this highly verbally skilled patient was considerably lessened by the consistent use of self-facilitating behaviors and, presumably, by the functional compensation entailed by the passage of time. In spite of this, alexia was still present and its most conspicuous aspect was an overall, still abnormal slowness in reading.

A CT scan performed 1 month post-stroke showed (Figure 1) a low-density area in the left occipital region involving part of the posterior and inferior aspect of the left temporal lobe—most likely, an infarct in the left posterior cerebral artery territory.

Case 4. A 59-year-old right-handed janitor with 5 years of schooling suddenly developed inability to read with relative preservation of writing. Language evaluation was performed 2 months post-stroke. While the standard language examination failed to show remarkable reading disorders, the special reading battery detected an abnormal performance on the phonological, audiovisual subtest (partly due to slowness, partly to self-corrected errors) and on the reading of entire texts, which was particularly slow (from 240 to 480 sec). Facilitations were very effective.

A CT scan performed 80 days post-stroke showed an infarct in the occipital lobe in the territory of the left posterior cerebral artery (Figure 2).

Case 5. A 69-year-old retired clerk with 17 years of schooling and a history of myocardial infarction had a transient episode of tingling and weakness of the right limbs, accompanied by a permanent right homonymous hemianopia and a reading defect with relatively well-preserved spontaneous writing. He complained of some word-finding difficulties for names of persons and streets. The standard language examination performed in the acute stage (1 week post-stroke) confirmed both the reading difficulties and the anomias. At the special battery for reading, administered 2 months post-onset, the patient fell below cutting score on the perceptual test, on all the phonological subtests, and in the reading of entire texts. The two former tests were impaired *both* by slowness in giving the correct response *and* by actual errors. Texts were read very slowly (range

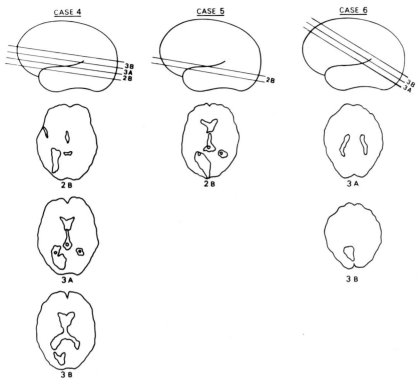

Figure 2. CT scan lesions in patients with mild alexia without agraphia (cases 4 and 5) and one without alexia (Case 6).

265–360 sec, mean 303 sec) and with obvious effort. The patient often complained that he could not remember the meaning of what he had read. Facilitations were very effective.

Several CT scans consistently showed a left hemisphere infarct involving both the occipital and the deep temporal lobe including the hippocampus (Figure 2).

A careful scrutiny of all CT scan records with left occipital lesions permitted us to pick up one more patient, who had escaped notice because he was neither aphasic nor alexic.

Case 6 (Figure 2) had suffered from an infarct in the left posterior cerebral territory that had brought about nothing more than a right homonymous field defect. Extensive language testing, including the special battery for reading, disclosed no defect whatsoever. The explanation, in our opinion, is that the left occipital lesion was located posterosuperiorly with respect to the preceding ones, thereby sparing the callosal fibers.

In summary, the site of the lesions shown by the CT scan in our cases of alexia without agraphia agrees quite well with that described by Dejerine in 1892. The infarct in all patients consistently belonged to the territory of the left posterior cerebral artery. It was so placed as to damage both the left occipital lobe and the callosal pathways from the intact right occipital lobe. Although the splenium as such was intact, the anterior extension of the left occipital lesion appeared to destroy the callosal fibers at the level of the forceps major.

The clinical picture ranged from a remarkably full-fledged, classical syndrome (Cases 1 and 2) to pictures in which the main symptom was an abnormal slowness of reading (Cases 3, 4, and 5). The reason for this difference remains obscure as it does not seem to be accounted for by differences either in the morphology of lesions or in the time elapsed from stroke.

Associated neuropsychological disorders were, on the whole, mild, and varied from one case to the next; there were anomias and verbal paraphasias, errors in the comprehension and expression of color names, and complaints about impairment of memory for ongoing events. These defects were not systematically investigated by means of formal testing. Although the small number of cases and the inherent limitations of the localizing method do not allow us to establish correlations between these concomitant defects and the exact site of the lesions, it seems likely that the word-finding difficulties were associated with damage of the posterior temporal lobe and the memory defects to damage of the inferior and mesial temporal lobe, both involving the left hippocampus.

As to the mechanism of this syndrome, the effectiveness of the somesthetic facilitation seems to favor the classic hypothesis of a visual–linguistic disconnection. At any rate, whatever the interpretation, the interruption of the callosal pathways (in addition to the left occipital lobe damage) seems to be crucial: it is significant that the only patient (Case 6) in whom the left occipital lobe damage did not bring about an isolated alexia had a very posterior lesion which did not interrupt the callosal fibers from the right occipital lobe to the language areas in the left hemisphere.

Isolated Agraphia

A disorder confined to writing may depend upon either apraxic or visuospatial defects or both; in addition, it may constitute an early symptom of mental confusion. In rare cases, however, one can observe a pure agraphia in which the defect seems to be primarily linguistic in nature, since paragraphias and neologisms are present, while there is little or no apraxia.

In Mazzocchi's and Vignolo's series (1979), one case out of 90 showed such isolated agraphia. The CT scan (Figure 3) showed two small areas of hypodensity in the upper parietal lobe. A previous study (Basso, Taborelli, & Vignolo, 1978) of pure agraphia in two surgical cases showed that lesions (due to excision of small congen-

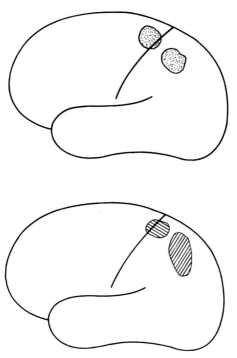

Figure 3. Lesions in patients with "pure" agraphia (redrawn): Top—CT scan lesions in one case of Mazzocchi and Vignolo (1979). Bottom—Drawing of lesions (post-surgery) in two cases of Basso et al. (1978).

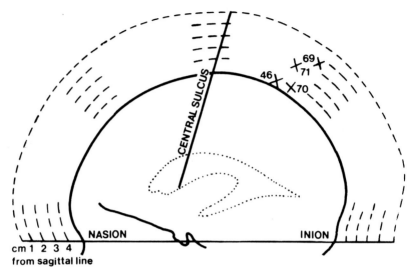

Figure 4. Position of wounds (*X*) on skull chart in four cases of Russel and Espir (1961) (redrawn).

ital malformations) were located approximately in the same region (Figure 3). These findings confirm the early observations of Russel and Espir (1961) in patients with penetrating missile wounds (Figure 4). They reported the "surprising" finding of a small group of gunshot wounds that caused relatively pure agraphia through deep parasagittal lesions of the left posterior parietal lobe, and pointed out that "this area of the brain is very much concerned with those correlations of body image and spatial orientation which may lead to apraxia and other remarkable parietal lobe syndromes."

Indeed, the association between agraphia without other language defects and lesions of the upper posterior parietal lobe is often found in the record of cases published as outstanding examples of other neuropsychological disorders—the patients with autotopoagnosia described by De Renzi and Faglioni (1963) and De Renzi and Scotti (1970). By contrast, it is interesting to observe that in the few published cases of fluent aphasia with relative sparing of writing (see Basso *et al.*, 1978, for a brief review), the posterior and superior marginal areas of the language zone in the parietal lobe are consistently spared. Therefore, we may hypothesize that the posterior superior left parietal lobule in man is crucial for the sensorimotor–linguistic integration needed for writing. This by no means implies that it is the only crucial place. The possibility that slight damage in other language zones may bring about the syndrome of isolated agraphia has been suggested by the CT case report of Rosati and De Bastiani (1979). Further anatomoclinical studies are needed to bear out this suggestion.

Appendix

The special battery for reading (Boccardi, Codini, & Vignolo, in press) consists of the following seven tests.

1. *Serial ordering of letters and numbers:* The patient is asked to put in the correct serial order 21 printed letters of the Italian alphabet and 21 numbers included between 1 and 100. The first and last element of each series are put on the table by the examiner as "anchors," and the patient must place the intermediate elements correctly. Performance on each series is scored separately. Scoring takes sequencing into account. Maximum score is 19, cut-off scores are 0 (letters) and 13.6 (numbers) (≤ 7 years of schooling) and 15.8 and 19 (> 7 years).

2. *Classification of graphic types:* Thirty-six white squares (cm 2×2)—on each of which either a letter of the alphabet, *or* an Arabic numeral, *or* a meaningless shape resembling a letter of the alphabet is handwritten—are given to the patient in succession. The patient must place each square in one of three boxes, labeled, respectively, with the letter *A*, the number *1*, and a letterlike form. Maximum score for right placements is 30; cut-off scores are 26 (≤ 7 years of schooling) and 28 (> 7 years); cut-off scores for total time spent to place the items are 191 sec and 101 sec, respectively.

3. *Perceptual test: visual discrimination of perceptually similar printing types:* The patient is presented with 40 cards in succession; on each, the top row displays a stimulus letter, syllable, or word; this is shown on the six lower rows in almost similar types of printing. The patient is asked to point out the *one* alternative choice which is, printwise (that is, perceptually) identical to the stimulus. Score: 2 points for each exact answer within 5 sec, 1 point for wrong answers self-corrected within 5 sec. Maximum score is 80, and cut-off scores are 19.8 (≤ 7 years of schooling) and 48.4 (> 7 years of schooling).

4. *Phonological test: identification of phonemically similar written logatomes:* Forty cards with a stimulus letter, syllable, or word and six alternative choices, but varying in terms of some small phonemical differences, are shown to the patient in succession. The patient must point out the one of the six alternative choices that is phonemically identical to the stimulus. There are three subtests with different modalities of stimulus and responses: (a) both stimulus and multiple choices are written in small printing typefaces; (b) the stimulus is handwritten in small letters; the responses are handwritten in block letters. In both (a) and (b), the patient silently reads both stimulus and responses before choosing; (c) the stimulus is given orally; the multiple choices are printed. Scoring for all subtests is analogous to that adopted for the perceptual or visual discrimination test. Maximum score is 80; normal cut-off scores for (a) are 48.9 and 72.3; (b) 53.2 and 69.0; (c) 62.8 and 75.

5. *Comprehension of written language:* (a) The patient is asked to read a half-page-long murder story and to indicate the suspected murderer among four alternative names. Score: 2 points for immediately correct answer, 1 point for incorrect answers spontaneously self-corrected within 5 sec. Nonbrain-damaged subjects usually score 2 on this subtest. (b) The patient is administered a 14-item Token Test (after De Renzi & Vignolo, 1962) in which written commands are given rather than oral. Score: 1 point for each correctly performed command.

6. *Reading aloud of entire written texts:* This tests speed and accuracy of reading in mildly impaired patients. The patient is asked to read aloud three 100-word texts. Two are typewritten and both are written either in single columns of 19 cm length or in 3 columns of 4 cm length each. The third text is an excerpt from an authentic newspaper article. The time employed to read aloud each test is recorded. Cut-off scores vary from 54 sec to 180 sec, according to instructional level and task difficulty.

7. *Facilitations:* The tests investigate the facilitations for reading that are classically described in these patients, in comparison with the absence of facilitation. Reading aloud three series of words of increasing length (i.e., 2, 3, and 4 letters) is compared under four conditions: (a) Visual, not Guided: The test word, made up of plastic block letters 10 cm high, is presented visually to the patient; providing a baseline condition without any facilitation (except perhaps the large size of the letters). (b) Visual, Guided: The test word is written by the examiner on a white sheet of paper in block letters 10 cm high. The patient simply is asked to watch and to read out loud the test word as soon as the examiner has finished writing it. (c) Somesthetic, not Guided: the test word, made up of plastic block letters 10 cm high, is put on the table in front of the blindfolded patient who is asked to feel it with both hands and to read it aloud after exploring it tactually. (d) Somesthetic, Guided: The patient is blindfolded and the test word is written by the examiner on the table in block letters about 10 cm high, using the patient's right index finger "as a pencil." The patient is asked to feel the movement of his finger (on the table) and to "read" out loud the test word as soon as the examiner has finished writing it. The responses must be given within 5 sec. Maximum score is 32; cut-off scores are 32 for (a) and (b), 23.7 for (c), and 15.7 for (d) (≤ 7 years of schooling), and 32 for (a) and (b), 27.5 for (c), and 27.7 for (d) (>7 years).

References

Basso, A., Taborelli, A., & Vignolo, L. A. (1978). Dissociated disorders of speaking and writing in aphasia. *Journal of Neurology, Neurosurgery and Psychiatry, 41,* 556–563.

Boccardi, E. & Vignolo, L. A. (1983). L'alessia pura. *Archivio di Psicologia, Neurologia e Psichiatria* (in press).

Boccardi, E., Codini, M. G., & Vignolo, L. A. (1983). L'esame dei disturbi della lettura: Valori normativi. *Archivio di Psicologia, Neurologia e Psichiatria.*

Dejerine, J. (1892). Contribution à l'étude anatomo-pathologique et clinique des différentes variétés de cécité verbale. *Memoires de la Societe de Biologie, 4,* 61–90.

De Renzi, E., & Faglioni, P. (1963). L'autotopoagnosia. *Archivio di Psicologia, Neurologia e Psichiatria, 24,* 1–34.

De Renzi, E., & Scotti, G. (1970). Autotopagnosia: Fiction or reality? *Archives of Neurology (Chicago), 23,* 221–227.

De Renzi, E., & Vignolo, L. A. (1962). The Token Test: A sensitive test to detect receptive disorders in aphasia. *Brain, 85,* 665–678.

Mazzocchi, F., & Vignolo, L. A. (1978). Computer assisted tomography in neuropsychological research: A simple procedure for lesion mapping. *Cortex, 14,* 136–144.

Mazzocchi, F., & Vignolo, L. A. (1979). Localisation of lesions in aphasia: Clinical-CT scan correlations in stroke patients. *Cortex, 15,* 627–654.

Rosati, G., & De Bastiani, P. (1979). Pure agraphia: A discrete form of aphasia. *Journal of Neurology, Neurosurgery and Psychiatry, 42,* 266–269.

Russel, W. R., & Espir, M. L. E. (1961). *Traumatic aphasia.* London: Oxford University Press.

15

Localization of Apraxia-Producing Lesions

Kenneth M. Heilman,
Leslie Rothi,
and Andrew Kertesz

Introduction

This chapter concentrates on the pathological anatomy of apraxic disorders. However, before discussing the anatomic aspect of a variety of apraxic disorders, we first define apraxia and discuss how it is assessed. The reader can find a detailed discussion of the neuropsychology and pathophysiology of apraxia in recent reviews (e.g., Heilman, 1979).

Apraxia is the inability to properly execute a learned skilled movement. Many neurological defects can interfere with the performance of a skilled movement, and apraxia is defined partly by excluding the other neurological defects that may impair motor activity. For example, disorders of skilled movements caused by weakness, deaf-

LOCALIZATION
IN NEUROPSYCHOLOGY

ferentation, abnormality of tone or posture, and abnormal movements are not termed "apraxia."

Limb apraxia refers to the inability to perform skilled movements with the arm and hand.

Oral or buccofacial apraxia consists of the inability to perform skilled movements with the muscles of the face, lips, tongue, pharynx, and larynx.

Apraxic agraphia is a writing disorder induced by an inability to execute the learned skilled movement required by writing (Heilman, Coyle, Gonyea, & Geschwind, 1973). Writing is a complex motor activity that requires linguistic and visuokinesthesic motor skills. We do not discuss apraxic agraphia in this chapter (see Heilman, 1979).

Visuoconstructive disorders have been termed "constructional apraxia." These usually are not considered "true apraxias." We will not discuss the gait disorders, which have been termed "apraxia of gait," and the dressing disorders, which have been termed "dressing apraxia." Lastly, Johns and Darley (1970) refer to some motor programming disorders of speech as "apraxia of speech." As we discuss in the section on buccofacial apraxia, Broca's aphasia commonly coexists with buccofacial apraxia; however, apraxia of speech is a complex issue, beyond the scope of this chapter.

Apraxia Testing

Traditionally, when testing for limb apraxia, the examiner requires the patient: (1) to pantomime acts (e.g., "Make believe you have a key in your hand. Now open a door with that key.") and perform gestures (e.g., "Show me how you hitchhike."); (2) to *imitate* pantomimed acts and performed gestures; and (3) to use actual objects. A patient's ability to perform a series of acts in the proper order should also be tested (e.g., cleaning a pipe, putting tobacco in the pipe, and then lighting the pipe).

Tests for buccofacial apraxia should be similar to those described for limb apraxia, but unlike such tests, these should test the ability of the face, lips, tongue, pharynx, larynx, and respiratory muscles to make skilled learned movements. As in testing for buccofacial apraxia, the examiner should ask the patient to pantomime acts ("How would you suck on a straw?"), perform gestures ("Blow a kiss."), imitate, and use actual objects. The examiner should also note the nature of the apraxic errors.

Pantomime recognition tasks may be used to explore the comprehension and perception of skilled movements. For example, we ask our patients which of three acts represents flipping a coin. The examiner pantomimes opening a door with a key, flipping a coin, and using a hammer. Similarly, we test their ability to discriminate between correctly and incorrectly performed acts. To do this, we may ask a patient which of three movement sequences represents the correct method of using scissors. We then (1) pantomime, using body parts as objects (the fingers are used as scissor blades); (2) move a hand correctly; and (3) perform wrong movements (e.g., flexing and extending an index finger at the metacarpophalangeal joint so that when flexed it meets the thumb).

Classification System

The terms used to classify the varieties of apraxia may be confusing because most classification systems—rather than being purely anatomic, physiologic, or even eponymic—are based on a combination of factors including theoretical postulates as to the underlying mechanisms. In this chapter, we divide the apraxias into two major groups based on the portion of the body involved (i.e., limb apraxia and buccofacial apraxia). Although we would like to classify apraxia by the major behavioral signs, apraxic disorders are often associated with a constellation of signs. Therefore, we divide the apraxias, using the classical nomenclature of Liepmann (1908)—that is, *ideomotor, limb kinetic,* and *ideational* apraxia. Liepmann's classification system, however, does not correspond to all varieties of apraxia that can be seen in the clinic; therefore, we elaborate on his system.

Limb Apraxia

IDEOMOTOR APRAXIA

Patients with ideomotor apraxia make a variety of spatial and temporal errors when performing learned skilled movements. They may use a body part as an object. For example, instead of putting the hand into the position of holding a key, they may use an index finger as if it were the key. When patients with ideomotor apraxia do not make such errors, they may move their finger (or fingers), hand, or arm incorrectly in space or incorrectly with respect to other parts of their body (spatial errors). For example, if they position the hand as if it were holding a key, they may flex and extend the wrist rather than making a rotary movement. Patients with ideomotor apraxia may also sequence their movements improperly. For example, they may rotate the hand before inserting the key; or, if a correct movement requires the contraction of muscle Group *A* before Group *B*, they may contract these muscle groups in the wrong order (temporal or sequential errors).

There are at least three forms of ideomotor apraxia: (1) the form associated with lesions of the corpus callosum; (2) the form associated with anterior dominant (for handedness) hemisphere lesions; and (3) the ideomotor apraxia associated with posterior dominant (for handedness) hemisphere lesions. Each of these three types of ideomotor apraxia have somewhat different signs and symptoms; therefore, we discuss each individually.

CALLOSAL APRAXIA (UNILATERAL LIMB APRAXIA)

Callosal apraxia is an unusual syndrome characterized by an inability to carry out verbal commands with the left hand with a preserved ability to carry out these same commands with the right hand.

There appear to be two clinical forms of callosal apraxia—impaired imitation and normal imitation. Liepmann and Maas (1907), who first noted that apraxia could be induced in a patient by a callosal disconnection, also noted that these patients were unable to imitate pantomimed acts with their left hand and were clumsy when using actual objects. Geschwind and Kaplan (1962) and Gazzaniga, Bogen, and Sperry (1967) noted, however, that although their patients with callosal lesions could not correctly carry out commands with their left hand, they could imitate and use actual objects correctly.

Liepmann and Maas (1907) postulated that in one of their patients, the left hemisphere contained both language and motor engrams that controlled the skilled movement of both hands. A callosal lesion, therefore, disconnected these language and motor (space–time) engrams from the right hemisphere that innervates the spinal motor neuron pool projecting to the muscles of the left hand. In those cases of callosal apraxia where patients are able to imitate and use actual objects, the motor engrams probably are less lateralized.

There are left-handed patients with motor engrams in the right hemisphere and language in the left hemisphere (Heilman *et al.*, 1973; Valenstein & Heilman, 1979). If those patients had a callosal section, the right hand would be deprived of motor engrams; consequently, the hand would perform poorly to commands, imitation, and in the use of actual objects. The left hand would perform well to imitation and use of the actual objects; however, because that hand is disconnected from language, it would perform poorly to command.

As can be seen from this discussion, the type of apraxic disturbance after a callosal lesion or section depends on the patterns of language and motor dominance of the individual patient. The variety of both real and potential disturbances of praxis that could be induced by callosal section is listed in Figure 1. A diagrammatic rep-

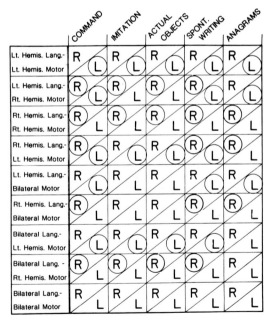

R -Right Limb
L -Left Limb
◯-Apraxia

Figure 1. Types of callosal apraxia.

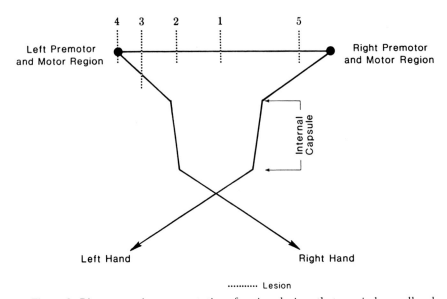

Figure 2. Diagrammatic representation of various lesions that may induce callosal lesions and anterior ideomotor apraxia: (1) Callosal lesion involving ideomotor apraxia of the left hand without hemiparesis; (2) left hemisphere white matter lesion inducing ideomotor apraxia of the left hand without hemiparesis; (3) subcortical left hemisphere lesion inducing ideomotor apraxia of the left hand and right hemiparesis; (4) left cortical lesion inducing ideomotor apraxia of the left hand and right hemiparesis; (5) right hemisphere subcortical lesion inducing ideomotor apraxia of the left hand without hemiparesis.

resentation of the various lesions that may induce callosal and anterior ideomotor apraxia is shown on Figure 2.

Patients with callosal agenesis do not have limb apraxia (Sheremata, Deonna, & Romanul, 1978). They may be using their anterior commissure to transfer their motor and language engrams, but these patients are also more likely to have stronger ipsilateral projections.

The most common natural lesions that induce callosal apraxia are infarctions in the distribution of the anterior cerebral artery. In these cases, most of the genu and body of the corpus callosum are damaged; however, the splenium is usually spared. Recently Watson and Heilman (in press) described a right-handed patient who was not able to carry out purposeful movements with the left hand on command, imitation, or actual object use. Her right-hand performance was normal. The patient had an infarction of the anterior corpus callosum (Figure 3). Callosal apraxia can be caused by

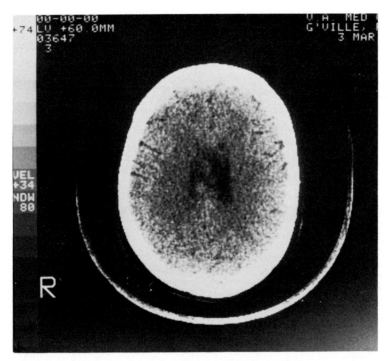

Figure 3. This high CT cut of a patient with unilateral ideomotor apraxia shows a lesion between the two ventrices in the body of the corpus callosum.

trauma or tumor, by diseases such as cystic degeneration of the corpus callosum (Marchiafava–Bignami disease), or by demyelinating diseases. Callosal apraxia can also be induced by cerebral commissurotomy for the treatment of intractable seizures.

APRAXIA INDUCED BY ANTERIOR HEMISPHERIC
LESIONS

As we discussed in the preceding section, according to Liepmann (1908) a lesion that affects the corpus callosum (Figure 2, Lesion 1) induces left-sided apraxia (in righthanders) or hemiapraxia because the left hemisphere visuokinesthetic motor engrams do not have access to the right hemisphere motor areas that control movement of the left hand. The right hand, however, would not be paralyzed or apraxic. Liepmann (1908) noted that a variety of other lesions may produce similar disturbances. A lesion in the left hemisphere that affects the callosal fibers where they separate from the common white matter (the roof of the left lateral ventricle) could also induce an apraxia of the left hand (Figure 2, Lesion 2). Many of the lesions would also induce a right hemiparesis since, in the centrum semiovale, the descending pyramidal fibers are in close proximity to the callosal fibers (Figure 2, Lesion 3 and Figures 4, 5, and 6). Lesions of the premotor and motor cortex would also induce a similar picture; that is, paresis of the right hand and apraxia of the left (Figure 2, Lesion 4, and Figures 7, 8, and 9). Theoretically, a lesion of

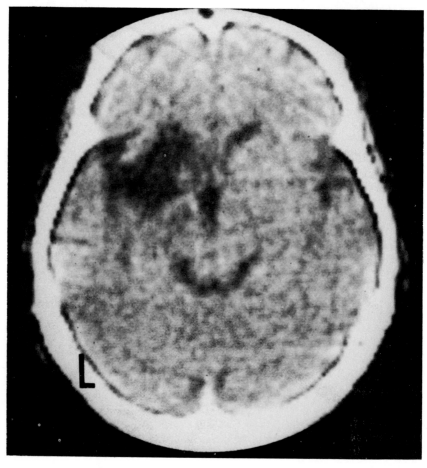

Figure 4. Case 1—Subcortical lesion with apraxia.

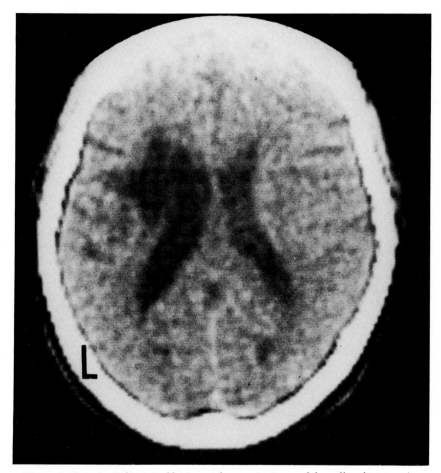

Figure 5. Case 1—Subcortical lesion with apraxia. Some of the callosal connections are affected by this lesion, as well as descending pyramidal fibers.

the right hemisphere that interrupts the callosal fibers on their way to the premotor cortex but does not involve the descending pyramidal fibers (Figure 2, Lesion 5) should also induce an apraxia of the left arm. We know, however, of no verified cases with a lesion in this distribution.

Case Illustrations

Case 1 is that of a 65-year-old housewife who presented with a severe right hemiplegia and aphasia. She was initially assessed 6

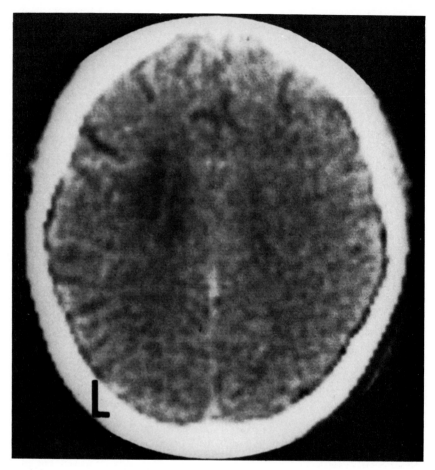

Figure 6. Case 1—Subcortical lesion with apraxia. Mainly callosal fibers are affected disconnecting the visuokinesthetic motor engrams in the left hemisphere from those in the right.

days after her stroke when she did not respond to any conversational questions, although she had a few whisper responses on the repetition and naming tasks. Her comprehension was moderately impaired for yes–no questions, word discrimination tasks, and sequential commands. She demonstrated a moderately severe apraxia, scoring $\frac{81}{120}$ on a modified scoring of the Western Aphasia Battery (Kertesz, 1982). A breakdown of the apraxia scores according to the type of praxis was as follows:

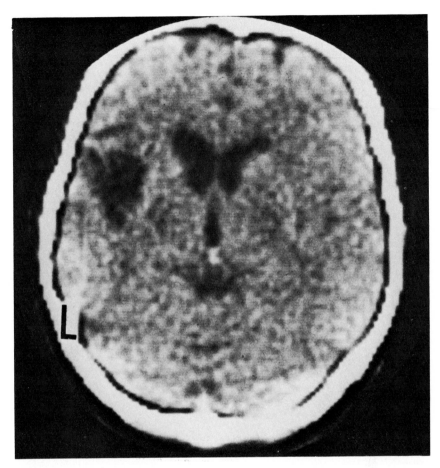

Figure 7. Case 2—A cortical lesion with severe persisting apraxia and Broca's aphasia.

Type of praxis	Command	Imitation
Intransitive movements	$\frac{12}{15}$	$\frac{15}{15}$
Buccofacial	$\frac{14}{15}$	$\frac{14}{15}$
Transitive movements	$\frac{0}{15}$	$\frac{9}{15}$
Complex movements	$\frac{6}{15}$	$\frac{11}{15}$

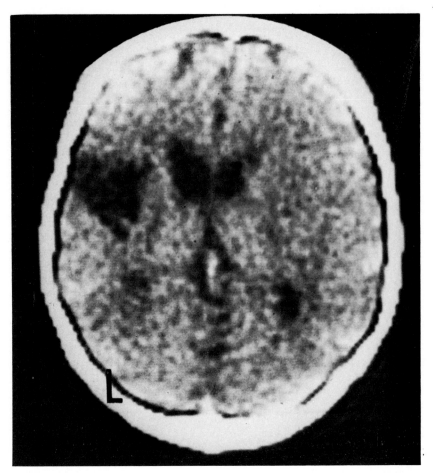

Figure 8. Case 2—A cortical lesion with apraxia. Posterior portion of the third frontal convolution and the frontal operculum of the insula as well as the precentral gyrus
are affected.

This indicated that the patient had more difficulty with transitive
and complex movements. She also demonstrated the phenomenon
of using body parts for objects such as when she was asked to show
how to brush her teeth, use a spoon, or comb her hair. She put her
fist in front of her nose when she was asked to sniff a flower. Some
of her proximal movements improved on imitation. She used verbalization for some of the tasks instead of performing them. She also

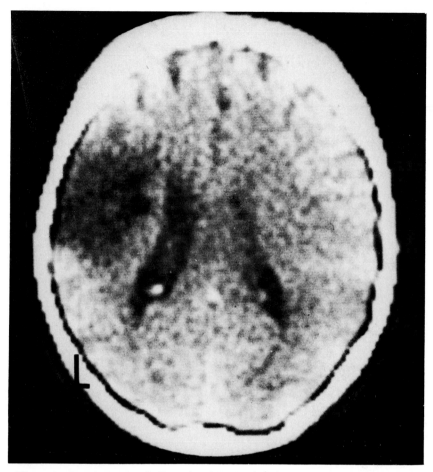

Figure 9. Case 2—Posterior frontal and central lesion with some extension in the subcortical white matter.

showed some breakdown on using the actual object on one occasion only.

Her lesion is shown on the CT scan, Figures 4, 5, and 6, indicating a substantial subcortical lesion that, presumably, disconnected the callosal connections to the right hemisphere but spared the cortical motor engrams (equivalent to Lesion 3 in Figure 2). The relatively mild degree of apraxia compared to her severe hemiplegia suggests that, in fact, some of the callosal fibers were spared because the lesion was relatively inferior and lateral to the lateral ventricle. At 3 months post-onset, she improved considerably and was only mildly apractic with a few errors on the performance of movements on command. This deficit remained stable on a 4-year post-stroke examination.

Case 2 is that of a 50-year-old right-handed woman who was initially mute after a stroke with a right hemiplegia. Her comprehension, repetition, and naming were also impaired, and she was considered to be globally aphasic on an examination 1 week after her stroke. On praxis testing, she was very slow with a great deal of perseveration. Of the responses, she had more difficulty performing on command but improved on imitation and with actual object use. The following indicates her scores on the Western Aphasia Battery (Kertesz, 1982):

Type of praxis	Command	Imitation
Intransitive movements	$\frac{6}{15}$	$\frac{13}{15}$
Buccofacial	$\frac{9}{15}$	$\frac{14}{15}$
Transitive movements	$\frac{0}{15}$	$\frac{5}{15}$
Complex movements	$\frac{5}{15}$	$\frac{11}{15}$

The total praxis score was $\frac{60}{120}$ (modifed scoring). She continued to be apractic at 3- and 9-month follow-up visits. She evolved to Broca's aphasia. Her lesion shows a destruction of the cortical area for language and motor engrams (Figures 7, 8, and 9). On the diagram on Figure 2, this would be equivalent to Lesion 4.

APRAXIA INDUCED BY POSTERIOR HEMISPHERIC
LESIONS

By using a neural model similar to that used by Wernicke (1874) to explain language processing, Geschwind (1965, 1975) proposed that language elicits motor behavior in the following manner: Auditory stimuli reach Heschl's gyrus and undergo auditory analysis, then are processed in Wernicke's area (the posterior portion of the superior temporal gyrus), which appears to be important in language comprehension. Wernicke's area is connected to the premotor areas or motor association cortex by the arcuate fasciculus, and the motor association area on the left is connected to the primary motor area on the left. When someone is asked to carry out a command with his right hand, he uses this pathway. If one wishes to carry out commands with the left hand, a similar neural substrate is used, except that information is carried from the left motor association cortex to the right motor association cortex and then to the right motor cortex.

Geschwind (1965, 1975) suggested that disruptions in certain portions of Wernicke's arc and its connections to the right motor association cortex may explain most of the apraxic disturbances. When patients with lesions in Heschl's gyrus and Wernicke's area fail to carry out verbal commands, their difficulty usually is not caused by a defect in skilled movement, but rather, by a comprehension defect. Callosal lesions produce the type of apraxia that we have already discussed. Lesions that destroy the left motor association cortex (also discussed) are usually associated with a right hemiparesis, but they also destroy the callosal pathway going from the left motor association cortex to the right motor association cortex.

According to Geschwind's schema, lesions in the region of the arcuate fasciculus and supramarginal gyrus should disconnect posterior language areas—important in language comprehension—from the motor association cortex—important in programming movements. Therefore, patients with lesions in this area should be able to comprehend commands with difficulty in performing motor skills to command. Unlike gesture-to-command that requires left hemisphere language processing, imitation of gesture should not require language processing. Because most right-handed apraxic patients do not have a right hemisphere lesion, they should be able to imitate, but cannot.

To explain this discrepancy, Geschwind (1965) proposed that the left arcuate fasciculus is dominant for these visuomotor connections. An alternative hypothesis that may help to explain these patients' inability to carry out skilled movements to both command and imitation is that visuokinesthetic motor engrams are stored in the dominant parietal lobe. These engrams are necessary to program the motor association cortex to make the correct movements. In turn, the motor association cortex connects to the motor cortex.

We wished to distinguish between dysfunction caused by destruction of the parietal areas, where these acts may be programmed, and the apraxia induced by a disconnection of this parietal area from the motor association cortex. We tested the ability of patients with dominant (left hemisphere) parietal lesions to differentiate a correctly performed skilled act from a poorly performed one. We found that such patients had more difficulty making these discriminations than do patients with anterior lesions (Heilman, Rothi, & Valenstein, 1982). Patients with posterior left hemisphere lesions often fail to comprehend language. In spite of an intact right hemisphere, they also fail to comprehend gestures. Their inability to comprehend gestures may be related to the destruction of the visuokinesthetic motor engrams.

Apraxia with Meaningless Gestures

Kimura (1982), using relatively meaningless gestures divided into single and multiple oral and hand movements, found differences in intrahemispheric organization of motor function. A left anterior-lesioned group was more impaired in single oral movements and a left posterior group in single hand postures. With multiple movement there was less localization. In the study by Kolb and Milner (1981) on a population of epileptics at the Montreal Neurological Institute, complex, meaningless arm movements were impaired mostly with left parietal lobe excisions, but facial movements were impaired more after frontal lobe excisions on either side. These patients, however, had no difficulty with symbolic gestures and few were aphasic. Meaningless movements differ in many respects from symbolic or purposeful movements traditionally tested in apraxia and each type of movement may be processed in a substantially different manner.

Limb Kinetic Apraxia

Patients with this disorder have a unilateral (contralesional) disturbance of movement that can be seen when these patients are asked to pantomime acts, to imitate, or to use actual objects. Patients with limb kinetic apraxia do not improve as much with imitation and actual object use as do patients with ideomotor apraxia. Unlike the patients with ideomotor apraxia who use body parts as objects, sequence their movements incorrectly, or move their hands and fingers incorrectly in space, patients with limb kinetic apraxia may have a reduced number of movements or move slowly or imprecisely (overshoot and undershoot). Usually, this disorder maximally affects movements of the hand. Liepmann (1908) and Hécaen and Albert (1978) consider that limb kinetic apraxia (melokinetic apraxia) represents a form of movement disorder intermediate between paresis and apraxia. Kleist (1912) thought that this disorder resulted from an inability to correctly link independent muscle groups that have a separate innervation.

The precise anatomic localization of lesions that induce limb kinetic apraxia has not been determined. Liepmann (1908) thought that the seat of the disturbance is probably the cortex of the central convolutions. He also thought that the neighboring areas may also be important. Pyramidal lesions of monkeys (Lawrence & Kuypers, 1968) may induce a clumsiness of the contralateral extremity that cannot be completely accounted for by weakness or changes in tone or posture. Although patients with lesions in motor and premotor cortex often have clumsy movements of the contralateral hand, they often have spasticity and weakness and tend to assume a hemiparetic posture. Consequently, it is often difficult to be certain that they are truly apraxic.

VERBAL—MOTOR DISASSOCIATION APRAXIA

In previous papers and chapters, this form of apraxia had been termed "ideational apraxia" (Heilman, 1973, 1979). This was an unfortunate choice of terms because this syndrome is not the same as the ideational apraxia described by Pick (1905) and Liepmann (1908).

As previously discussed, patients with ideomotor apraxia who fail to pantomime correctly often may improve their performance with imitation and the use of actual objects. However, when compared with nonapraxics, ideomotor apraxics perform poorly on imitation and, at times, even in their use of actual objects. As previously discussed, patients with limb kinetic apraxia also often fail to imitate correctly and use actual objects. Heilman (1973) described three patients who were unlike others with ideomotor and limb kinetic apraxia; although they performed poorly with either hand to command, their performance on imitation and use of actual objects with either hand was excellent. Although these patients had fluent aphasia, they showed both verbally and nonverbally (by picking out the correct act performed by the examiner) that they comprehended the commands.

Liepmann (1908) thought that the presence of preserved copying ability may suggest that the patients had lesions posterior to those that induced ideomotor and limb kinetic apraxia. He postulated that patients with preserved imitation were unable to arouse the time–space–form picture of the movement. Similarly, Heilman (1973) proposed that patients with this form of apraxia had a disconnection between the areas decoding language and those containing visuo-kinesthetic motor engrams. Only one of the three patients described by Heilman (1973) had a positive radioisotope brain scan. This scan was abnormal in the region of, and deep to, the angular gyrus.

IDEATIONAL APRAXIA

Marcuse (1904), Pick (1905), and Liepmann (1908) described patients who had difficulty achieving a goal when it required a series of acts in a specific temporal order. For example, we may place an empty pipe, tobacco, and a match before a patient with ideational apraxia. To follow a request to smoke the pipe, the patient may light the match, attempt to light the empty bowl, put out the match, and then fill the bowl with tobacco.

Although patients with ideational apraxia may incorrectly sequence a series of acts, the individual acts may be correctly performed. In contrast, patients with ideomotor and limb kinetic apraxia may perform an act incorrectly but may be able to properly sequence a series of acts. Liepmann (1908) noted that these two syndromes often coexist in the same patient.

Ideational apraxia may be associated with difficulty in using actual objects correctly. As previously discussed, patients with ideomotor apraxia also may have difficulty with actual objects. Although patients with ideomotor apraxia (and limb kinetic apraxia) may make performance errors, they are usually able to discriminate what an object was designed to do. There are patients, however, who do not know the intended use of an object. They may not know what to do with it or may use it inappropriately (e.g., they may attempt to eat with a pencil). This form of disability has also been termed *ideational apraxia*. Although both agnostic and aphasic disturbances can masquerade as an apraxic disturbance, we suspect that an inability to recognize the intended use of an object is caused by a defect at a conceptual level. Patients with ideational apraxia usually have bilateral cerebral involvement such as infarcts, tumors, or Alzheimer's disease. Frequently, the CT scan in these patients will show profound cortical atrophy, or, at times, bilateral posteriorly placed infarcts or unilateral tumors or very large strokes.

Buccofacial Apraxia (Oral Apraxia)

Buccofacial apraxia was described in detail by Jackson (see Taylor, 1932) and is defined as an inability to perform learned skilled movements of the lips, facial muscles, tongue, pharynx, larynx, and respiratory muscles. Usually, unlearned (automatic) movements like chewing are preserved. Most patients with buccofacial apraxia may improve somewhat with imitation, but their performance remains abnormal. The use of an actual object, like a straw, or even seeing a lighted match may dramatically improve their performance. Unlike those with facial diplegia, these patients may have only unilateral facial weakness or no weakness at all. When asked to pantomime a learned skilled movement (e.g., "Show me how you would blow out a match."), the patient makes the wrong movement in space and may also sequence the movement incorrectly. Buccofacial apraxia most often occurs with ideomotor limb apraxia; however, each of these forms of apraxia may occur independently. Buccofacial apraxia as noted by Liepmann (1908) often accompanies Broca's aphasia. DeRenzi, Pieczuro, and Vignolo (1966) noted that 90% of Broca's aphasics have buccofacial apraxia. However, because buccofacial apraxia may occur in the absence of aphasia and Broca's aphasia may occur in the absence of buccofacial apraxia, the relationship is not causal.

An extensive study of the localization of lesions that induce buccofacial apraxia has been done by CT scan by Tognola and Vignolo (1980). They studied 28 patients with buccofacial apraxia and found that the most crucial areas include the frontal opercula, central (Rolandic) opercula, first central convolution, and the anterior portion of the insula. Lesions that did not induce buccofacial apraxia were mainly posteriorly situated, spacing the frontal and central opercula and the anterior portion of the insula.

Kleist (1934) suggested that the posterior lesions may induce an ideomotor buccofacial apraxia and the anterior lesion may induce a kinetic buccofacial apraxia. Benson, Sheremata, Bouchard, Segarra, Price, and Geschwind (1973) and Geschwind (1975) proposed that buccofacial apraxia may accompany posterior lesions. We have seen cases of buccofacial apraxia in which the lesion was in the region of the supramaximal and angular gyrus and did not involve the critical areas of Tognola and Vignolo (1980). In a study of apraxia and aphasia, Kertesz (1979) found that although buccofacial apraxia was more prominent with Broca's aphasia, it was present with Wernicke's aphasia and other fluent aphasias.

Conclusions

The inability to carry out learned skilled movements can be induced in righthanders by a variety of left hemispheric periSylvian lesions. Lesions in the premotor or motor cortex or both may induce a contralateral clumsy extremity (limb kinetic apraxia). Lesions in the corpus callosum and the left motor association cortex may disconnect the neurons in the right motor cortex from the visuokinesthetic motor engrams encoded in the posterior portion of the left hemisphere and produce an ideomotor apraxia of the left hand. Lesions in the region of the supramarginal and angular gyrus may destroy these visuokinesthetic motor engrams. Destruction of these engrams not only induces a bilateral ideomotor apraxia but also may induce a receptive disability. Lesions in and deep to the angular gyrus induce a verbal–motor apraxia in which the patient has difficulty carrying out skilled movements to command but flawlessly uses actual objects and imitates. Finally, patients with extensive cortical lesions may fail to correctly sequence a series of acts or recognize the use of objects (ideational apraxia).

References

Benson, F., Sheremata, W., Bouchard, R., Segarra, H. M., Price, D., & Geschwind, N. (1973). Conduction aphasia: A clinico-pathological study. *Archives of Neurology, (Chicago), 28*, 339–346.

DeRenzi, E., Pieczuro, A., & Vignolo, L. A. (1966). Oral apraxia and aphasia. *Cortex*, *2*, 50–73.

Gazzaniga, M., Bogen, J., & Sperry, R. (1967). Dyspraxia following division of the cerebral commissures. *Archives of Neurology (Chicago)*, *16*, 606–612.

Geschwind, N. (1965). Disconnexion syndromes in animals and man. *Brain*, *88*, 237–294, 585–644.

Geschwind, N. (1975). The apraxias: Neural mechanisms of disorders of learned movements. *American Scientist*, *63*, 188–195.

Geschwind, N., & Kaplan, E. (1962). A human cerebral disconnection syndrome. *Neurology*, *12*, 675–685.

Hécaen, H., & Albert, M. L. (1978). *Human neuropsychology*. New York: Wiley.

Heilman, K. M. (1973). Ideational apraxia: A re-definition. *Brain*, *96*, 861–864.

Heilman, K. M. (1979). Apraxia. In K. M. Heilman & E. Valenstein (Eds.), *Clinical neuropsychology*. London & New York: Oxford University Press.

Heilman, K. M., Coyle, J. M., Gonyea, E. F., & Geschwind, N. (1973). Apraxia and agraphia in a left-hander. *Brain*, *96*, 1–28.

Heilman, K. M., Rothi, L. J., & Valenstein, E. (1982). Two forms of ideomotor apraxia. *Neurology*, *32*, 342–346.

Johns, D. F., & Darley, F. L. (1970). Phonemic variability in apraxia of speech. *Journal of Speech and Hearing Research*, *13*, 556–583.

Kertesz, A. (1979). Apraxia. *Aphasia and associated disorders*. New York: Grune & Stratton.

Kertesz, A. (1982). *The western aphasia battery*. New York: Grune & Stratton.

Kimura, D. (1982). Left-hemisphere control of oral and brachial movements and their relation to communication. *Philosophical Transactions of the Royal Society of London, Series B*, *298*, 135–149.

Kleist, K. (1912). Der gang und der gegenwurtige Stand der Apraxie-forschung. *Ergebnisse der Neurologie und Psychiatrie*, *1*, 342–452.

Kleist, K. (1934). *Gehirnpathologie*. Leipzig: Barth.

Kolb, B., & Milner, B. (1981). Performance of complex arm and facial movements after focal brain lesions. *Neuropsychologia*, *19*, 491–503.

Lawrence, D. G., & Kuypers, H. G. J. M. (1968). The functional organization of the motor systems in the monkey. *Brain*, *91*, 1–36.

Liepmann, H. (1908). *Drei Aufsatze aus dem Apraxie-gebiet*. Berlin: Karger.

Liepmann, H., & Maas, O. (1907). Fall von limksseiter Agraphie und Apraxie bei rechtsseitiger Lahmung. *Zeitschrift fuer Psychologie und Neurologie*, *10*, 214–227.

Marcuse, H. (1904). Apraktische Symptome bei einem Fall con senlier Demenz. *Zentralblatt fuer Nervheilkunde Psychiatrie*, *27*, 737–751.

Monakow, C. von (1914). *Die Lokalization im Grosshim und der Abbau der Funktionen durch corticale Herde*. Wiesbaden: Bergmann.

Pick, A. (1905). *Studien uber motorische Apraxie und ihre nahestehende Erscheinungen*. Leipzig: Deuticke.

Sheremata, W. A., Deonna, R. W., & Romanul, F. C. (1978). Agenesis of the corpus callosum and interhemispheric transfer of information. *Neurology*, *23*, 390.

Taylor, J. (Ed.) (1932). *The writings of John Hughlings Jackson*. London: Hodder & Stoughton.

Tognola, G., & Vignolo, L. A. (1980). Brain lesions associated with oral apraxia in stroke patients: A clinico-neuroradiological investigation with the CT scan. *Neuropsychologia, 18,* 257–272.

Valenstein, E., & Heilman, K. (1979). Apraxic agraphia. *Archives of Neurology (Chicago), 36,* 506–508.

Watson, R., & Heilman, K. (in press). Callosal ideomotor apraxia. *Brain.*

Wernicke, C. (1874). *Der aphasische Symptomenkomplex.* Breslau: Cohn & Weigart.

16

The Anatomical Basis
of Visual Agnosia

*Michael P. Alexander
and Martin L. Albert*

Introduction

Visual agnosia is a rare clinical disorder. Despite arguments to the contrary, it is also a specific disorder. Cogent attempts to discredit the concept of agnosia have been made periodically (Bender & Feldman, 1972; Critchley, 1964), however, there is no doubt that there exist specific syndromes of disordered visual identification that fit even a strict definition of agnosia. *Visual agnosia* may be defined as an impairment in visual recognition of objects (or other categories of stimuli such as faces or colors) despite visual acuity, visual fields, visual scanning, language function, and general mental abilities that

393

LOCALIZATION
IN NEUROPSYCHOLOGY

are adequate for the task. In the precise prose of Critchley (1964), "vision alone is powerless to evoke meaning . . . objects are detected, but not identified . . . [even though] the agnosic patient [has] no visual defect which might preclude him from seeing the object clearly; nor any inadequacy within his mental equipment."

To dispense with questions about the existence of visual agnosia, it is sufficient to make a few observations. First, Bay (1953) has argued that visual agnosia is reducible to a primary visual deficit if proper testing is utilized (adaptation times, flicker fusion frequencies, for example), but others have shown no relationship between the deficits in functional vision and the presence or absence of agnosia (Ettlinger, 1956; Levine, 1978). Second, Bender and Feldman (1972), among others, have claimed that agnosia is reducible to a primary visual defect combined with some general cognitive impairment. Perusal of the case material on which such claims are based reveals a flaw in that argument. They describe no patients with specific focal lesions (as described here in the section, "Associative Agnosias"); instead, all their patients apparently have diffuse or multifocal disorders. They argue, correctly, that a combination of visual and cognitive disorders may produce ostensibly agnosic behaviors. This observation is, however, of uncertain relevance to those cases with specific focal lesions. Third, surveys of large populations of brain-damaged individuals that attempt to identify patients with agnosia have not been a useful mechanism to uncover the rare, meaningful individual cases (Hécaen & Angelergues, 1962; DeRenzi & Spinnler, 1966). The primary source for study of visual agnosia is the individual case report with thoroughly examined, clearly defined deficits. It is also within that small, but illuminating, population that useful information about the neuroanatomical bases for agnosia will be found.

In this chapter we consider several relevant syndromes. We begin with a brief listing of those disorders that are probably best considered language disturbances limited to the visual modality: pure alexia, color anomia, and optic aphasia. This is followed by the major focus of the text, the associative agnosias (i.e., object agnosia and prosopagnosia). We conclude with a review of apperceptive agnosia, a disorder which rightfully may be considered a primary visual disorder. Each syndrome is defined, with its typical findings enumerated, its anatomical localization emphasized, and its psychophysiological nature briefly considered.

Language Deficits Limited
to the Visual Modality

There are three syndromes, not truly agnosic, that may be confused with visual agnosia and, therefore, require definition to set them clearly off from agnosia. These three syndromes are pure alexia (also called "alexia without agraphia"), color anomia (also called "color agnosia"), and optic aphasia. Patients with visual agnosias commonly have impaired reading, impaired color naming, and impaired object naming to visual presentation, but these findings alone are *not* sufficient to establish a diagnosis of agnosia as defined here.

Patients with *pure alexia* have normal spoken language, normal auditory comprehension, and normal written language, at least within the limits of writing without meaningful visual–verbal feedback. Reading is severely impaired initially, but in most cases numbers, many letters and some short words can be read (Geschwind, 1965). The range of eventual severity and outcomes may be quite wide (Johannsen & Fahlgren, 1979). The neuropathological basis of pure alexia, at least in right-handed adults, is an extensive left occipital lesion; many different etiologies have been reported.

The neuropsychological mechanism(s) is/are not known with certainty. Geschwind (1965) has re-emphasized the traditional theory of a visual–verbal disconnection, but other investigators have stressed either a visual processing disturbance (Levine & Calvanio, 1978) or a disruption of specific cortical centers (Hécaen & Albert, 1978). Some authors (Oxbury, Oxbury, & Humphrey, 1969) have noted that in the severe case of pure alexia, patients are unable to demonstrate recognition of letters and thus might be said to have an agnosia for letters, but because there are no other purely visual recognition disturbances, we have not included pure alexia as a form of visual agnosia.

Color anomia is primarily a disturbance in the use of color names, not a disturbance in the use of colors themselves independent of their names. When asked to name saturated colors, incorrect color names are produced, and when asked to point to a named color from among several choices, incorrect colors are selected. Tasks which are purely verbal ("What color is grass?" "What color represents cowardice?") are handled normally. Tasks that are purely visual (sorting by colors, hue discrimination, pseudoisochromatic plates) are usually normal. Occasional patients with color anomia do not use colors normally in coloring tasks (Lhermitte & Beauvois, 1973).

The neuropathological basis of color anomia is also a left occipital lesion, most commonly infarction. In patients with left occipital lesions but with preservation of the dorsal corpus callosum, color naming is normal. Furthermore, damage to limited portions of the interhemispheric visual pathways may produce a color-naming disturbance for colors presented to the left visual field only (Damasio, Chui, Corbett, & Kassel, 1980; Zihl & von Cramon, 1980). These observations suggest that the interhemispheric connections for color information are quite specific. The psychophysiologic mechanism is more clearly determined than that of alexia without agraphia. In color anomia, purely visual color tasks and purely verbal color tasks are normal (Damasio, McKee, & Damasio, 1979). Only tasks which require both aspects are abnormal. This observation has been interpreted as evidence for a visual–verbal dysconnection; functionally, it is a defect in the use of color names. This disorder in color naming is sometimes called "color agnosia," but we believe that this name causes confusion with the syndrome of achromatopsia in which the defects in color recognition are more clearly agnosic.

Optic aphasia is a disorder of object naming using vision alone, when naming is normal through other sensory modalities. When asked to name an object presented to vision, patients with optic aphasia primarily make aphasic errors, that is, the incorrect response is within the same semantic class as the target object (cup for glass, for example). Some errors are visual, that is, based on the visual shape or morphology of the object, not the class or category of the item (Lhermitte, Chedru, & Chain, 1973). Selecting a named object from among a group is much better although not normal.

The neuropathological basis of optic aphasia is also a left occipital lesion (Caplan & Hedley–White, 1974; Lhermitte and Beauvois, 1973). Oxbury and others (1969) have suggested that only very extensive infarctions in the left posterior cerebral artery territory, which includes the inferior lateral convexity of the temporal lobe, will produce optic aphasia. The psychophysiologic mechanism is apparently similar to that of color anomia. Only tasks which require the use of visual information to evoke a verbal label are abnormal. Several reviews of agnosia have not clearly distinguished between this naming disorder and a recognition disorder (Nielsen, 1937, for instance). Patients with optic aphasia are able to indicate normal recognition (descriptive gestures, circumlocutions, etc.) and thus are not agnosic. It is an important distinction; patients with visual agnosia cannot indicate recognition through any output modality.

Pure alexia, color anomia, and optic aphasia are all disorders of language limited to the visual modality. Although the distinctions may be arbitrary at times (as described for pure alexia), for the reasons given, we do not believe it useful to consider these three disorders as partial syndromes of visual agnosia. Collectively, they represent one boundary of associative agnosia.

One last cautionary remark concerns potential confusion between aphasia and agnosia. Visual agnosia is a disorder in visual recognition of one or more specific categories of items. All patients with aphasia have defects in word finding. The difficulty in word finding is an integral element of the larger language disorder. It may encompass proper names, object names, body part names, and so forth, but there is little or no difference in word retrieval ability with different modalities of object presentation, such as visual or tactile (Goodglass, Barton, & Kaplan, 1968). Despite impaired naming, aphasic patients can demonstrate normal recognition (circumlocution, gesture, etc.). A patient with agnosia cannot demonstrate recognition (naming, circumlocution, description of use, pantomime, etc.), but items presented through other intact sensory modalities are recognized and identified. The differences between aphasia and agnosia should be clear, but in patients with left parietotemporal lesions and fluent aphasias, distinguishing them may require more than a casual examination.

Associative Agnosia

Visual associative agnosias are those disorders in which (1) visual acuity, visual fields, visual scanning, and mental capacity are adequate for perception; (2) adequate perception can be demonstrated through normal copying or description; but (3) *recognition* does not take place. This is not an aphasic naming defect but an impairment in recognition through the visual modality. To reemphasize, we reject the notion that these disorders are secondary to a deficit in primary visual function combined with a vague decrease in general mental abilities (Ettlinger, 1956; Ettlinger & Wyke, 1961). Associative visual agnosias are specific syndromes; we review object agnosia and, briefly, prosopagnosia.

OBJECT AGNOSIA

Patients with visual agnosia typically complain that there is a problem with their eyes, but they do not complain of visual loss and are unable to provide insight into the nature of their disability (Geschwind, 1965). By definition, visual acuity is normal or near normal. Visual field defects are seen, but no particular pattern dominates. In the reported cases where optokinetic nystagmus is specifically mentioned, generally, it has been normal. There are no deficits on the neurologic examination outside the visual system.

There are associated visual deficits. Reading has been variously affected: severe alexia is the rule (Rubens & Benson, 1971) although some cases have mild or no alexia (Albert, Reches, & Silverberg, 1975; Mack & Boller, 1977). Prosopagnosia is uniformly severe. *Achromatopsia* (a defect in hue discrimination and color recognition, not merely color naming) has been variously affected: severe achromatopsia (Lhermitte, Chain, Escourolle, Ducarne, & Pillon, 1972; Mack & Boller, 1977) to normal color discrimination (Rubens & Benson, 1971). Topographic memory defects have not invariably been assessed, being present in some cases (Albert *et al.*, 1975) but not in others (Lhermitte *et al.*, 1972).

Visual agnosia for objects is manifested in several ways. Recognition of real-life objects is not completely lost but there may be variability in performance from session to session. Unambiguous items are recognized whereas uncommon and complex objects are not. Pictures are often more difficult than real objects, and complex pictures may be the most fragile category for recognition (Lhermitte *et al.*, 1972; Rubens & Benson, 1971). Analysis of errors reveals a preponderance of morphological (i.e., visual) errors not semantic (i.e., aphasic) mistakes (Lhermitte & Beauvois, 1973; Mack & Boller, 1977). Perseverative errors based on an initial morphological mistake or, at times, even on an initially normal response, are common. Uncertainty and rejection of correct answers are also common; for example, the patient will say, "Is it a comb?" or "That's not a watch."

The patient can demonstrate adequate perception in several ways: matching identical objects (Albert *et al.*, 1975), drawing a presented object (Rubens & Benson, 1971), or copying a presented picture (Mack & Boller, 1977; Rubens & Benson, 1971) even when the object or picture has not been recognized. All visual recognition tasks are performed slowly and deficits are magnified by restricting the exposure time. Recognition difficulties are reduced if the patient is given categorical information about an object or if he sees it in its natural use. Selecting a named item from an array is less difficult. Patients followed for months/years have shown considerable improvement in object recognition, but complex pictures and familiar faces have remained difficult to identify.

In 1937, Nielsen reviewed all the autopsied cases to that time (13 in number) and concluded that the "center" for object recognition was the posterior inferior occipital convexity on the left. Unilateral superficial lesions in that region or deep left occipital lesions disrupting input from both calcarine regions produced agnosia. Review of the 13 cases leaves little doubt that they are *not* suitable for anatomical–clinical correlations for one or more reasons: inadequate testing, inappropriate pathologies (i.e., brain tumors with mass effect), failure to separate naming from recognition disturbances, and unsubstantiated assertions about cerebral dominance.

The anatomical localization of associative visual agnosia is a relatively recent accomplishment. The clinical setting in which visual associative agnosia has been best described is stroke: one- or two-step ischemic events in the posterior cerebral artery territories. Three representative cases have come to post-mortem study (Albert, Soffer, Silverberg, & Reches, 1979; Benson, Segarra, & Albert, 1974; Lhermitte *et al.*, 1972). The patient of Lhermitte *et al.* (1972) had infarcts in the posterior right hippocampus, the subcortical white matter of the right fusiform and lingual gyri, the cortex and subcortical white matter of the left fusiform gyrus, and the left angular gyrus (an older lesion). The patient of Benson *et al.* (1974) had infarcts in the cortex and subcortical white matter of the left fusiform and hippocampal gyri, the deep white matter of the right fusiform gyrus, and the ventral half of the splenium (Figure 1). The patient of Albert *et al.* (1979) had infarcts in the deep white matter of the right hippocampal and lingual gyri, the white matter of the left hippocampal gyrus, the cortex and subcortical white matter of the left fusiform gyrus, and the left lingual gyrus (Figure 2). The case of Mack and Boller (1977) had CT scanning performed, and infarcts were seen in the left posterior cerebral artery territory, the right, inferior occipital, and occipitotemporal region, including the deep white matter.

The psychophysiologic mechanisms of associative agnosia are implicit in the clinical and anatomical observations we have made. The errors are visual, not aphasic, and difficulty is influenced only by visual manipulations, such as using objects which are morpho-

(A)

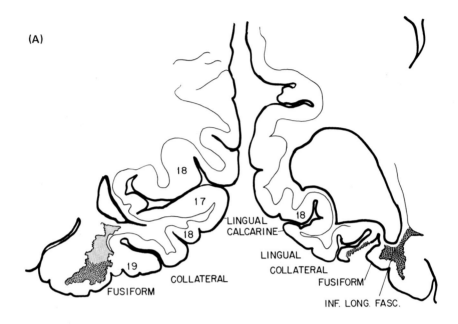

Figure 1. Pathologic anatomy in one case of visual agnosia and prosopagnosia. The figure represents three coronal sections which are 1 cm posterior to posterior callosal splenium (1A), at posterior splenium (1B), and 1 cm further anterior (1C). Gyri and Brodman's areas are indicated. Lesions in nearly symmetrical regions of fusiform gyri and ventral callosal splenium are indicated by stippling. From Benson, Segarra, and Albert (1974). Reprinted by courtesy of *Archives of Neurology,* © 1974, American Medical Association.

logically similar, displaying items out of their usual context, and using drawings which are visually complex. The difficulty is not simply a failure in visual perception because even adequately perceived stimuli may fail to evoke meaning and recognition. Associative visual agnosia is, apparently, a disruption of functional connections between visual processing or discrimination and memory systems: a visual–limbic disconnection (Albert *et al.*, 1979). Bilateral damage to the white matter association pathways (the inferior longitudinal fasciculus) from occipital association cortex to medial temporal lobe is the pathologic substrate.

Recently, Ross (1980a) has described memory disturbances limited to a specific sensory modality. He has speculated, in a manner parallel to ours, that disruption of pathways from visual systems to

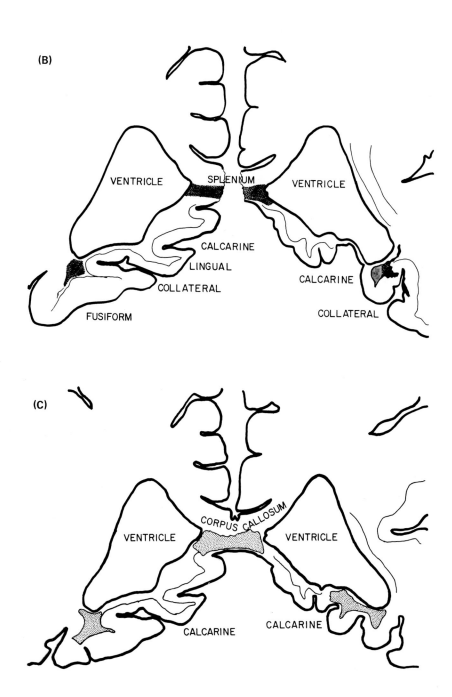

(B)

(C)

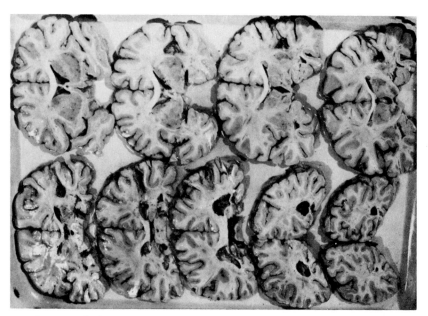

Figure 2. Pathologic anatomy in a case of visual agnosia and prosopagnosia. General sections are in posteroanterior view, from occipital (lower right) to anterior temporal-midfrontal (upper left). The bilateral areas of old infarction in the parahippocampal gyri with extension into the subjacent white matter destroying the inferior longitudinal fasciculus. There is a small infarction in the left occipitotemporal gyrus. Figure from Albert ML, Soffer D, Silverberg R, Reches A (1979), reprinted courtesy of *Neurology*.

hippocampus blocks access of the visual system to memory systems. He has further (Ross, 1980b) suggested that many deficits attributed to an agnosia should more accurately be considered modality-specific memory deficits. We do not consider any mnestic explanation adequate for the clinical phenomenon of failure to recognize long-familiar objects with unlimited time (Albert, 1980). It is probable that patients with visual agnosia *also* have new learning deficits specific to visual material, perhaps on the same pathological basis.

The associated findings may be explained by a similar review of the relevant anatomy. The uniformly present prosopagnosia probably is a result of the same lesions and might be simply a more sensitive measure of visual discrimination–visual memory connections. In those cases with alexia, the lesion also disrupts functional connections between visual association cortex bilaterally and the left language zone: a large, left medial occipital lesion with splenial involvement (Benson et al., 1974) or deep, left parietal damage (Lhermitte et al., 1972). In some cases, preserved reading is accounted for by preservation of either the more lateral left occipito–angular connections, or the splenium, or both (Albert et al., 1979). Impaired verbal (Wapner, Judd, & Gardner, 1978) or visual (Albert et al., 1979) memory reflects anterior extension of the lesion into the medial temporal regions.

Discussed in detail elsewhere (Chapter 17), a brief word here on prosopagnosia will clarify these anatomical issues. Prosopagnosia is impaired visual recognition of familiar faces. Patients are aware of this problem and complain of it, but the patient's subjective assessment of his disability rarely provides helpful insight into the nature of the visual or visual–memory disorder. On examination, visual acuity and mentation are adequate. Visual field deficits are common. In a thorough review, Meadows (1974) analyzed the visual fields in all reported cases and demonstrated a preponderance of left hemifield and upper quadrant defects, superior altitudinal defects being most common. Highly trained visual discrimination (and memory) skills are lost in parallel. These skills may be idiosyncratic; for instance, the ability of a farmer to distinguish his cows (Bornstein, Sroka, & Munitz, 1969) or of an electrician to distinguish different wiring panels (personal case experience).

The psychophysiologic mechanism of prosopagnosia is not known, but there is some evidence identifying neuropsychologic deficits that are not sufficient to explain prosopagnosia. Simple visual discrimination of faces is not the relevant difficulty. Several patients with prosopagnosia have been studied for their ability to distinguish small visual differences in unfamiliar faces (lighting, angulation, etc.); in three cases, this visual discrimination skill was normal (Assal, 1969; Benton & Van Allen, 1972; Rondot, Tzavaras, & Garcia, 1967), in one case, it was abnormal (DeRenzi, Faglioni, & Spinnler, 1968). Milner (1968) has shown that patients with right parietal lesions have impaired discrimination of unfamiliar faces but none of these patients had prosopagnosia.

Furthermore, memory disturbance alone is insufficient to account for prosopagnosia. Patients with Korsakoff's disease do not have prosopagnosia despite a severe impairment in memory. Milner (1968) demonstrated that patients with right medial temporal lesions have impaired short-term memory for unfamiliar faces, but again, none of her patients had prosopagnosia. That prosopagnosia occurs in patients with normal (or at least adequate) memory suggests that impaired recognition of familiar faces is caused by a disconnection between visual processing and visual memory (Rubens & Benson, 1971). Thus, prosopagnosia would be an associative disorder because of the deficit in associating normal perception with normal memory: a visual–limbic disconnection.

All patients with visual object agnosia have prosopagnosia; the reverse is not always true, and prosopagnosia is much more common than object agnosia. The neuropsychological mechanisms are closely related. The pathologic anatomy of the two disorders is very similar (Chapter 17). We believe that patients with prosopagnosia alone have a milder form of exactly the same disorder as patients with both object agnosia and prosopagnosia.

Apperceptive Agnosia

In the traditional dichotomy of higher-level visual processes (see Rubens & Benson, 1971), associative agnosias were those disorders in which visual perception is adequate, but recognition does not take place. *Apperceptive agnosias* are those in which there is demonstrable visual function with poor perception. Logically, recognition could be no better than perception. It is reasonable to consider apperceptive agnosia as a form of visual impairment and not a higher-level processing or recognition deficit, but the clinical syndrome of apperceptive agnosia is sufficiently different from peripheral visual loss and from cortical blindness that separate clinical identification is warranted. The clinical syndrome has been described in two distinctive settings: carbon monoxide poison and bilateral structural occipital damage due to stroke or trauma.

There are two case reports of carefully studied patients with visual problems after carbon monoxide injury; their disorder is quite specific (Adler, 1944; Benson & Greenberg, 1969). Both patients were young adults who suffered acute carbon monoxide intoxications with subsequent confusional states; one patient (Benson & Greenberg, 1969) had more evidence of diffuse brain injury. Both complained of visual loss from the outset and were, ostensibly, blind for several days. Both had nearly normal acuity. One patient could not be tested with the usual techniques, but detection of small dots on a white background was used to compute acuity. Visual fields were normal to a 3 mm white object. Optokinetic nystagmus was normal in the patient tested. Extraocular movements were not entirely normal: Visual fixation fatigued and eye movements were erratic and constricted.

Both patients could name saturated colors and detect light–dark differences and movement. All other visual tasks were impaired. Alexia was severe, including for letters, although one patient (Adler, 1944) learned to trace letters in order to recognize them. Object recognition was severely impaired; picture recognition even more so, especially for black-and-white photographs. Facial recognition was also severely impaired. Geometric figures could not be distinguished at all. When attempting to recognize any visual target, the patients had erratic eye movements and seemed to detect only one feature of a stimulus at a time. There was severe topographical disorientation. Copying and matching of objects was also impaired.

The morbid anatomy of this unique disorder is not known with certainty; there are no postmortem data. The patient of Benson and Greenberg had bilateral posterior slowing on electroencephalography performed 7 months after injury; pneumoencephalography revealed bilateral posterior ventricular enlargement. Adler's patient had a normal electroencephalogram 3 weeks and, again, 4 months after injury. Basing their argument on the known neuropathology of carbon monoxide intoxication (Richardson, Chambers, & Heywood, 1959), Benson and Greenberg argued that calcarine neuronal laminar necrosis had occurred and that the degradation of visual information for contrast, margin, edge, and form occurred within the calcarine cortex. This argument is compatible with the putative cellular function of the calcarine cortex as a stepwise feature analyzer.

The remaining cases of apperceptive visual agnosia are heterogeneous. A few include both adequate anatomical information and detailed test procedures, and illustrate apperceptive agnosia with focal structural brain lesions (Kertesz, 1979; Levine, 1978; Tyler, 1967). The etiology was severe closed head injury, tumor compression and surgical manipulation, and bilateral posterior cerebral artery ischemia, respectively.

In these three cases, visual acuity was normal or near normal ($\frac{20}{20}$ to $\frac{20}{30}$); nevertheless, two patients complained of visual loss. Visual fields were abnormal in all three cases: extremely rapid adaptation of the entire peripheral fields (Tyler, 1967); left hemianopia, right upper quadrantanopia and diminished flicker fusion in the preserved quadrant (Levine, 1978); and constricted fields with abnormal adaptability (Kertesz, 1979). All patients had severe gaze disturbance with inability to maintain fixation and impaired ocular pursuit. Two had severely impaired visually guided hand movements (optic ataxia). All three had simultanagnosia: inability to analyze more than a single feature of a complex stimulus at one time, combined with erratic eye movements. Visual processing was sensitive to the duration of stimulus exposure on tachistoscopic presentation. Letters, objects, pictures and faces were all poorly identified. With objects and pictures, copying was severely impaired but matching was nearly normal.

Further testing revealed different responses in the three cases. Kertesz concluded that improved visual identification with auditory facilitation argued for an associative mechanism in his patient. Levine contended that normal copying, given unlimited time, was not evidence for an associative mechanism and that more basic visual disorders (diminished feature extraction and slow feature processing) were responsible. Tyler dismissed associative–apperceptive arguments and asserted that a combination of primary visual disorders (deficits in feature analysis and processing time) combined with faulty visual search and fixation produced his patient's problem. We repeat our initial observation that this syndrome has elements resembling a primary visual disorder, but that it is sufficiently different from peripheral visual disorders and from cortical blindness to warrant independent clinical status.

The specific neuroanatomical basis of this complex syndrome of visual identification is not known; postmortem data are not available and the clinical material is heterogeneous. The neuroophthalmologic data support more extensive bilateral damage to optic radiations and/or calcarine cortex than in the cases of the associative agnosia. One clinical setting is the bilateral posterior cerebral artery territory infarction sparing the most posterior calcarine regions. The other is trauma with either direct occipitotemporal contusions or increased intracranial pressure causing tentorial herniation and secondary posterior cerebral artery territory ischemia (Keane, 1980; Kertesz, 1979; Levin & Peters, 1976). There is, however, a related neuropsychologic syndrome about which some neuroanatomical data exist: Balint's syndrome.

Balint's syndrome consists of three specific disturbances: (1) psychic paralysis of fixation of gaze: an inability to voluntarily look toward a point in the peripheral fields; (2) optic ataxia: an inability to carry out accurate hand and arm movements under visual control; and (3) diminished visual attention: only single, central, and powerful stimuli are noticed. Only a few cases of Balint's syndrome are in the literature (Hécaen & de Ajuriaguerra, 1954). The pathology has rarely been helpful for specific clinicoanatomic correlations, but all cases have had bilateral lesions of the parietal–occipital regions, affecting cortex and portions of the subcortical white matter (Hécaen & de Ajuriaguerra, 1954), presumably damaging occipitofrontal connections. The medial and basilar temporo-occipital structures and connections are not involved (Tyler, 1967). There is also evidence that the individual elements of Balint's syndrome are caused by occipitofrontal disconnection. For instance, several case studies (Auerbach & Alexander, 1981; Damasio & Benton, 1979) have demonstrated that unilateral optic ataxia (more accurately called "impaired visually guided hand movement") is seen with small lesions in the contralateral superior parietal lobule and the underlying white matter. Damage to these white matter pathways produces inaccurate reaching in monkeys (Haaxma & Kuypers, 1975). Perhaps, in patients with apperceptive agnosia, there is sufficient injury to the occipital regions that the cells of origin for the long (occipitofrontal via parietal lobe) and the short (occipitotemporal) association tracts are damaged. As a result, both Balint's syndrome and agnosic syndromes are seen.

Case Examples

E. S. This 33-year-old, right-handed man was found unconscious in a burning home. He remained unconscious for 2 days. Soon after awakening, he noticed visual problems that he described as being able to see far but not near objects, and not being able to recognize faces. After discharge, he also became aware of memory problems. He was evaluated at the Boston Veterans Administration Medical Center 7 months after his initial injury. Neurologic examination was normal except for fleeting, small amplitude, shifting myoclonic jerks of the limbs at rest. Language (excluding visual presentation) and verbal reasoning were normal. Memory (verbal) was severely impaired (verbal IQ—WAIS 90; memory quotient—WMS 60). Oral calculations were impaired, but right–left orientation and finger recognition were intact. Drawing to command (eyes opened or closed) was exceedingly poor with failure of line closure, overdrawing, and omissions; he often would be unable to tell what he had done and thus be unable to finish. Writing was similarly impaired.

Visual acuity could not be measured, but he gave ample evidence of being able to see very small objects if the objects were alone and moving (e.g., identifying birds or planes flying at a great distance or easily detecting a 1-mm white object at a 2-m distance). Visual fields were normal to 1 mm white object at 2 m. Extraocular movements were normal except that he could not maintain fixation and, if he lost fixation, he could no longer see the object at which he had been looking. There was bilateral impairment of visually guided hand movements. Colors were named as were most real objects, but all other visual tasks were severely impaired: reading letters or numbers, identifying faces, geometric figures, or complex pictures. He could not draw or copy any of these items (Figures 3a and 3b). He examined complex stimuli one element at a time.

Electroencephalogram was normal. Pattern shift visual evoked responses demonstrated no occipital potentials. CT scanning revealed moderate enlargement of cortical sulci. There was no important change over an additional 15 months of followup.

We concluded that E. S. had an apperceptive agnosia with the characteristic impairments of cortical damage secondary to carbon monoxide intoxication. Because his damage involved neurons

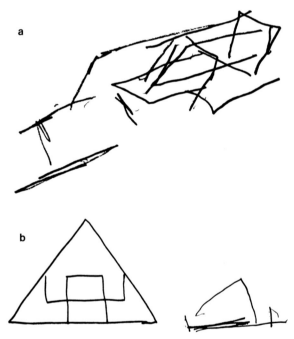

Figure 3. a. Copy of a line drawing made by E. S. in perspective of a house, which he did not recognize. b. Attempt to copy a geometric figure.

throughout the occipital regions, he had extensive disturbances in function including visual attention, visual perception, visual recognition and the use of vision to guide limb movements. We repeat that this disorder is not simply agnosic, but that it is clinically unique and clearly differs from cortical blindness or associative agnosia. Recognition of distinctive syndromes may be the first step to accurate diagnosis and prognosis.

G. H. This 47-year-old right-handed man suffered from severe depression and alcoholism. While intoxicated he fell, struck his forehead, and was taken to a local hospital where he evidenced a widespread bleeding disorder: melena, hemarthroses, ecchymoses, and grossly bloody spinal fluid, all believed secondary to alcohol induced thrombocytopenia. CT scanning revealed bilateral occipitotemporal intracerebral hematomas (Figure 4a). Initially, he had a fluent aphasia with impaired comprehension and naming but normal repetition and severe alexia. He rapidly developed progressive hydrocephalus, and a ventriculoperitoneal shunt was placed. After surgery, his language and memory improved dramatically (verbal IQ—WAIS 101; memory quotient—WMS 99). He was discharged with major problems in reading and writing.

Detailed neuroophthalmologic assessment 5 months after injury revealed normal visual acuity, bilateral partial peripherial upper quadrant field defects (greater on the right), normal optokinetic nystagmus, and normal extraocular movements except for a subtle right superior oblique palsy. Visually guided hand movements were normal. Repeated evaluations over 1 year after injury revealed persistent difficulties in reading; a letter-by-letter approach allowed recognition of most words, but reading was inefficient. Spelling was poor, aloud or written. Color naming was normal, and the Ishihara plates were read correctly. Faces, personally familiar or famous, were poorly identified.

The patient underwent extensive re-evaluation 15 months post-injury. Neuroophthalmologic findings were unchanged. Language remained normal except for impaired spelling and mildly impaired naming through all modalities. Reading was laborious: All numbers and most letters were correctly identified, but words were read with a slow letter-by-letter approach. Memory was normal for verbal tasks, but severely impaired for nonverbal tasks. Right–left orientation, finger recognition, and oral calculations were normal. Proverb interpretations were adequate.

Visual testing revealed no evidence of real object agnosia but recognition of pictures was impaired. Complex, colored pictures were

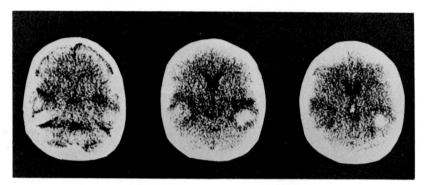

Figure 4a. Consecutive 10 mm, unenhanced CT scans performed 3 weeks postonset, demonstrating the resolving bilateral inferior temporal hematomas and surrounding edema. At the time of this scan, the patient had severe object agnosia, prosopagnosia and alexia, and moderate anomia. Hemorrhagic lesions are centered in the subcortical white matter of the fusiform gyrus and inferior temporal gyrus bilaterally; right-sided lesion extends somewhat higher than the left-sided lesion.

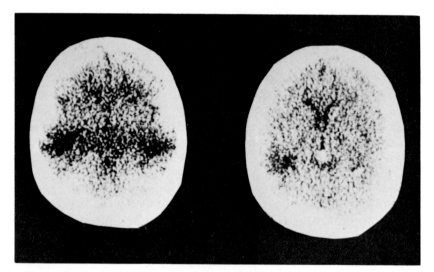

Figure 4b. Consecutive 10 mm, unenhanced CT scans performed 15 months post-onset, which demonstrating the residual areas of diminished densities in the inferior temporo-occipital junctions. At the time of this scan, the patient had severe pro-sopagnosia and alexia, agnosia for complex pictures (see text), and mild anomia. Lucent areas are in the deep white matter of the occipitotemporal junctions. At this time, the lucency in the left hemisphere extends more superiorly than on the right. (Lesions localized with the technique of Gado, Hanaway, & Frank, 1979.)

particularly difficult. Prosopagnosia was still prominent (seven of 22 correct, and five of those by paraphernalia of dress). Recognition of common animals in complex pictures was similarly impaired (five of 16 correct). Identification of familiar elements in the landscape (e.g., sunrise, Grand Canyon, Crater Lake, a windmill, the Statue of Liberty, etc.) was very poor (4 out of 12 correct). Pictures of people involved in sports events were much better identified (16 out of 20). He could copy well (Figure 5) including some drawings that he could not identify. There were several characteristic errors in these identification tasks: (1) mistakes were morphological; (2) he analyzed one item of a picture at a time. Sometimes identification of one element of a picture might be sufficient for recognition (e.g., tennis racket), but usually was not; (3) many answers revealed that he had only seen a portion of the picture (e.g., men in water with snorkels were described as swimming, and he denied seeing the snorkels); (4) he did not synthesize sequential elements (e.g., a montage of one woman in various steps of a waterskiing jump was identified as many women skiing in single file). A CT scan at 15 months post-onset revealed bilateral areas of lucency in inferior occipitotemporal junction, greater on the left (Figure 4b).

We concluded that G. H. had an associative agnosia. This was most apparent in the recognition of familiar faces and in the analysis of complex pictures. He also had a severe alexia, and we discussed the merits of considering occipital alexia to be a form of associative agnosia.

Although we cannot make subtle clinico-anatomic correlations on CT data alone, the available evidence suggests that calcarine cortical regions were not involved. The superior visual field defects were secondary to partial damage to the temporooccipital visual radiations. Visual agnosia was secondary to damage to the temporooccipital junctions; the absence of achromatopsia in this and other cases of prosopagnosia indicates that these disorders have close but not identical pathologic anatomy. The preserved verbal memory suggests that the left temporo-occipital damage did not extend into the left hippocampus. Preservation of parietooccipital structures accounts for the absence of any elements of Balint's syndrome.

Conclusions

1. The clinical syndromes of agnosia are distinct and have specific morbid anatomies.
2. Damage to calcarine cortex or to extensive portions of the oc-

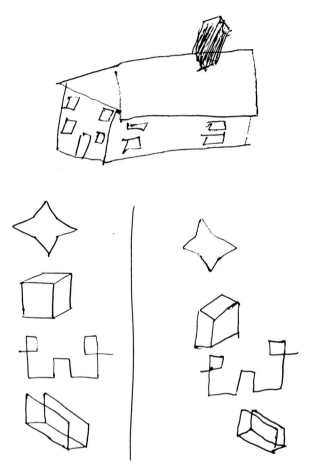

Figure 5. Copy of a line drawing made by G. H., perspective of a house which he recognized (top). Copies of several geometric figures (model on left) (bottom).

cipital visual radiations produces a disorder in visual perception in which visual identification of all categories of objects is impaired (possibly excepting color) and all occipital- fugal association functions are impaired (recognition, visually guided hand movements, etc.)
3. Bilateral damage to parietal lobe that includes the white matter and thus the superior coursing pathways from occipital association cortex to frontal motor and oculomotor cortex results in Balint's syndrome.

4. Bilateral damage to the inferior temporo-occipital junction that includes the subjacent white matter pathways; thus, the inferior coursing pathways from occipital association cortex to medial temporal regions results in the various forms of associative agnosia.

5. Injury to inferior occipital association cortex produces achromatopsia in the contralateral visual field. Injury to the dorsal splenial interhemispheric connections produces impaired color naming in the left visual field. If combined with a right hemianopia, color anomia will be seen, representing defective visual–verbal connections.

6. Injury to the ventral splenial interhemispheric connections in combination with a right hemianopia produces a visual–verbal dysconnection and pure alexia.

7. The usual cerebrovascular setting for the associative agnosias is posterior cerebral artery territory infarctions. Variability in collateral circulations and in border zone supply may account for the specific stroke syndromes.

8. The rarity of these syndromes is due to two factors: the optic radiations may be damaged by infarcts of somewhat greater size, thus producing visual field defects instead of agnosias; and precise bilateral lesions are required for the majority of these syndromes, an unusual occurrence.

References

Adler, A. (1944). Disintegration and restoration of optic recognition in visual agnosia: Analysis of a case. *Archives of Neurology and Psychiatry, 51,* 243–259.

Albert, M. L. (1980). Reply to Ross. *Neurology, 37,* 110.

Albert, M. L., Reches, A., & Silverberg, R. (1975). Associative visual agnosia without alexia. *Neurology, 25,* 322–326.

Albert, M. L., Soffer, D., Silverberg, R., & Reches, A. (1979). The anatomic basis of visual agnosia. *Neurology, 29,* 876–879.

Assal, G. (1969). Regression des troubles de la reconnaissance des physionomes et de la mémoire topographique chez un malade opere d'un hématome intracérébral pariéto-temporal droit. *Revue Neurologique, 121,* 184–185.

Auerbach, S. H., & Alexander, M. P. (1981). Pure agraphia and unilateral optic ataxia. *Journal of Neurology, Neurosurgery and Psychiatry, 44,* 430–432.

Bay, E. (1953). Disturbances of visual perception and their examination. *Brain, 76,* 515–530.

Bender, M. B., & Feldman, M. (1972). The so-called "visual agnosias." *Brain, 95,* 173–186.

Benson, D. F., & Greenberg, J. P. (1969). Visual form agnosia. *Archives of Neurology (Chicago), 20,* 82–89.

Benson, D. F., Segarra, J., & Albert, M. L. (1974). Visual agnosia-prosopagnosia. *Neurology, 30,* 307–310.

Benton, A. L., & Van Allen, M. W. (1972). Prosopagnosia and facial discrimination. *Journal of the Neurological Sciences, 15,* 167–172.

Bornstein, B., Sroka, H., & Munitz, H. (1969). Prosopagnosia with animal face agnosia. *Cortex, 5,* 164–169.

Caplan, L. R., & Hedley-White, T. (1974). Cuing and memory dysfunction in alexia without agraphia: A case report. *Brain, 97,* 251–262.

Critchley, M. (1964). The problem of visual agnosia. *Journal of the Neurological Sciences, 1,* 274–290.

Damasio, A. R., & Benton, A. L. (1979). Impairment of hand movements under visual guidance. *Neurology, 29,* 170–178.

Damasio, A. R., Chui, H. C., Corbett, J., & Kassel, N. (1980). Posterior callosal section in a non-epileptic patient. *Journal of Neurology, Neurosurgery and Psychiatry, 43,* 351–356.

Damasio, A. R., McKee, J., & Damasio, H. (1979). Determinants of performance in color anomia. *Brain and Language, 7,* 74–85.

Damasio, A. R., Damasio, H., Van Hoesen, G. W. (1982). Prosopagnosia: Anatomic basis and behavioral mechanisms. *Neurology, 32,* 331–341.

DeRenzi, E., & Spinnler, H. (1966). Visual recognition in patients with unilateral cerebral disease. *Journal of Nervous and Mental Disease, 112,* 515–525.

DeRenzi, E., Faglioni, P., & Spinnler, H. (1968). The performance of patients with unilateral brain damage on face recognition tasks. *Cortex, 4,* 17–34.

Ettlinger, G. (1956). Sensory deficits in visual agnosia. *Journal of Neurology, Neurosurgery and Psychiatry, 19,* 297–301.

Ettlinger, G., & Wyke, M. (1961). Defects in identifying objects visually in a patient with cerebrovascular disease. *Journal of Neurology, Neurosurgery and Psychiatry, 24,* 254–259.

Gado, M., Hanway, J., Frank, R. (1979). Functional anatomy of the cerebral cortex by computed tomography. *Journal of Computer Assisted Tomography, 3,* 1–9.

Geschwind, N. (1965). Disconnection syndromes in animals and man. *Brain, 88,* 239–294, 585–644.

Goodglass, H., Barton, M. I., & Kaplan, E. (1968). Sensory modality and object-naming in aphasia. *Journal of Speech and Hearing Research, 3,* 257–267.

Haaxma, R., & Kuypers, H. (1975). Intrahemispheric cortical connections and visual guidance of hand and finger movements in the rhesus monkey. *Brain, 98,* 239–260.

Hécaen, H., & Albert, M. I. (1978). *Human neuropsychology.* New York: Wiley, pp. 54–58.

Hécaen, H., & Angelergues, R. (1962). Agnosia for faces (prosopagnosia). *Archives of Neurology 7,* 24–32.

Hécaen, H., & de Ajuriaguerra, J. (1954), Balint's syndrome (Psychic paralysis of visual fixation) and its minor forms. *Brain, 77,* 373–400.

Johansson, T., & Fahlgren, H. (1979). Alexia without agraphia: Lageral and medial infarction of left occipital lobe. *Neurology, 29,* 390–393.

Keane, J. R. (1980). Blindness following tertorial herniation. *Annals of Neurology, 8,* 186–190.

Kertesz, A. (1979). Visual agnosia: The dual deficit of perception and recognition. *Cortex, 15,* 403–419.

Levin, H. S., & Peters, B. H. (1976). Neuropsychological testing following head injuries; prosopagnosia without visual field defect. *Diseases of the Nervous System,* 68–71.

Levine, D. N. (1978). Prosopagnosia and visual object agnosia: A behavioral study. *Brain and Language, 5,* 341–365.

Levine, D. N., & Calvanio, R. (1978). A study of the visual defect in verbal alexia-simultanagnosia. *Brain, 101,* 65–81.

Lhermitte, F., & Beauvois, M. F. (1973). A visual-speech disconnexion syndrome: Report of a case with optic aphasia, agnosic alexia and colour agnosia. *Brain, 96,* 695–714.

Lhermitte, F., Chain, F., Escourolle, R., Ducarne, B., & Pillon, B. (1972). Etude anatomo-clinique d'un cas de prosopagnosie. *Revue Neurologique, 126,* 329–346.

Lhermitte, F., Chedru, F., & Chain, F. (1973). A propos d'un cas d'agnosie visuelle. *Revue Neurologique, 128,* 301–322.

Mack, J. L., & Boller, F. (1977). Associative visual agnosia and its related deficits: The role of the minor hemisphere in assigning meaning to visual perceptions. *Neuropsychology, 15,* 345–349.

Meadows, J. C. (1974). The anatomical basis of prosopagnosia. *Journal of Neurology, Neurosurgery and Psychiatry, 37,* 489–501.

Milner, B. (1968). Visual recognition and recall after right temporal lobe excision in man. *Neuropsychology, 6,* 191–209.

Nielsen, J. M. (1937). Unilateral cerebral dominance as related to mind blindness. *Archives of Neurology and Psychiatry, 38,* 108–135.

Oxbury, J. M., Oxbury, S. M., & Humphrey, N. K. (1969). Varieties of colour anomia. *Brain, 92,* 847–860.

Richardson, J. C., Chambers, R. A., & Heywood, P. M. (1959). Encephalopathies of anoxia and hypoglycemia. *Archives of Neurology (Chicago), 1,* 178–190.

Rondot, P., Tzavaras, A., & Garcia, R. (1967). Sur un cas de prosopagnosie persistant depuis quinze ans. *Revue Neurologique, 117,* 424–428.

Ross, E. D. (1980). Sensory-specific and fractional disorders of recent memory in man: I: Isolated loss of visual recent memory. *Archives of Neurology, 37,* 193–200.

Ross, E. D. (1980). The anatomic basis of visual agnosia. *Neurology, 30,* 109–110.

Rubens, A. B., & Benson, D. F. (1971). Associative visual agnosia. *Archives of Neurology (Chicago), 24,* 305–316.

Tyler, H. R. (1967). Abnormalities of perception with defective eye movements (Balint's syndrome). *Cortex, 3,* 154–171.

Wapner, W., Judd, T., & Gardner, H. (1978). Visual agnosia in an artist. *Cortex, 14,* 343–364.

Zihl, J., & von Cramon, D. (1980). Colour anomia restricted to the left visual hemifield after splenial disconnexion. *Journal of Neurology, Neurosurgery and Psychiatry, 43,* 719–724.

17

Localization of Lesions in Achromatopsia and Prosopagnosia

Antonio R. Damasio
and Hanna Damasio

The occurrence of acquired defects in color perception (achromatopsia) and facial recognition (prosopagnosia) was discovered at the end of the nineteenth century by Verrey (1888) and Wilbrand (1892), respectively. They described not only the fundamental clinical features but also an accurate anatomical localization. However, neither author has received appropriate credit (Verrey, in particular, has received little more than casual reference) and few defects of higher-brain function have remained as misunderstood and controversial. Indeed, the very existence of these disorders was denied for a long time and the early evidence from anatomical correlations was neglected for decades.

There are many reasons to explain the eventful history of achromatopsia and prosopagnosia. Perhaps the principal one is the rel-

LOCALIZATION
IN NEUROPSYCHOLOGY

ative rarity with which either disorder occurs. As a result, many researchers lack personal experience of the phenomenon, but both disorders have come to be recognized in recent years.

With respect to achromatopsia, Critchley (1965) acknowledged the existence of defects of color vision produced by lesions of the central nervous system; Meadows (1974) reviewed the literature in detail, and, in a series of recent papers, Albert, Reches, and Silverberg (1975), Green and Lessell (1978), Pearlman, Birch, and Meadows (1979), and Damasio, Yamada, Damasio, Corbett, and McKee (1980) provided fresh case material, correlated with radionuclide scan, computerized tomography (CT), and cerebral evoked potentials. Nevertheless, few textbooks of ophthalmology and neurology even mention achromatopsia. It is fair to say that not many neurologists investigate this condition to help their evaluation of a case.

The fate of prosopagnosia has been somewhat more fortunate. Bodamer (1947) coined an appropriate term for what had been known until then as *facial agnosia* (from the Greek *prosop* signifies face and *gnosis* signifies knowledge). It became easier to distinguish the phenomenon from the equally controversial *global visual agnosia*, of late designated as *visual object agnosia*. Furthermore, a large number of psychological studies in both normal and brain-damaged subjects approached the question of the mechanisms underlying the learning and recognition of human facial patterns. Such studies have contributed to the understanding of prosopagnosia, although they are also responsible for the erroneous and currently widespread notion that facial recognition is, somehow, a "right hemisphere task."

Another line of studies has clearly established that prosopagnosia is related to a defect in processing familiar faces, concomitantly, that the perception of previously unknown faces need not be impaired (Benton, 1979). But the most controversial chapter in the history of prosopagnosia relates to anatomical localization of the defect. Some authors (cf. Hécaen & Angelergues, 1962; Whitely & Warrington, 1977) suggested that prosopagnosia might result from a single lesion located in occipital or parietal lobe structures of the right hemisphere.

This notion clashes with the records of the 11 cases of prosopagnosia that have come to autopsy, as all such cases had bilateral lesions (see tabular matter, this chapter). Other authors, while agreeing that prosopagnosia is unlikely to result from unilateral lesion, have suggested that the lesion located in the right hemisphere is the crucial one, whereas almost any lesion in the left hemisphere might be the complement necessary for the defect to arise (Benton,

1979; Meadows, 1974). Our contention is not only that prosopagnosia requires a bilateral lesion but also that the lesions must
occur in visually related structures (Damasio, Damasio, & Van Hoesen, 1982).

Achromatopsia

Central achromatopsia is defined as an acquired failure to perceive
colors, in part or in the whole of the visual field, due to central nervous system (CNS) disease, and in the absence of retinal disease.
Visual acuity and depth perception are normal in the achromatopsic
field. The patient with achromatopsia is able to see well-formed images—in correct perspective—but only in shades of gray.

The essential anatomical correlate of achromatopsia was established by Verrey on the basis of a case in which only one field was
involved (hemiachromatopsia).

Verrey reported the case of a 60-year-old woman who suddenly
had lost the ability to perceive colors in the right visual field. In
addition, there was a 15° concentric restriction of the whole visual
field and a mild decrease in visual acuity in the right field. But the
patient did not have other neurologic signs, namely, no defect of
higher nervous function. The autopsy revealed an infarct in the left
occipital lobe. Verrey writes,

> The infarct extends from the white matter immediately above the lateral
> ventricle into the white matter of the third occipital gyrus continuing into
> the white matter of the occipital portion of the lingual and fusiform gyri
> and into the inferior caudal extreme of the cuneus. Towards the base of
> the brain it gets close to the mesial surface of the occipital lobe without
> completely destroying it.

Verrey concluded that "the center for the chromatic sense is located
in the most inferior portion of the occipital lobe, probably in the
posterior area of the lingual and fusiform gyri." He was entirely
correct. Nine decades later, we can applaud the observation and interpret it in terms of modern physiology of the nervous system.

Ten years after Verrey's initial case, MacKay and Dunlop (1899)
described a patient with complete achromatopsia. The brain of their
patient, a 62-year-old man, showed bilateral occipital lesions. In the
right hemisphere, the infarct involved both gray and white matter
in the temporo-occipital convolution (fusiform gyrus). There was involvement of the lower portion of the optic radiations but none of
the calcarine regions. In the left hemisphere, the infarcted area involved the temporo-occipital gyrus, extended into the lower portion

of the optic radiations, and moved deeper to involve a small portion of the gray substance of the calcarine fissure. Mackay and Dunlop concluded that the complete loss of color sense was "associated with a bilateral lesion of the fusiform gyrus, so well defined and symmetrical that it becomes difficult to avoid the conclusion that the gray matter of that convolution is probably concerned in the perception of colors."

The few modern cases in which some anatomical localization has been possible—by means of radionuclide or CT scanning—have reaffirmed Verrey's original discovery (Damasio *et al.*, 1980; Green and Lessell, 1977). One of our cases is a close behavioral and anatomical replica of Verrey's, although involving the opposite hemisphere.

The patient was a 49-year-old man, right-handed, who lost all color sense in the left visual field, suddenly and permanently (for a complete description, see Case 1 in Damasio, *et al.*, 1980). A careful neurologic and ophthalmologic examination disclosed only a 10° left homonymous defect, superior and quadrantic. The patient was unable to name or match colors in his left visual field, but as soon as the color stimulus passed the vertical meridian and came into the right visual field, naming became normal, as did color matching. In the left visual field itself, there was no deficit other than color perception: The patient was able to see and name even small objects.

The CT scan of this patient revealed a lesion involving the ventromedial quadrant of the right occipital lobe. It is likely that both the lingual and fusiform gyri were involved, but not the calcarine region that sits at a higher level (Figure 1). This localization is in keeping with the ophthalmological findings.

It is apparent that lesions of the inferior visual association cortex, of either the left or right hemisphere, will impair color perception, provided they compromise a crucial region of the fusiform gyrus. In the instance of a unilateral lesion, hemiachromatopsia will result; in that of a bilateral lesion, there will be complete achromatopsia.

For achromatopsia to appear, the lesion needs to be fairly circumscribed and low lying. If either the optic radiations or the primary visual cortex are involved to any considerable extent, a blind area of the field will develop, obviously precluding achromatopsia. That accounts for the rarity of achromatopsia. Most lesions of the lower occipital lobe will produce hemianopic field defects and patients report a blind field, not a color-deprived one.

It is interesting to note that lesions of the superior visual association cortex—related to the upper lip of the calcarine fissure—do

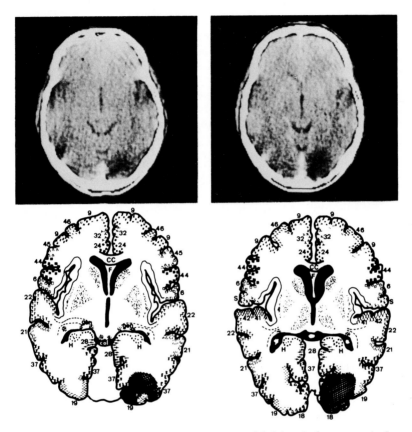

Figure 1. CT scan and templates of a patient with left hemiachromatopsia. Low-density area corresponds to infarct in the right occipital lobe, below the calcarine region, and involves the inferior visual association cortex.

not produce achromatopsia. This fact is of the highest interest. It supports the notion of parcellation of the visual association cortex in subregions capable of processing different features of visual information. The anatomical subregion specializing in color processing is located in the inferior visual association cortex; from there, it controls the chromatic information of the *entire* opposite hemifield. In all likelihood such a region is functionally and, perhaps, anatomically homologous to areas of maximal color coding described (Zeki, 1973, 1977) in the monkey (some controversy surrounds the studies of color processing in nonhuman primates; see De Monasterio and Schein, 1982). But the inferior occipital location of these lesions is interesting for yet another reason. It answers the question: why an observer as careful and astute as Gordon Holmes failed to encounter and even denied central achromatopsia. Lesions of the inferior visual association cortex were conspicuously absent in his war-injured patients (Damasio, 1981).

Prosopagnosia

Prosopagnosia is a distinct form of visual agnosia that, notably, affects the recognition of familiar human faces. Most patients also have difficulty in recognizing previously familiar stimuli that are part of a visually ambiguous class (e.g., cars, clothes, food utensils and ingredients, buildings). But a patient who is unable to recognize a given familiar face does know that a face is a face and can, if requested, point to its several components. The same patient, unable to recognize his own car, will know, however, that a car is a car and generically name or identify it as such. In other words, prosopagnosia compromises the recognition of a previously well-known, specific member within a visual class, although the recognition of the class in itself is not impaired.

On the other hand, patients with visual object agnosia fail even to recognize the class to which a certain stimulus belongs. When shown one of their belongings, they will not only fail to identify the object as their own but also will not recognize the general class to which it pertains. (For instance, they will be unable to name or identify a book, or a telephone.) Prosopagnosia and visual object agnosia can coexist. In fact, visual object agnosia is, in our experience, always accompanied by prosopagnosia. But prosopagnosia frequently is seen *without* visual object agnosia. Prosopagnosia is often, but not always, accompanied by achromatopsia, that affects some part, or all, of the intact visual field. (For additional details on the neurobehavioral mechanisms of prosopagnosia, see Damasio *et al.*, 1982.)

Prosopagnosia is an acquired condition, almost always of acute onset, most frequently consequent to infarctions in the territory of *both* posterior cerebral arteries. The defect almost invariably is permanent. Rarely, prosopagnosia can result from bilateral occipital tumors or from a seizure focus. In the latter case, the defect is paroxysmal.

Eleven cases of prosopagnosia have come to autopsy. In eight, the condition was due to stroke and the material lends itself appropriately to anatomical analysis.

The first case is that of Wilbrand, in 1892. He described a 63-year-old woman who suddenly became unable to recognize her friends, her relatives, and even the streets of her home town. She had bilateral field defects, particularly marked on the left. This patient died several years later from another cerebrovascular insult; her postmortem showed bilateral occipital lesions, involving the inferior temporal and temporo-occipital gyri, more extensively on the right side.

All other autopsied cases have demonstrated bilateral occipital lesions, mainly involving the lingual or fusiform gyri. There is no reported case of a unilateral lesion, in either right or left hemisphere, capable of causing prosopagnosia. Pertinent details of the eight cases are tabulated as follows, ordered by date of publication.

	Left hemisphere	Right hemisphere
Wilbrand (1892)	Cortical lesion is between 1st and 2nd occipital gyri but damage extends anteriorly to destroy the white matter of the whole lobe.	Fusiform gyrus. Cuneus (posterior portion). Cortex of calcarine fissure.
Heidenhain (1927)	Striate cortex. Extends anteriorly into mesial and inferior portions of the occipital lobe. Third occipital gyrus is destroyed. Involvement of lingual gyrus as well as inferior lip of calcarine cortex.	Identical to the left side but larger at the occipital pole.
Pevzner, Bornstein, and Loewenthal (1962)	The core of the lesion is in angular gyrus but it extends into the occipitoparietal sulcus.	Lower lip of calcarine fissure.
Gloning and Gloning (1970)	Lingual gyrus and fusiform gyri. There is involvement of optic radiations and extension into occipital pole.	Fusiform an lingual gyri. Lesion extends into supramarginal gyrus and involves optic radiations.
Lhermitte et al. (1972)	Cortex of fusiform gyrus. Lesion extends into occipital horn.	Fusiform and lingual gyri, predominantly the latter. Lesion extends into inferior lip of calcarine fissure and into hippocampus.
Benson et al. (1974)	Parahippocampal cortex. Anterior third of fusiform gyrus. Lesion extends to posterior periventricular white matter and to cingulate gyrus. (Lesion is much larger on the left.)	Cyst in fusiform gyrus.

(continued)

	Left hemisphere	Right hemisphere
Cohn *et al.* (1976)	Case 1: Upper and lower lip of calcarine fissure (spares polar portion of area). Caudal portion of hippocampal gyrus. Fusiform and lingual gyrus.	Upper and lower lip of calcarine fissure all the way to occipital pole. Lower portion of cingulate gyrus and precuneus. Caudal portion of hippocampal gyrus. Fusiform gyrus.
	Case 2: All of lingual and fusiform gyrus (the lesion is much larger than on the right).	Lingual and fusiform gyri close to the pole of the occipital lobe.

It is apparent that involvement was bilateral in all patients, and that damage compromised structures of the central visual system bilaterally also. Anatomically, the lesions were not necessarily a mirror image of each other. But in terms of the functional system affected, with one exception, the lesions were symmetric. The exception is the case of Pevzner *et al.* (1962); it should be noted that his patient was not a typical case of prosopagnosia. The facial recognition defect had improved remarkably and so had the achromatopsia. The course and exact nature of the disease were never clarified. Finally, the pathological findings were puzzling regarding *both* the left and the right lesions: A lesion of the inferior lip of the calcarine fissure on the right should not have produced more than an upper quadrantic field cut (that was the extent of the patient's defect at the time of death), whereas the lateral parieto-occipital lesion on the left is not typically associated with prosopagnosia. Obviously, additional structures must have been dysfunctional at the time the patient was prosopagnosic and achromatoposic. On balance, this case should be given limited weight in a discussion of the anatomical basis of prosopagnosia.

The three additional patients in whom autopsy was performed had tumors. Although tumor material is generally not appropriate for anatomical localization, it is interesting to note that all had bilateral lesions too, and that the lesion involved occipital lobe structures in all.

Computerized tomography has further contributed to the understanding of the anatomical correlates of prosopagnosia. In three of our cases (all due to vascular disease) we were able to obtain CT scans. The neuroradiological findings encountered in our study are tabulated as follows.

	Left hemisphere	Right hemisphere
Case 1 64-year-old man	Lesion involves Cortex of areas 17 and 18, and White matter subjacent to areas 17, 18, 19 and 37. Forceps major, optic radiations and inferior occipital bundle are compromised, too.	Lesion is lower and smaller than on left. It compromises white matter of occipitotemporal junction and inferior occipital lobe. Cortical involvement appears minimal.
Case 2 60-year-old woman	Lesion involves White matter of occipito-temporal junction and occipital lobe. Possible cortical involvement of areas 19, 20, 36 and 37.	Lesion is symmetrically placed but smaller than on the left. White matter of occipitotemporal junction is involved. Possible cortical involvement of areas 20 and 36.
Case 3 75-year-old man	Lesion involves White matter of occipital lobe subjacent to areas 17, 18, 19 and 37. Optic radiations as well as forceps major are damaged.	Lesion is lower and smaller than on the left, involving white matter subjacent to areas 17, 18 and 37.

All the described lesions either compromise cortex of fusiform and lingual gyri, or impair connections to and from those structures.

The conclusion is inescapable: Prosopagnosia requires bilateral damage to the mesial and inferior visual association cortex. The localization is grossly comparable to that of achromatopsia, except that a unilateral lesion does not produce any sensible defect in facial recognition. Patients with unilateral left or right damage at approximately the same location develop hemiachromatopsia but not prosopagnosia, as previously noted (Damasio, *et al.*, 1982).

The notion that, in the context of a bilateral lesion, the right hemisphere lesion might be the crucial one for the appearance of prosopagnosia (see Meadows, 1974) cannot be supported on the basis of postmortem or CT scan findings. Nor are there clinical grounds to support this contention, as visual field information cannot be a reliable guide to the presence or absence of damage in the lower sector of the occipital lobe. For instance, the well-known cases of Hécaen and of Benson failed to show right or left visual field defects indicative of lesions. Lesions were present but were only discovered at postmortem. We suggest that facial recognition generally depends on bilateral cerebral function, with each hemisphere contributing a qualitatively different stage in the operation. However, each isolated hemisphere, with its own different strategy, will be able to perform facial recognition. That is the reason a unilateral lesion in

phasized the elusiveness of frontal lobe deficits, suggesting that even minor modifications in test administration may determine whether a deficit is demonstrated. The necessary emphasis on test procedure and method of response is not always present in frontal lobe research. Additionally, it has been difficult to translate theoretical concepts into experimental paradigms capable of localizing prefrontal function.

Finally, the greatest impedance to knowledge of localized frontal lobe function in man is the unavailability of well-defined frontal pathology to serve as an independent variable by which psychological functions could be differentiated. The animal literature on frontal lobe pathology did not have this problem and gradually differentiated some specific functional–anatomical correlations. For example, a functional distinction between the dorsolateral and ventrolateral–orbitofrontal areas has long been described (Iversen, 1973; Iversen & Mishkin, 1970; McEnaney & Butter, 1969; Mishkin, Vest, Waxler, & Rosvold, 1969; Oscar–Berman, 1975, 1978). The literature based on human clinical data, however, does not yield the same definitive pathological differentiation. Closed head injury, although often implicating significant frontotemporal damage (Ommaya & Gennarelli, 1976), produces diffuse pathology. Localized prefrontal lobe strokes are uncommon, and often confounded by language disability. Frontal lobe tumors frequently go unrecognized until massive and/or bilaterally situated (Hécaen & Albert, 1978).

Some localizing frontal lobe pathology is available through patients who have undergone central nervous system (CNS) surgical intervention for various reasons. Pathology is demarcated and specific and the extent and location of the damage now may be outlined precisely by computerized tomographic (CT) scan. Such material, however, is subject to criticism that the psychological functions are contaminated by premorbid pathology such as epilepsy or psychiatric disease. Nevertheless, at present, research based on prefrontal surgery—using adequate control groups and cautiously interpreted—provides useful localizing information.

This review compares patients with frontal lobe pathology in two separate areas secondary to neurosurgical intervention and who have subsequently undergone extended psychological assessment. One group has dorsolateral damage, secondary to surgical treatment of epilepsy. The comparison group consists of leucotomized schizophrenics with pathology in more anterior orbitomedial white matter. Examples of lesion localization are illustrated and described, and specific neuropsychological functions will be compared. Emphasis is on localization of function in man and results of animal research are used only as a parallel.

Examples of Localization of Frontal Pathology

DORSOLATERAL FRONTAL DAMAGE

Frontal lobectomies have been used to treat epilepsy. Milner (1964) reported 18 patients with unilateral frontal lobectomies (10 left, 8 right); a composite figure based on her presentation provides a schematic approximation of location and extent of lesion (see Figure 1). Lesion size varied, with maximum pathology in the superior frontal area, in Brodmann areas 9, 10, 11, 46, 47, and 32. Although considered dorsolateral, there was obvious extension of the excision to medial cortex. Orbitofrontal areas, however, appear to be spared.

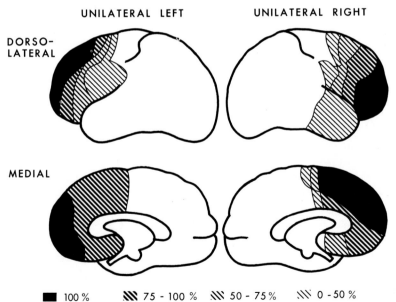

Figure 1. Schema approximating location of frontal ablations for epilepsy from Montreal Neurological Institute Series (see Milner, 1964): Eighteen patients had left unilateral frontal ablations, 10 right. Schema shows percentage of patients having damage in a given area.

ORBITOFRONTAL PATHOLOGY

In the 1940–1950s, apparently uncurable psychopathology often was treated by frontal psychosurgery. The lesions were defined and limited and the effects of the frontal lobe damage can be assessed by using proper control groups. Long-term follow-up of 16 leucotomized schizophrenics, divided into three groups based on degree of clinical recovery, and two control groups have been reported (Benson, Stuss, Naeser, Weir, Kaplan, & Levine, 1981; Naeser, Levine, Benson, Stuss, & Weir, 1981; Stuss, Kaplan, Benson, Weir, Naeser, & Levine, 1981). Schematic illustrations approximating the location and extent of the lesions in these individuals are presented in Figure 2.

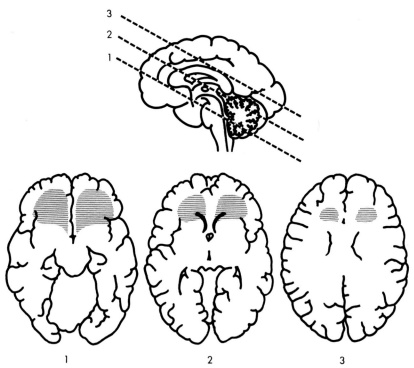

Figure 2. Schema approximating location of frontal leucotomy lesions for Schizophrenia from Northampton VA Medical Center Series: All 16 patients had bilateral lesions involving anterior medial–frontal white matter with the greatest involvement at the lowest section.

Lesion size varied from small to very large. The lesions were located in the white matter deep to the superior and medial frontal gyri. The most consistent lesions were inferior. There was little lateral extension or involvement of additional structures. The degree of recovery correlated with volume of tissue destroyed, particularly in the low orbitofrontal areas. Although asymmetry of lesion size was noted, all lesions were bilateral.

COMPARISON OF THE TWO PATHOLOGIES

There are obvious disadvantages in these groups for localization study. The dorsolateral group has unilateral damage, the orbitofrontal patients bilateral pathology, and both groups suffer significant presurgical abnormality. Irrespective of this, they do provide a basis for discussion of localization of function in the human frontal lobes. In the original reports, both groups were compared to control groups to minimize the effects of presurgical pathology. The lesions are relatively discrete and localizable and, more importantly, the localization of pathology is notably different in the two groups. Neuropsychological tests administered are sufficiently similar to allow some comparison of function. Finally, the two groups provide a global approximation to some of the localizing information available in the animal literature.

When possible, specific neuropsychological functions are compared. If such comparison is not possible, deficit noted with either lesion will be presented as baseline information for future comparisons.

Language and Spontaneous Initiation of Behavior

FLUENCY

Frontal lobe damage may produce language disturbances which are not definitely aphasic in nature. Clinically, this is manifested as a decrease in the spontaneity of speech (Bonner, Cobb, Sweet, & White, 1951; Zangwill, 1966). Closely allied is the demonstration of impaired generation of word lists [the word fluency test of Milner (1964)]. In this test, the patient produces a list of words in a requested category (i.e., beginning with a specific letter), and responses may be written or verbal, with little alteration of results (Jones–Gotman & Milner, 1977).

Comparison of the two frontal patient groups suggests that the dorsolateral cortex is more essential to the generation of word lists. Milner (1964) suggested that defective generation of written lists occurs after frontal lobectomy of the dominant hemisphere. The most critical area appears to be inferior and lateral frontal cortex, anterior to Area 44 (Broca's area). Supporting evidence for the localization of this function to the lateral cortex is derived from the negative results on word generation following pathology in the inferior medial white matter. The leucotomized patients were given the F-A-S test (Spreen & Benton, 1969); most performed within normal limits, with no significant difference compared to normal control subjects.

Specific clarifications have been made. The frontal lobe deficit occurs primarily with verbal (letter of the alphabet) rather than semantic (e.g., lists of animals) fluency (Newcombe, 1969), suggesting that different fluency tests may be tapping different abilities (Guilford, 1967; Jones–Gotman & Milner, 1977). Right frontal dorsolateral lobectomy did not influence word fluency significantly (Milner, 1964). Although this left frontal predominance has been replicated, some clarifications in the localization of function have been suggested in other studies (Benton, 1968; Perret, 1974; Ramier & Hécaen, 1970). Left medial supplementary motor pathology may also result in decreased ability to generate lists of words (Alexander & Schmitt, 1980). Either left or right frontal pathology can cause defective performance ability (Benton, 1968; Ramier & Hécaen, 1970). The percentage of the patients demonstrating the word fluency deficit was 70% of those with left hemisphere damage, 38% right, and 71% bilateral (Benton, 1968). Ramier and Hécaen (1970) proposed a two-component feature to verbal fluency: a deficit in action initiation would result after lesion of either frontal lobe; a linguistic component would be left hemisphere sensitive. None of these latter studies were restricted to surgical ablation cases, however, and the question of bilaterality remains. A later study reported that localization of lesion within the frontal lobes had little effect on verbal fluency measures (Hécaen & Ruel, 1981). However, there was an insufficient number of patients with focal orbitofrontal pathology for statistical comparison.

There is an apparent hemispheric asymmetry in nonverbal fluency. Jones–Gotman and Milner (1977) compared design fluency, that is, the ease of production of drawings, in right and left frontal lobe patients. The right frontal and right frontocentral patients were significantly inferior in comparison to either normal subjects or left frontal subjects but the performance of the left frontal group was between the normal and the right frontal patients.

Thus there is suggestion that a deficit in fluency indicates a problem in frontal lobe regions. Part of this deficit may be based on a general difficulty in initiation of behavior (Hécaen & Albert, 1975; Ramier & Hécaen, 1970). False positives are possible, however. Deficits in word generation occur in both aphasic syndromes and dementia, and design fluency impairment was noted after lesions in several cortical areas.

In summary, this particular language deficit appears primarily with frontal lobe damage. If dorsolateral, the necessary lesion appears to be anterior to Brodmann Area 44. The left supplementary motor area has also been implicated. The negative results with the leucotomy lesions suggest that orbitofrontal pathology does not influence fluency. Material (verbal versus nonverbal) hemispheric specificity has been noted, although the asymmetry was not overwhelming.

VERBAL REGULATION OF BEHAVIOR

A disturbance of the regulative role of speech has been described after frontal lobe damage (Luria, 1966, 1973; Luria & Homskaya, 1964; Luria, Pribram, & Homskaya, 1964). Frontal lobe patients can understand speech and remember the verbal formulations of a test, but fail to guide their action according to the verbal instructions. The loss of verbal regulation can occur with any symbolic instructions, not just verbalized statements. For example, if asked to say "press" and actually press to a specific cue, the frontal lobe patient may remember the verbalized aspect and correctly continue to say "press" while the actual motor act stops, indicating that verbalization has lost its signaling function. If asked to tap once when the examiner taps twice and vice versa, patients with frontal lesions often deteriorate into an echopractic (mirror) reaction. There is dissociation between words and deeds (Luria, 1973; Zangwill, 1966).

The dorsolateral patients just described (see Figure 1) frequently and spontaneously verbalized the abstraction requirements of a sorting task but failed to use this verbalized knowledge to guide their behavior (Milner, 1964). Luria suggested that this deficit primarily was seen with frontal convexity pathology, especially the left, although some right frontal lobe patients with this dysfunction have also been reported (Luria, 1960, 1966, 1969). Patients with orbitofrontal leucotomies, on the other hand, had little difficulty in the 1 tap–2 tap tests in which the cue stimulus appeared to conflict with the verbal instruction (Benson & Stuss, 1982). Other tests designed to have them verbalize while performing responses did not reveal any action–behavior dissociation. This suggests a possible differentiation of function between dorsolateral-frontal and orbitofrontal cortex.

In summary, defective verbal regulation of behavior and verbal–action dissociation would appear to be a good indicator of prefrontal cortex damage. Patients with posterior lesions, even in premotor zones, usually improve in performance with verbal self-regulation while patients with prefrontal lobe lesions do not (Luria & Homskaya, 1964). Drewe (1975) suggested that this deficiency in the regulation of motor behavior by overt verbalization was not as general as suggested by Luria (1973). Such results may reflect the size of pathology of particularly massive frontal tumors (Luria, 1966; Luria & Homskaya, 1964). There is some evidence suggesting a lateral convexity predominance, especially on the left (Luria, 1969; Milner, 1964). Negative results after orbitofrontal lesions tend to corroborate this suggestion. However, such precise localization cannot be conclusively made from present information.

FRONTAL LOBE APHASIC SYNDROMES

Several language dysfunctions have been localized to frontal cortical areas. These include the syndromes of Broca aphasia, aphemia, and transcortical motor aphasia as well as the output disturbance secondary to supplementary motor area damage. (These are described elsewhere in this volume and will not be reviewed here but their importance is obvious.)

Cognitive Functions

This section reviews several psychological functions that can be loosely grouped under the generic term "cognitive abilities."

IQ TESTS

Does frontal lobe pathology affect general intellectual functioning? The answer is muddled by undefined factors such as the definition of intelligence and localization of the pathology. Comparison of the two groups with localized pathology is also hindered by incomplete information. Pre- and postoperative comparison of the dorsolateral-frontal group revealed a mean loss of 7.2 IQ points (Milner, 1964). Mean IQ, however, remained within average limits (102.9, with a range of 71–123). Those patients with left temporal or left parietal lobe excisions showed the greatest loss. No pre- and postoperative comparisons were available in the group of leucotomized schizophrenics; most had been too psychotic for reliable testing in the preoperative period. The five patients with good recovery were not significantly different from the normal control subjects and scored within the average range ($\overline{X}$ IQ = 99.8, SD = 13.1) (Stuss, Kaplan, Benson, Weir, Naeser, & Levine, 1981). The IQ appeared to be affected considerably by the present level of schizophrenic symptomatology. It should also be noted that the larger the lesion in the orbital area, the greater the degree of recovery and the greater the subsequent level of IQ.

These results firmly replicate the common observation that little or no deficit in results, as measured by standard tests of "intelligence," are seen in frontal lobe patients. Frontal lobe lesions have less effect on IQ than pathology in posterior cortical areas (Black, 1976; Feuchtwanger, 1923; Hebb, 1939, 1945; Pollack, 1960; Smith, 1966; Teuber, 1964; Weinstein & Teuber, 1957); these studies also indicate that the negative results were independent of the etiology of frontal lobe pathology.

Observation of deficits in intelligence test results in patients with frontal lobe damage, when they do occur, almost exclusively indicate dorsolateral cortical lesions, not pathology in orbitomedial areas (Girgis, 1971; Malmo, 1948; Petrie, 1952; Smith & Kinder, 1959). The negative results of detailed testing in the leucotomized patients corroborate the negative results with orbitofrontal pathology. This apparent avoidance of IQ deficits is one reason that led psychosurgeons to focus on medial–inferior structures (Freeman & Watts, 1950; Greenblatt & Solomon, 1953). However, there is some suggestion that left frontal pathology has a greater influence on IQ scores. Smith (1966), subdividing his frontal tumor patients into those with left or right pathology, found that the left frontal patients had significantly lower mean IQ scores and his reexamination of Pollack's (1960) data confirmed the finding. This asymmetry has not been carefully reevaluated; it may reflect only the heavy emphasis that standard IQ tests give to verbalization in both test administration and response.

In summary, the most striking feature of IQ measures in patients with prefrontal pathology is negative. The frontal lobes are not primarily involved in the functions being measured in standard tests of intelligence and this seems most true for orbitofrontal lesions. There are, however, some suggestions of dorsolateral–orbitofrontal differences in cognitive activities as well as hemispheric asymmetry.

ABSTRACTION

The frontal lobes were deemed to be important for abstract thought. However, experimental proof of this hypothesis has been difficult and controversial. Part of the difficulty evolves from a lack of vigorous operational definition of "abstraction." Goldstein (1944) criticized Brickner (1936) for not distinguishing between thinking abstractly and using abstract words. Goldstein and Sheerer (1941) attempted to clarify this issue by listing eight characteristics of abstract attitude but the characteristics do not clearly separate abstract attitude from other frontal lobe functions.

Abstraction was addressed only indirectly in the dorsolateral group. Milner (1964) reports that the frontal lobe patients had no difficulty "abstracting" the criteria required to successfully complete the sorting task. They could verbalize the "color, shape, or number" but could not use this information consistently in performing the task. The leucotomy study looked further at abstraction ability by administering a number of tests designed to probe abstraction (Stuss, Kaplan, & Benson, 1982). In the visual metaphor test (Winner & Gardner, 1977), a sentence with metaphorical quality ("he has a heavy heart") was read aloud; the subject selected one of four possible responses presented pictorially: metaphorical, literal, nominal, or adjectival and described why that response was chosen. In another test, the subject was presented with a series of cards, each having four objects, three of which could be placed in two different categories or concepts (Feldman & Drasgow, 1960). The subject was required to note three objects that were alike in some way,

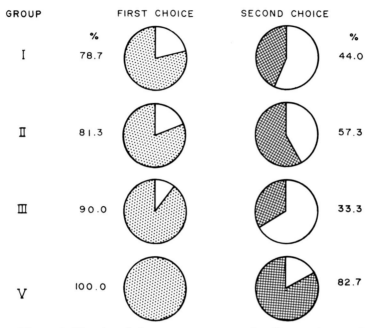

Figure 3. Visual–verbal correct responses for first and second response choice.

The nonleucotomized schizophrenic group is not illustrated, since they were unable to complete this task of abstraction. Percentage of correct responses in relationship to total possible correct is noted for first and second response choice. Task demands are explained in the test. For the first choice, all groups performed well. For the second choice, performance for the normal control group remained relatively constant, whereas the three leucotomized groups significantly deteriorated. This was interpreted as a difficulty in shifting set.

and then how three of the four were alike in some other way. Results from these tests (see Figure 3) demonstrated that orbitofrontal pathology does not interfere with the ability to respond abstractly but specific differences, nevertheless, were noted. The quality of the verbalization of the reason for a choice was inferior and the ability to switch mental sets was impaired as demonstrated by difficulty in selecting a second concept from the four objects.

In summary, information on the localization of abstraction in the frontal lobes is far from definitive. It would appear that the ability to abstract is not seriously impaired by frontal lobe pathology but other functions dependent on the utilization of abstracting ability may be impaired. These would include difficulty in shifting set and decreased ability to describe abstract thought. Considerable more research is necessary to define both the specific psychologic factors and the possible localization of abstraction performance in frontal lobe damage.

SORTING BEHAVIOR AND DEFICIENCIES IN INHIBITION

The concept that "intellectual" deficiencies following frontal lobe pathology reflects a loss of executive ability rather than loss of IQ is supported by the performance of frontal lobe patients on sorting tasks such as the Wisconsin Card Sorting Test (WCST) (Grant & Berg, 1948). In this test, the patient is presented four stimulus cards, varying in three dimensions: color, shape, and number of shapes. The patient is requested to sort 128 similar cards by placing them in front of one of the four stimulus cards. Unknown to the patient, the examiner has selected one of the three dimensions as a correct sorting criterion. The patient is informed of this only through feedback as to whether the sort is right or wrong. The criterion is changed, without warning to the subject, after 10 consecutive correct responses and the patient must again use feedback to learn the second correct sorting criterion and so on.

Milner first demonstrated a striking impairment of her dorsolateral frontal patients on this test (1963, 1964, 1966). Even prior to the lobectomy, patients with dorsolateral epileptogenic lesions did worse than those with foci elsewhere. The deficit was greater postoperative with all the frontal lobe patients deteriorating to a marked impairment whereas the control group showed minor improvement. The dorsolateral frontal group, both right and left, made more errors and made fewer sorting categories. They had difficulty in shifting to meet changing demands. Responses became inflexible and perseverative. The required lesion appeared to be dorsolateral rather than orbital, as a control group with combined lesions of orbitofrontal and temporal cortex were comparatively efficient.

Results from the leucotomized patients both corroborated and disagreed with Milner's results (Stuss, Benson, Kaplan, Weir, Naeser, & Ferrill, 1981). The test was divided into two halves (64 cards in each), the second half preceded by a statement of the required abstractions. In the first half, many orbitofrontal patients performed as well as the normal control subjects, suggesting that dorsolateral lesions were indeed required. In the second half, however, after being offered additional information, all orbitofrontal patients regardless of IQ or level of recovery were significantly impaired while the normal control Ss improved. These results suggest that orbitofrontal lesions, even after apparent recovery, can cause significant impairment on sorting tasks. The nature of the deficit appeared different, an inability to maintain extended sequences of correct behavior being more prominent than perseveration of previously reinforced response modes.

The quantitative and qualitative deficits seen in sorting tasks are thought to be typical of frontal lobe dysfunction (as opposed to other cortical areas), particularly in the presence of normal IQ scores (Damasio, 1979; Drewe, 1974). There is controversy over the precise frontal lobe localization that underlies the sorting deficit. It has been suggested that, although both left and right frontal pathology affects sorting, left frontal damage might be selectively more sensitive (Drewe, 1974; Milner, 1966) and, within one hemisphere, the dorsolateral convexity was suggested as the critical area (Milner, 1964). This latter concept was apparently buttressed by the reports of other intellectual impairments following dorsolateral but not orbitofrontal excisions (Malmo, 1948; Petrie, 1952; Smith & Kinder, 1959). Moreover, early animal literature revealed delayed alternation and delayed response deficits after dorsolateral but not ventromedial lesions (Mishkin, 1957; Pribram, Mishkin, Rosvold, & Kaplan, 1952). Drewe (1974), however, suggested that the critical area may be medial and not dorsolateral convexity and that orbital damage may not be detrimental to sorting behavior. If left frontal damage patients also had orbital lesions, they achieved more categories than if frontal damage did not affect this region (Drewe, 1974). However, the very clearly defined orbitofrontal leucotomy lesions had impaired performance on this test (Stuss, Benson, Kaplan, Weir, Naeser, & Ferrill, 1981). Furthermore, more recent animal studies, using a task superficially similar to card sorting, demonstrated greater impairment after orbital than dorsolateral frontal lesions (Mishkin, 1964).

Two factors are evident in the examination of this controversy.

First, there is a continuing problem in defining localized frontal lobe pathology in humans, confounded by differing terms used to describe the location. Many of Milner's (1964) dorsolateral group also had medial cortex pathology (see Figure 1). Use of the term "medial" to represent Mishkin's orbital animals (Milner, 1964, Discussion) is not equivalent to the way Drewe (1974) used the term in opposition to orbital damage. Only the leucotomy patients have pre-cisely localized lesions and these are variable between patients.

Second, work is needed to specify aspects of the sorting task that appear to measure both general dysfunction (i.e., impaired results regardless of localization of frontal lobe damage) and specific dys-function (dependent on localized pathology for elicitation). Mishkin (1964) formulated such a hypothesis to explain his results. Orbital lesions lead to impairment in "perseveration of central sets," whereas dorsolateral pathology results in two deficits: a lesser but similar impairment in perseveration of central sets plus a spatial disturbance.

Whereas the WCST probes both the ability to sort and inhibit, other tests are sensitive to deficiencies in inhibition. One measure of the ability to inhibit interference and maintain constant behavior is the Stroop Test (Stroop, 1935) in which the essential subtest es-tablished a conflict of categories. Three color words (red, blue, green) are printed in a color different than the actual word, causing interference. Subjects must inhibit reading of the word to name the color of print.

Most leucotomy patients had little difficulty with the Stroop Test, which was not used with the localized dorsolateral group. This sug-gests that the orbitofrontal area is not essential to the ability to sep-arate categories within a single stimulus by suppressing one of the categories (Stuss, Benson, Kaplan, Weir, & Della Malva, 1981). Be-cause these same patients had difficulty on the WCST, comparison of the two tests may suggest localization of function. Perret (1974) reported that all left-hemisphere-damaged patients were more im-paired on the Stroop Test than those with homologous right hemi-sphere lesions, and that left frontal involvement caused the most impairment. This was interpreted as suggesting a two-factor theory: a verbal left hemisphere factor, superimposed on a general "cate-gorical" factor, resulting in inability to adapt to unusual situations, similar to the inertia of initial or central sets described by Mishkin (1964). A problem again exists in that most patients in this (Perret's) study had large tumors.

Although there is some parallel in interpretation of these different studies, confusion remains. At least two lessons can be extracted. First, localization of frontal lobe function requires control of many variables including recovery status, task difficulty, and test instruc-tion. Second, bifactor or multifactor influences must be considered.

Motor Functions

Control of motor functions is an important ability of the frontal lobe. Unfortunately, the parallel between the two groups is incomplete as many aspects were not specifically tested in the dorsolateral group. The orbitofrontal leucotomized subjects had little difficulty in a series of Luria's and other "frontal motor" tests, including two- and three-step motor sequences, go/no go tasks with either hand, tasks requiring response alternation between left and right hand, "conflicting" motor tasks in which the subject had to tap once when the examiner tapped twice and vice versa, finger tapping, three loop drawings, and sequential production of the written letters "mn" (Benson & Stuss, 1982; Luria, 1966, 1973; Luria & Homskaya, 1964; Luria et al., 1964). These negative results with orbitofrontal lesions suggest that involvement of dorsolateral cortex and/or basal ganglia must be present for impairment in these actions. Moreover, none of the leucotomy patients exhibited frontal neurological signs such as the snout or palmomental reflex.

Other data suggest that the dorsolateral–orbitofrontal differences may indeed exist for motor function. In general behavioral terms, frontal lobe patients are divided into two main types. Some patients are slow, apathetic, lethargic, lack initiative and spontaneity, and tend to have pathology maximal in the dorsolateral convexity (Blumer & Benson, 1975; Goldstein, 1944; Kleist, 1934; Lishman, 1968). This behavioral syndrome is most typical of massive frontal lobe damage (Luria, 1973). In contrast, patients who are restless, impulsive, explosive, and hyperkinetic more often have pathology involving the orbital area. The leucotomized patients, with pathology in orbitofrontal areas, resembled the hyperkinetic type. They were apathetic, however, in the sense that they would do nothing until instructed.

Luria (1973) divided motor deficits in a posterior–anterior fashion. Lesions in premotor areas resulted in deficits of dexterity in tests such as rhythm tapping. If the lesion was sufficiently deep to involve basal ganglia, the patient correctly performed an action but could not cease the behavior, resulting in compulsive repetition of the initiated behavior. Pathology involving prefrontal areas resulted in disturbance of the actual motor program. There was no compulsive repetition of an initiated act but difficulty in completing sequences or in inhibiting inappropriate responses (as in the go/no go task) was present.

Other localizing motor signs have been suggested. Unimanual deficits in strength and finger-tapping speed may indicate a lesion in the contralateral precentral–postcentral gyri (Swiercinsky, 1978). Buccolinguo-facial apraxia most often is reported after lesions involving the left premotor cortex (Geschwind, 1965). Sympathetic or ideomotor apraxia often indicates pathology at the origin of the callosal motor connection in the left hemisphere (Geschwind, 1965; Heilman, 1979). Kinetic apraxia of the magnetic type is said to be secondary to pathology in the medial frontal cortex (Denny-Brown, 1958).

In summary, motor tests seem to be useful indicators of frontal lobe dysfunction. Comparatively precise localization appears possible, either in a rostral–caudal fashion, or in separation of dorsolateral and orbital lesions.

Attention and Memory

ATTENTION

Deficits in attention after frontal lobe pathology are commonly reported (see Chapter 20 for inattention). Although much of the evidence comes from the animal literature (Buffery, 1967; Isaac & De Vito, 1958; Malmo, 1942; Orbach & Fischer, 1959), research and observation of attentional deficits in humans comes from tumor (Hécaen, 1964), trauma (Goldstein, 1944), and frontal lobotomy (Angelergues, Hécaen, & Ajuriaguerra, 1956; Rylander, 1939). "From the very first examination of the (frontal lobe) patient, the disorder of attention is noticeable: It is necessary to repeat questions and orders several times to obtain a response" (Hécaen & Albert, 1978).

The dorsolateral patients did not appear to have attentional deficits. Even when they failed a task, they clearly could understand and remember the instructions, as well as attempt the task. The orbitofrontal leucotomized patients were administered a test battery to measure attention, sustained mental activity, and mental flexibility (Stuss, Benson, Kaplan, Weir, & Della Malva, 1981). The most striking observation: Leucotomized subjects with very large orbital lesions were not significantly different from normal control subjects; many performed as well or better than these control subjects. The major effect appeared to be the degree of psychopathology.

These results strongly suggest that frontal lobe lesions in these locations do not result in impaired attention.

Several reasons may be postulated for these negative results. Lesion location is one obvious aspect. Whether the damage involves the reticular activating system, the diffuse thalamic system, or isolated frontal lobe areas may be important. Variations in the definition of attention also play an important role. Frontal lobe lesions may lead to deficiencies only in "higher order" attention such as the selection of strategies of response (Luria, 1973; Moscovitch, 1979) whereas automatic performance of simpler tasks is unimpaired.

MEMORY

INTRODUCTION

The possibility of frontal lobe involvement in memory function has its origin in the animal attention literature. The observation that monkeys with frontal lobe damage could perform immediate discrimination but not delayed response tasks was first interpreted as a memory deficit (Jacobsen, 1935, 1936). Subsequent research suggested that the memory loss was apparent rather than real. It also appeared that human frontal lobe damage resulted in frontal amnesia. For instance, frontal lobe tumor patients were impaired in learning verbal paired associates (Hécaen, 1964) and frontal damage resulted in impaired nonverbal learning (stylus maze) (Milner, 1964). Careful analysis of test behavior and comparison with other test results eventually led to the same conclusion found in the animal literature.

INTERFERENCE

Milner (1964) suggested that the frontal lobe impairment was not a real memory loss but due to other disorders. Frontal lobe patients tended to break more rules and had more repetitive errors than patients with lesions in other areas. They were deficient in suppressing preferred modes of response and were not guided by external cues. Hippocampal-damaged patients, on the other hand, who had severe learning problems, had no difficulty in following rules. Another factor influencing memory function after frontal lobe pathology is interference. Prisko (Milner, 1964), using a delayed paired comparison technique, noted that the frontal lobectomy patients had impaired performance on three of four tests. That frontal lobe patients did well on other memory tests indicated an inability to inhibit the memory of previous trials in the delayed paired comparison. The interference effect of previous trials, not an actual loss of memory, resulted in impaired test performance in these dorsolateral patients.

Study of memory functioning in orbitofrontal leucotomized patients confirmed the frontal lobe effect of interference (Stuss, Kaplan, Benson, Weir, Chiulli, & Sarazin, 1982). No deficits were noted on commonly used tests of memory such as the Wechsler Memory Scale, the Rey–Osterreith Visual Memory Test, Ben Seltzer test of retrograde amnesia, and verbal and nonverbal recurring figures test. When given the consonant trigrams test, which has varying delays of interference between presentation of stimuli and recall of data (Cermak & Butters, 1972), these same patients now had significantly impaired performance, suggesting that interference was a crucial factor.

The observance of interference effects with either orbitofrontal or dorsolateral lesions suggests that a common frontal lobe factor is being assessed. This effect appears similar to the inflexible behavior and perseveration of central sets reported above. Fuster (1980), however, proposes an intrahemispheric localization of frontal lobe involvement in memory functions: "The operations for memorizing relevant elements seem accomplished primarily by dorsolateral cortex, whereas those for suppressing interfering memories seem accomplished by ventral and medial cortex" (p. 135).

RECENCY

Patients with frontal lobe damage are impaired in remembering the sequencing of events, despite apparently adequate encoding of actual facts (Làdavas, Umilta, & Provinciali, 1979; Milner, 1971, 1974). If given a series of facts and asked to recall which of two items was more recently presented, frontal lobe patients have difficulty. This has been termed "the recency effect" (Milner, 1971). There appears to be some hemispheric material-specificity for this recall. Left unilateral frontal lesions resulted in decreased recency judgment for verbal events whereas right unilateral pathology caused comparatively greater problems for nonverbal recency.

In summary, frontal lobe memory disorder does not appear to be a true amnesia. Clinically, the deficit is better described as a "forgetting to remember" (Hécaen & Albert, 1978). Deficits on memory tests appear to be more parsimoniously explained by other disorders such as inability to follow external cues and rules, problems with perseveration and sequencing, or susceptibility to the effects of interference. Precise localization of these specific deficits is presently unavailable, although some gradient of hemispheric material-specificity may be present in the recency deficit.

Personality

The main characteristics of the frontal lobe personality are well described and have been so frequently recorded that they are considered excellent indicators of frontal lobe pathology. Unfortunately, very little has been done to categorize or quantify these signs and they lack confirmation. Neither the studies of the dorsolateral- or orbitofrontal-lesioned patients contained quantified personality investigations. Attempts have been made to divide the frontal lobe personality changes into two types (Blumer & Benson, 1975; Kleist, 1934). A pseudoretarded or pseudodepressed group is characterized by apathy, lethargy, little spontaneity of behavior, unconcern, reduced sexual interest, little overt emotion, and inability to plan ahead. Although they appear retarded, IQ tests are at or near normal levels. Pathology in this group appears to be located dorsolaterally. The "pseudo-psychopathic" subgroup shows the typical *Witzelsucht* (puerile, jocular attitude), sexual disinhibition, increased motor activity, inappropriate social and personal behavior, self-indulgent attitude, and little concern for others. Pathology is most severe in the orbitofrontal areas. These two distinctly different frontal lobe personality syndromes appear to be based on anatomical (dorsolateral–orbital) localization and as such could be compared to other divisions of function within the frontal lobes. Most commonly, however, patients with large frontal lesions will show a mixture of both personality types resulting in the paradoxical description of frontal lobe personality as "apathetic, irritable, and euphoric" (Geschwind, 1977).

To date, no specific frontal lobe personality alterations have been reported on the basis of unilateral frontal lobe damage although the possibility has been considered (Blumer & Benson, 1975). Kolb and

Whishaw (1980) borrow Blumer and Benson's terminology to suggest that pseudodepressed patients would most likely occur after
left frontal damage while the pseudopsychopathic personality would
be most typical of right frontal damaged patients. No data was offered to support this suggestion.

In summary, specific personality changes long have been accepted
as good indicators of frontal lobe involvement. To date, this is limited to clinical observations, and there is an obvious need for quantified investigations of frontal personality disturbances.

Conclusion

Localization of psychologic function in the prefrontal cortex has
proven to be a difficult task, made more difficult by the fact that
frontal functions have been described as consisting of several basic,
nonlocalized abilities plus other more superimposed localized abilities. A selective review of functions associated with frontal lobe
pathology, nevertheless, indicates that some conclusions about localization can be reached.

First, it appears that certain psychologic functions can be localized to prefrontal cortex. The frontal lobe signs include specific personality changes, distinct aphasic and nonaphasic linguistic deficits,
impairment in spontaneous initiation of behavior, impaired response inhibition, specific disorders affecting memory—performance including difficulties in recency and inhibition of
interference—and characteristic motor problems. This list does not
include other functions such as personal orientation and deficits in
visual search.

Second, there is some indication of hemispheric material-specificity, with the left hemisphere more involved with verbal material,
the right hemisphere with nonverbal. This was most strongly suggested by tests of fluency and recency. It must be emphasized, however, that the hemispheric specificity of these frontal tests was not
absolute; there is evidence of overlap in the results.

Third and finally, there is indication of functional systems within
each frontal lobe. The animal literature suggests at least two functional systems: a dorsolateral system and an orbitoventral system.
Rosvold (1972) has demonstrated subcortical counterparts that fit
with each of the major anatomical–functional frontal lobe systems.
The dorsal system includes the dorsolateral prefrontal cortex, an-

terodorsal caudate, lateral pallidum, subthalamic nucleus, and hippocampus. The orbital system consists of the orbital prefrontal cortex, ventrolateral caudate, medial pallidum, centromedian nucleus, hypothalamus, and septal nuclei.

Do separate frontal functional systems exist in man? The first response must be that there is insufficient evidence to make a definite affirmation. Nevertheless, current evidence implies that functional systems comparable to those described in animals may indeed exist in man. Comparison of the altered functions following dorsolateral lobectomy and orbitofrontal leucotomy was the basis of this review and supports this suggestion. Differences were noted in motor ability, personality variables, fluency, IQ comparisons, sorting tests, and response inhibition.

Localization of function in human frontal cortex awaits much more rigorous research, especially in the definition of independent variables such as lesion localization and laterality, and the construction of more specific tests. One obvious avenue would be to extend Rosvold's (1972) cortical–subcortical animal studies by comparing psychologic functions in patients with distinct and separate pathology in cortical and subcortical areas.

Acknowledgments

Supported in part by Grant NS06209 from the National Institute of Health to Boston University School of Medicine, the Research Service of the Veterans Administration, University of Ottawa Faculty of Social Sciences Grant, the National Research Council of Canada, the Ontario Mental Health Foundation, and the Augustus S. Rose Endowment Fund. The library search assistance of Ms. Francine Sarazin is gratefully acknowledged. Ms. Diane Brazeau and Francine Lafrance are thanked for the preparation of the manuscript. Figures 1 and 2 were prepared by M. Emil Purgina, University of Ottawa, Health Sciences, Communication Services, and the Ottawa General Hospital Medical Communications Department.

References

Alexander, M. P., & Schmitt, M. A. (1980). The aphasia syndrome of stroke in the left anterior cerebral artery territory. *Archives of Neurology (Chicago)*, 37, 97–100.

Angelergues, R., Hécaen, H., & de Ajuriaguerra, J. (1956). Les troubles mentaux au cours des tumeurs du lobe frontal. *Annales Medico-Psychologiques, 113*, 577–642.

Benson, D. F., & Stuss, D. T. (1982). Motor abilities after frontal leukotomy. *Neurology, 32,* 1353–1357.

Benson, D. F., Stuss, D. T., Naeser, M. A., Weir, W. S., Kaplan, E. F., & Levine, H. (1981). The long term effects of prefrontal leukotomy. *Archives of Neurology (Chicago), 38,* 165–169.

Benton, A. L. (1968). Differential behavioral effects in frontal lobe disease. *Neuropsychologia, 6,* 53–60.

Black, W. F. (1976). Cognitive deficits in patients with unilateral war-related frontal lobe lesions. *Journal of Clinical Psychology, 32,* 366–372.

Blumer, D., & Benson, D. F. (1975). Personality changes with frontal and temporal lobe lesions. In D. F. Benson & D. Blumer (Eds.), *Psychiatric aspects of neurologic disease.* New York: Grune & Stratton, 151–170.

Bonner, F., Cobb, S., Sweet, W. H., & White, J. C. (1951). Frontal lobe surgery: Its value in the treatment of pain with consideration of post-operative psychological changes. *Research Publications—Association for Research in Nervous and Mental Disease, 31,* 392–421.

Brickner, R. M. (1936). *The intellectual functions of the frontal lobes.* New York: Macmillan.

Buffery, A. W. H. (1967). Learning and memory in baboons with bilateral lesions of frontal or inferotemporal cortex. *Nature (London), 214,* 1054–1056.

Cermak, L. S., & Butters, N. T. (1972). The role of interference and encoding in the short-term memory of Korsakoff patients. *Neuropsychologia, 10,* 89–95.

Damasio, A. (1979). The frontal lobes. In K. M. Heilman & E. Valenstein (Eds.), *Clinical neuropsychology.* London: Oxford University Press, 360–412.

Denny-Brown, D. (1958). The nature of apraxia. *Journal of Nervous and Mental Disease, 126,* 9–33.

Drewe, E. A. (1974). The effect of type and area of brain lesion on Wisconsin Card Sorting test performance. *Cortex, 10,* 159–170.

Drewe, E. A. (1975). An experimental investigation of Luria's theory on the effects of frontal lobe lesions in man. *Neuropsychologia, 13,* 421–429.

Feldman, M. J., & Drasgow J. (1960). *The visual–verbal test manual.* Beverly Hills, Calif.: Western Psychological Service.

Feuchtwanger, E. (1923). *Die funktionen des stirnhirns ihre pathologie und psychologie.* Berlin: Springer-Verlag.

Freeman, W., & Watts, J. W. (1950). *Psychosurgery in the treatment of mental disorders and intractable pain* (2nd ed.). Springfield, Ill.: Thomas.

Fuster, J. M. (1980). *The prefrontal cortex. Anatomy, physiology, and neuropsychology of the frontal lobe.* New York: Raven Press.

Geschwind, N. (1965). Disconnection syndromes in animals and man. *Brain, 88,* 237–294, 585–644.

Geschwind, N. (1977). Lectures in Neurobehavior, Harvard University School of Medicine, Boston.

Girgis, M. (1971). The orbital surface of the frontal lobe of the brain. *Acta Psychiatrica Scandinavica, Supplementum, 222,* 1–58.

Goldstein, K. (1944). The mental changes due to frontal lobe damage. *Journal of Psychology, 17,* 187–208.

Goldstein, K., & Scheerer M. (1941). Abstract and concrete behavior: An experimental study with special tests. *Psychological Monographs, 43,* 1–151.

Grant, A. D., & Berg, E. A. (1948). A behavioral analysis of reinforcement and ease of shifting to new responses in a Weigl-type card sorting problem. *Journal of Experimental Psychology, 38,* 404–411.

19

Right-Hemisphere Lesions in Constructional Apraxia and Visuospatial Deficit

Andrew Kertesz

Introduction

Cerebral organization can be measured in terms of symptoms or simple behaviors, or syndromes of distinct behaviors occurring together. On more detailed analysis, certain symptoms such as constructional apraxia are shown to have several basic components such as spatial neglect, spatial perceptual agnosia, and so forth. Even these components can be broken down to more elementary features depending on the tests used. Right hemisphere deficits, however, have shown less clustering into well-accepted syndromes and have been less clearly associated with a specific locus when compared to left hemisphere deficits. There is a suggestion based on clinical and experimental observations that the right hemisphere

LOCALIZATION
IN NEUROPSYCHOLOGY

functions are less focally organized than those in the left (Semmes, 1968).

It is the purpose of this chapter to review the available evidence for or against the association of certain deficits and the localization of lesions in the right hemisphere. There are relatively few functions exclusively the domain of the right hemisphere. However, clinical and subsequently experimental observations have indicated that the right hemisphere may, in fact, be dominant for spatial relationships, pattern recognition, facial recognition, spatial construction, drawing ability, dressing praxis, emotional expression, perception of emotions, humor, tonal discrimination, subtleties of discourse, and attentional arousal. These functions are complex behaviors that were observed to be impaired predominantly with right hemisphere lesions. Their number grows as clinicians become aware of them and they become subjects to experimentation. Very few represent isolated or pure functions in any sense, and most are mixtures of clinical syndromes approached from various experimental angles. There is a great deal of functional and conceptual overlap among them, such as between visuospatial neglect and hemi-inattention, or constructional apraxia and dressing apraxia. Furthermore, the testing of these functions is widely varied and inadequately standardized, creating a source of disagreement among investigators. Many group studies had no localization of lesions other than noting the hemispheric side.

Constructional Apraxia

The most often tested deficit with a postulated right hemispheric dominance is constructional apraxia (CA). The term originated with Kleist (1923), but it is considered a misnomer by many because it draws undue attention to the executory or motor aspects of the disorder. Investigators such as Ajuriaguerra, Angelergues, & Hécaen (1960) clearly demonstrated the dissociation of construction difficulties from ideomotor apraxia, although they are often associated in left hemisphere lesions. Kleist conceived CA as a cognitive deficit between visuospatial perception and execution.

Initially, constructional difficulties were described as part of the general deficit of intelligence with aphasia and left hemisphere lesions (Poppelreuter, 1917), but Lange (1936), Paterson and Zangwill (1944), and subsequently, many others, associated it with right-sided lesions. Dide (1938) established the syndrome of the right parietal lobe as anosognosia, constructional apraxia, and spatial disorientation. The distinction of CA from other visuoperceptual difficulties is often unclear. Many patients will have both, although patients with pure CA have been shown to have adequate visual perception, discrimination, and ability to localize objects in space. Visuoperceptual difficulties are often measured on a matching task, from multiple choice to a sample, while constructional tasks involve putting parts together such as assembling blocks or drawing.

The term is used for right and left hemisphere deficits on these tasks but certain qualitative aspects are characteristic of the right hemisphere syndrome, such as the neglect of the left side of the design, perseveration, and lack of articulation whereas lack of perspective, loss of detail, and inappropriate angles are seen more in left-sided lesions. These qualitative differences in constructional performance are difficult to measure, and the production of the patients is not considered sufficient to differentiate the laterality of the lesions (Piercy & Smyth, 1962). In right hemisphere damage, CA may be related to visuoperceptual defects as matching tasks are often impaired (visuospatial agnosia). Furthermore, CA due to right brain damage does not improve on copying, in contrast to left-sided damage (McFie, Piercy, & Zangwill, 1950). Most investigators hold that CA is more severe in right hemisphere damage and that the right parietal lobe may have a special role.

Various tests of CA have demonstrated different abilities to distinguish between right or left hemisphere lesions. Benton (1967) found that three-dimensional block building and copying designs were impaired more than twice as frequently in right- than left-hemisphere-damaged patients, but defective performance on the WAIS block design test was equal. Unfortunately, lesion size has not been controlled for in many of these studies. An exception is that of Benson & Barton (1970) who estimated lesion size on the brain scan and found it did not account for the laterality difference.

The strategies of solving certain tasks may be different in each hemisphere. Duensing (1953) suggested that left hemisphere lesions produce an executive deficit while right sided deficits a perceptual one. When non-verbalizable perceptual tasks such as a form assembly (Mack & Levine, 1981) are used, the right sided deficit is more frequent and more severe.

Intrahemispheric Locus

The location of lesions producing right-hemisphere deficit has not been extensively investigated. Only few studies exist where the intrahemispheric locus of the lesion was considered. Piercy, Hécaen, and Ajuriaguerra (1960) concluded that the lesions in CA were more restricted in location to the parietotemporal and parieto-occipital area in the right hemisphere than in the left. Similarly, DeRenzi & Faglioni (1967) found that CA occurred with right posterior (i.e., with visual field defect (VFD)) and not with anterior lesions, in contrast to the left hemisphere where the presence or the absence of VFD did not matter. They suggested a more restricted localization for CA with right-sided than left-sided lesions. The results were somewhat different for visuospatial copying and matching tasks in patients with CA. Those without VFD (anterior lesions) on the right side had poor scores as did those with VFD (posterior lesions), but those on the left had visuospatial impairment only with VFD.

Benson & Barton (1970) used radioisotope brain scans to localize lesions to one of the four quadrants of the brain in patients with CA as measured by drawing to memory and copy, puzzle construction, stick–pattern reversals, template matching, visual and auditory reaction times, and token patterns. Drawing and puzzle scores were not significantly different in either location. Caudal lesions produced more reversal deficit in the left posterior group but on template matching and pattern omission right anteriors are worse. They also estimated lesion size in some of their subjects and this did not correlate with reaction times. Unfortunately, lesion size, a potentially important factor, was not correlated with the other measures.

Petrovici (1972) found no CA in tumors which were in the frontotemporal and temporal lobes. Block design impairment is considered to be greatest with parietal lobe involvement, but it is also seen with right frontal and temporal lobe lesions. Taylor and Warrington (1973) did not find significant differences among the right posterior, anterior, and temporal groups in visual discrimination and block design, but the right posterior group was much worse on spatial position discrimination.

Black and Strub (1976) studied CA in Vietnam veterans with penetrating missile wounds, using WAIS block design, object assembly, and Bender Gestalt scores. Their findings suggested a stronger effect for the anterior–posterior locus of the lesion than for laterality. The performance was worse in retro-Rolandic lesions. The generally low incidence of CA in their study indicates good recovery of CA in some of their patients who were examined 3–4 months after their head injury. Costa (1976) showed that patients with posterior right hemisphere lesions had poorer performance on Raven's Colored Progressive Matrices (RCPM) subtests than did those with anterior or left-sided lesions. However, the borders of these posterior and anterior lesions were not specifically defined, and the posterior groups included extensive hemispheric lesions as well.

Hier, Mondlock, and Caplan (1982) found that spatial neglect on drawing and constructional apraxia correlated with right parietal damage, but with motor impersistence, neglect, and anosognosia structures outside the parietal lobe were also affected. They found no correlation between lesion size and constructional apraxia or neglect on drawing, in agreement with our studies (Kertesz & Dobrowolski, 1981). Extinction, motor impersistence, and denial of illness tended to occur in larger strokes.

Table 1 attempts to summarize the selected studies that address the issue of localization of lesions in CA. This table cannot claim to be comprehensive, but it serves to highlight the complexity of tasks versus localizing findings. Clearly, many important studies concerning CA are omitted, but most of those with localization data were considered.

We studied lesion localization in CA in the right hemisphere (Kertesz, Harlock, & Coates, 1979). We grouped lesions according to the presence or absence of CA as defined on the drawing and block design scores (Figures 1 and 2). These lesion locations do not show significant antero–posterior or size differences. Those with CA appear somewhat more subcortical than those without CA. We continued to explore the interhemispheric localization of various right hemisphere functions, including CA in a population of stroke patients examined 2–6 weeks after a stroke (Kertesz & Dobrowolski, 1981).

We chose an acute population, because when acute and chronic patients are grouped together, the factor of recovery alters performance, accounting for a significant portion of the variability. We decided to group the lesions according to the anatomical area involved and examine the distribution of deficits for each area. The lesions were traced on standardized templates by a radiologist, who was unaware of the type or extent of behavioral deficit.

Five groups were formed (again independently from the test scores) where the lesions appeared to be on a similar location on the CT or isotope scans. These groups were (1) Frontal, Figure 3

TABLE 1

Constructional Apraxia with Localization

Task	Author	Lesion Localization
Copying and drawing	McFie *et al.* (1950)	Copying does not improve RBD[a]
	Piercy *et al.* (1960)	Right parietotemporal > left only post-Rolandic lesions tested
	Arrigoni & DeRenzi (1964)	RBD more frequent
	DeRenzi & Faglioni (1967)	No hemispheric difference
	Kertesz & Dobrowolski (1981)	No difference between frontal, central parietal, occipital, or deep lesions
Copying with cues	Hécaen & Assal (1970)	LBD[b] helped by cues
	Gainotti *et al.* (1977)	No hemispheric difference for cuing but spatial agnosia in RBD
Block building	Benton & Fogel (1962)	RBD more frequent
	Arrigoni & DeRenzi (1964)	RBD : LBD = 2:1 (involvement)
	Benson & Barton (1970)	Anterior, posterior same
Object assembly	Piercy & Smyth (1962)	RBD more severe
Token construction	Arrigoni & DeRenzi (1964)	RBD is more severe (R.T.[c])
Form assembly	Mack and Levine (1981)	RBD > LBD (in severity and incidence)
	Petrovici (1972)	Right parietal, not temporal or frontal
Block design (Wechsler)	Taylor & Warrington (1973)	No differences between right posterior anterior and temporal groups
	Black & Strub (1976)	Retro-Rolandic lesions worse
	Kertesz & Dobrowolski (1981)	No differences for frontal, parietal, central, occipital, and subcortical groups

[a] RBD = Right brain damage (patients).
[b] LBD = Left brain damage (patients).
[c] Reaction times.

(anterior to the rolandic sulcus); (2) Central, Figure 4 (posterior frontal, superior temporal, and inferior parietal); (3) Subcortical, Figure 5 (deep central); (4) Parietal, Figure 6 (postrolandic supra-Sylvian); and (5) Occipital, Figure 7 (confined to a 20° wedge medially). The central lesions were larger but the lesion size, as measured by digitizing the outline of the lesions with a computer (Kertesz *et al.*, 1979), did not correlate with the deficits except in the case of per-

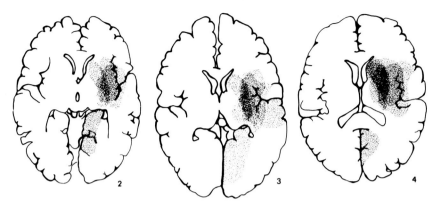

Figure 1. The overlap of nondominant hemisphere lesions with constructional apraxia. From Kertesz, Harlock, and Coates (1979).

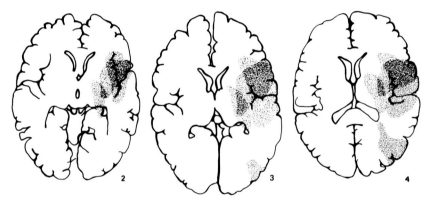

Figure 2. The overlap of lesions without constructional apraxia in the right hemisphere. From Kertesz, Harlock, and Coates (1979).

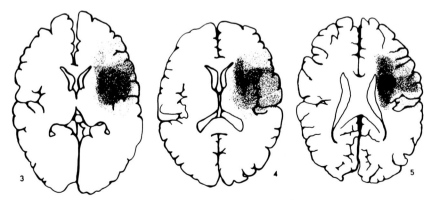

Figure 3. The overlap of frontal lesions anterior to the Rolandic sulcus ($N = 9$). From Kertesz and Dobrowolski (1981).

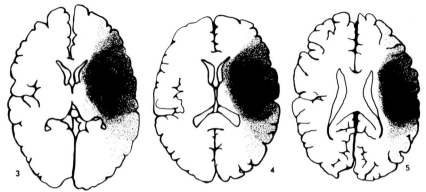

Figure 4. The overlap of central lesions involved in the posterior frontal, superior temporal and inferior parietal (*N* = 12). From Kertesz and Dobrowolski (1981).

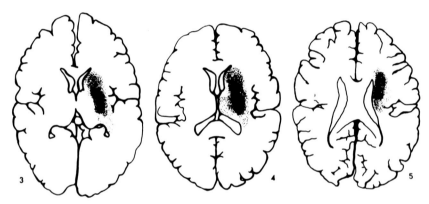

Figure 5. The overlap of subcortical lesions that were deep and central (*N* = 6).

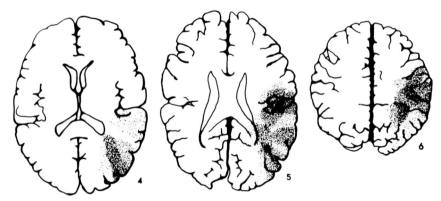

Figure 6. The overlap of parietal lesions that were post-Rolandic and supra-Sylvian (*N* = 7). From Kertesz and Dobrowolski (1981).

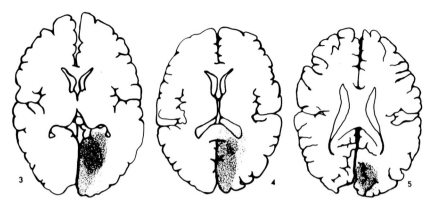

Figure 7. The overlap of occipital lesions ($N = 3$). From Kertesz and Dobrowolski (1981).

severation. The greatest impairment was seen in the frontal and central cortical regions, in block design, the drawing task of the Western Aphasia Battery (WAB), measures of neglect on drawing, and perseveration. Central and parietal lesion groups scored worst on perspective. The frontal and central groups also made significantly greater deviations to the right on a task of line bisections. However, the intergroup differences in overall drawing and block design were not significant.

The findings were different from the traditional association of CA, neglect and visuospatial deficit with right parietal or at least retro-Rolandic lesions. The exclusivity of this location could not be confirmed even if the lesion size differences and relatively small n-s in some of the lesion groups were considered. Although some of the tasks were complex (Raven's matrices) and may require diverse areas for processing and even hemispheric interaction, others were more elementary (e.g., drawing from an example or line bisection), suggesting that complexity alone cannot explain interference with function from widely spread lesions.

The groups that were formed on the basis of similar anatomical involvement do not follow lobar boundaries such as may be seen in neurosurgical populations, but conform to the reproducibility of the vascular territories seen in stroke.

A purely stroke population eliminates the confounding distance and growth effects of tumors, and the difficulty in localizing traumatic brain damage. This study is restricted to acute strokes to eliminate the confounding effects of recovery when the relatively mild residual deficit in the chronic stage is correlated with a relatively large lesion.

We interpret the results to indicate that right hemisphere functions may be more diffusely distributed than expected on the basis of previous knowledge. This notion has received more recent confirmation in a study presented by Whitely and Warrington (1982).

Visuospatial Defects

At the end of the nineteenth century, clinicians began to study patients who had difficulty finding their way, orienting themselves on maps, or recognizing directions in space. Jackson (1876) described a patient with a large right temporo-occipital tumor who had facial agnosia, dressing apraxia, and was lost in familiar surroundings. Badal's (1888) case also showed spatial disorientation in the visual, auditory, and sensory modalities. Many of these cases were bilateral posterior brain injuries such as the case of Dunn (1895) who thought the right hemisphere lesion was responsible for the topographical memory loss. Holmes and Horrax (1919) found disturbances in orientation, size and distance estimation, and occular fixation with gunshot wounds of the occipital parietal and temporal lobes. "Optic apraxia" became a popular term, and was applied widely to a host of tasks requiring placing objects in space, copying designs, or any action requiring visual guidance.

Spatial abilities were recognized to be part of general intelligence and, rather early in this century, they were standardized, such as the Porteus mazes (1918), in conjunction with verbal tests of intelligence. Various components of spatial skills such as discrimination of location or direction, ability to perceive relation or reversal, or the relationship of the observer to space were intensively investigated. Hundreds of tests of spatial ability were devised during the 1940s and 1950s. They were correlated with mathematical and geometrical skills, information processing, and general intelligence.

Information concerning the localization of lesions that cause spatial deficit was slow to accumulate. Brain (1941) reported three patients with posterior right hemisphere disease who appeared to have visuospatial agnosia for the left side of the space. They seemed to neglect turning to the left on a familiar route. The role of the right hemisphere in visual space perception was further elaborated by Paterson and Zangwill (1944).

Benton (1969) distinguished the following types of spatial disorders:

1. Localization of stimuli in extrapersonal space. This is often measured by dot localization, or crossing out lines.
2. Short-term memory for spatial location. An example of this would be Wechsler's visual memory test.
3. Route finding. This can be tested with tactile and visual mazes as well as ad hoc real routes of the patient to work or to the hospital.
4. Topographical memory. This is tested by finding locations and directions on maps. The deficit appears to be that of revisualization.
5. Visuoconstructive abilities (discussed previously).
6. Simultaneous recognition. The simultanagnosia of Wolpert (1924).
7. Reading and counting. Paralexic errors mainly due to neglect of the left side of a word. "Spatial dyscalculia" also falls in this category.

Each of these impairments may result from different mechanisms; for example, visuoconstructive difficulty may be caused by unilateral neglect or spatial disorientation or each of these basic mechanisms may appear under different clinical labels. Thus, neglect may be described under defective stimulus localization or reading disability.

Newcombe and Russel (1969) in the Oxford head injury population found a difference in localization between the right hemisphere group that was most impaired in the visual perceptual closure task and those most impaired in the maze learning tasks. The visual perceptual impairment seemed to be associated with right-temporo–occipitoparietal lesions and the maze learning deficit with higher parietal or parieto-occipital lesions on the right side. The memory and perceptual components of visuospatial performance may be differentially impaired after right temporal and parietal damage (Warrington & James, 1967; Warrington & Rabin, 1970). DeRenzi, Faglioni, and Scotti (1970), using a visual search and a tactile maze task, found no significant hemisphereic asymmetry in the exploration of extrapersonal space. However, the majority of failures occurred in the group with right hemisphere post-Rolandic lesions (localization extrapolated from the presence or absence of visual field defect).

Topographic orientation is an often-mentioned example of visuospatial ability. The first systematic study is that of Hécaen and Angelergues (1963) who found defective localization of geographical locations on a map in 21% of right hemisphere and 4% of left hemisphere lesions, and loss of topographical memory (inability to describe familial surroundings and routes) in 6% of right hemisphere and 1% of left hemisphere lesions. Benton, Levin, and Van Allen (1974) studied geographical orientation with a verbal and nonverbal pointing mode. A vector score indicated a sense of direction on a familial map. Education was the most important factor, but the vector scores were shifted most in right-hemisphere-damaged patients.

DeRenzi (1978) summarized spatial behavior under the headings of: (1) spatial exploration and localization; (2) spatial perception; (3) intelligent elaboration of spatial information; and (4) spatial memory. After reviewing several experiments, he postulated (a) a supramodal mechanism guiding the sensory–motor neuronal networks

TABLE 2

Visuospatial Defects in Localized Lesions

Task	Author	Localization
Spatial memory	Semmes et al. (1955)	Both parietal lobes worse
Map location	Hécaen & Angelerques (1963)	RBD worse
Perceptual maze (Elithorn)	Benton et al. (1963)	RBD worse
Maze learning	Milner (1965)	Right temporal, right parietal
	Newcombe & Russel (1969)	High posterior parietal
Pattern rotation	DeRenzi & Faglioni (1967)	Posterior, anterior same
Closure	Lansdell (1968)	Right temporal
	Newcombe & Russel (1969)	Right temporooccipital
	Orgass et al. (1972)	Right posterior (+ VFD)
Form board	DeRenzi et al. (1968)	Right posterior (+ VFD)
Template matching	Benson & Barton (1970)	Left anterior worst
Embedded figures (Gotschalk)	Orgass et al. (1972)	Aphasics worst
Progressive matrices (Raven)	Colonna & Faglioni (1966)	Posterior and Anterior same
	Costa (1976)	Right posterior worse
	Kertesz & Dobrowolski (1981)	Parietal, central, frontal same
Dot localization	Taylor & Warrington (1973)	Right posterior worse
	Hannay et al. (1976)	Posterior, anterior same
Visual discrimination	Taylor & Warrington (1973)	Posterior, anterior same
Geographical orientation	Benton et al. (1974)	RBD slightly worse
Spatial orientation	Semmes et al. (1963)	Diffusely represented in R

involved in scanning extrapersonal space; (b) each hemisphere is involved in scanning the contralateral half of space but damage to the right side of the brain impairs exploration of the left field more than damage to the left side impairs exploration of the right field, (c) neglect may be conceived as a cognitive defect of space representation as well as space exploration; (d) damage to the right retro-Rolandic area (as defined by the presence of visual field defects) produces the most disruption of extrapersonal spatial localization; (e) memory for position is partially independent from spatial perception and from general nonverbal memory, and is related to posterior damage regardless of the side affected; and (f) tactile spatial tasks were even more sensitive than visual ones. Table 2 attempts to summarize those studies that dealt with spatial perception in focal brain damage. These studies often require matching or choosing from a multiple choice, thereby eliminating the executive aspect required for CA.

Conclusion

The complexity and diversity of constructional and visuospatial abilities and tasks used to test them makes the comparison of localizing information even more difficult than that of language function. This underlies the continuing uncertainty concerning the localization of lesion causing these deficits. Much of the evidence so far points to the role of post-Rolandic parietotemporal and occipital region in visuospatial abilities and constructional performance. However, a growing body of studies, including ours as well as those summarized Chapter 20 of this book, indicate that more anterior portions of the right hemisphere are substantially involved.

The role of language and language impairment in the performance of these tasks by normals and brain-damaged patients cannot be ignored. Some of the tasks are easier to verbalize than others; some may utilize alternate verbal strategies for their solutions. Interhemispheric differences are confounded by this factor. For instance, exclusion of some aphasics from an interhemispheric comparison may result in an artificial increase in the incidence or severity of constructional apraxia in right hemisphere patients (DeRenzi, 1978). This could be related to differences in lesion size between the two groups—supported by greater EEG abnormalities on the right side (Costa & Vaughan, 1962)—and greater reaction times (DeRenzi & Faglioni, 1965).

It is assumed that some of the elementary components of visuo-spatial ability and constructional praxis have less verbal mediation than the complex tasks used in tests of "nonverbal" intelligence. It has been suggested that these elementary components of visuo-spatial ability indeed possess right hemisphere dominance and that they are focally organized. On the other hand, the more complex a task, the more structure it requires for its solution and this results in blurring the inter- and intrahemispheric differences.

The degree of focality or diffuseness of organization in the right hemisphere remains a contentious issue. On the basis of undisputably focal organization of language in the left hemisphere, it is assumed that the more dominant a function in a hemisphere, the more focally it is organized. It is possible that the more diffuse organization of the right hemisphere indicates relatively less dominance for these functions. This is compatible with the empirical impression that the right hemisphere is different in the relative paucity of clinical syndromes that could be unequivocally attributed to one or another location.

References

Ajuriaguerra, J. de, Hécaen, H., & Angelergues, R. (1960). Les apraxies, variétés cliniques et latéralisation lésionnelle. *Revue Neurologique, 102,* 494–566.

Arrigoni, G., & DeRenzi, E. (1964). Constructional apraxia and hemispheric locus of lesion. *Cortex, 1,* 170–197.

Badal, J. (1888). Contribution à l'étude des cecites psychiques: Alexie, agraphie, hemianopsie inférieure, trouble du sens de l'espace. *Archives d'Ophtalmologie (Paris), 8,* 97–117.

Benson, D. F., & Barton, M. I. (1970). Disturbances in constructional ability. *Cortex, 6,* 19–46.

Benton, A. L. (1967). Constructional apraxia and the minor hemisphere. *Confinia Neurologica, 27,* 1–17.

Benton, A. L. (1969). Disorders of spatial orientation. In P. J. Vinken & G. W. Brwyn (Eds.), *Handbook of clinical neurology* (Vol. 3). Amsterdam: Elsevier.

Benton, A. L., & Fogel, M. L. (1962). Three dimensional constructional praxis. *Archives of Neurology, 7,* 347–354.

Benton, A. L., Elithorn, A., Fogel, M. L., & Kerr, M. (1963). A perceptual maze test sensitive to brain damage. *Journal of Neurology, Neurosurgery & Psychiatry, 26,* 540–543.

Benton, A. L., Levin, H. S., & Van Allen, M. W. (1974). Geographic orientation in patients with unilateral cerebral disease. *Neuropsychologia, 12,* 183–191.

Black, F. W., & Strub, R. L. (1976). Constructional apraxia in patients with discrete missile wounds of the brain. *Cortex, 12,* 212–220.

Brain, W. R. (1941). Visual disorientation with special reference to lesions of the right cerebral hemisphere. *Brain, 64*, 244–272.

Colonna, A. & Faglioni, P. (1966). The performance of hemisphere-damaged patients on spatial intelligence tests. *Cortex, 2*, 293–307.

Costa, L. D. (1976). Intertest variability on the raven's coloured progressive matrices as an indication of specific ability deficit in brain-lesioned patients. *Cortex, 12*, 31–40.

Costa, L. D., & Vaughan, H. G. (1962). Performance of patients with lateralized cerebral lesions. 1. Verbal and perceptual tests. *Journal of Nervous and Mental Disease, 134*, 162–168.

DeRenzi, E. (1978). Hemispheric asymmetry as evidenced by spatial disorders. In M. Kinsbourne (Ed.), *Asymmetrical function of the brain.* Cambridge University Press.

DeRenzi, E., & Faglioni, P. (1965). The comparative efficiency of intelligence and vigilance tests in detecting hemispheric cerebral damage. *Cortex, 1*, 410–433.

DeRenzi, E., & Faglioni, P. (1967). The relationship between visuo-spatial impairment and constructional apraxia. *Cortex, 3*, 327–342.

DeRenzi, E., Faglioni, P. & Scotti, G. (1968). Tactile spatial impairment and unilateral cerebral damage. *Journal of Nervous & Mental Disease, 146*, 468–475.

DeRenzi, E., Faglioni, P., & Scotti, G. (1970). Hemispheric contribution to exploration of space through the visual and tactile modality. *Cortex, 6*, 191–203.

Dide, M. (1938). Les désorientations temporo-spatiales et la prépondérance de l'hémisphère droit dans les agnoso-akinésies proprioceptives. *Encephale, 33*, 276.

Duensing, F. (1953). Raumagnostische und ideatorisch—apraktische Stöung des Gestaltenden Handelns. *Deutsche Zeitschrift fuer Nervenheilkunde, 170*, 72–94.

Dunn, T. D. (1895). Double hemiplegia with double hemianopsia and loss of geographic centre. *Transactions of the College of Physicians of Philadelphia, 17*, 45–56.

Gainotti, G., Miceli, G., & Caltagirone, C. (1977). Constructional apraxia in left brain-damaged patients: a planning disorder? *Cortex, 13*, 109–118.

Hannay, H. J., Varney, N. R., and Benton, A. L. (1976). Visual localization in patients with unilateral brain disease. *Journal of Neurology, Neurosurgery & Psychiatry, 39*, 307–313.

Hécaen, H., & Angelergues, R. (1963). *La cécité psychique.* Paris: Masson.

Hécaen, H. & Assal, G. (1970). A comparison of constructive deficit following right and left hemispheric lesions. *Neuropsychologia, 8*, 289–303.

Hier, D. B., Mondlock, J., & Caplan, L. R. (1982). *Behavioral deficits after right hemisphere stroke.* Presented at the meeting of the American Academy of Neurology, Washington.

Holmes, G., & Horrax, G. (1919). Disturbances of spatial orientation and visual attention, with loss of stereoscopic vision. *Archives of Neurology and Psychiatry, 1*, 385–407.

Jackson, H. J. (1876). Case of large cerebral tumour without optic neuritis and with left hemiplegia and imperception. *London Ophthalmology Hospital Report, 8*, 434–442.

Kertesz, A., & Dobrowolski, S. (1981). Right-hemisphere deficits, lesion size and location. *Journal of Clinical Neuropsychology, 3*, 283–299.

Kertesz, A., Harlock, W., & Coates, R. K. (1979). Computer tomographic localization, lesion size and prognosis in aphasia and nonverbal impairment. *Brain and Language, 8*, 34–50.

Kleist, K. (1923). Kriegverletzungen des Gehirns in ihrer Bedeutung fur die Hirnlokalisation und Hirnpathologie. In O. von Schjerning (Ed.), *Handbuch der arztlichen Erfahrung im Weltkriege, 1914/1918* (Vol. 4). Leipzig: Barth.

Lange, J. (1936). Agnosien und Apraxien. In F. Bumke & O. Foerster (Eds.), *Handbuch der neurologie* (Vol. 6). Berlin: Springer-Verlag.

Landsdell, H. (1968). Effect of extent of temporal lobe ablations on two lateralized deficits. *Physiology & Behavior, 3,* 271–273.

Mack, J. L., & Levine, R. N. (1981). The basis of visual constructional disability in patients with unilateral cerebral lesions. *Cortex, 17,* 515–532.

McFie, J., Piercy, M. F., & Zangwill, O. L. (1950). Visual spatial agnosia associated with lesions of the right cerebral hemisphere. *Brain, 73,* 167–190.

Milner, B. (1965). Visually guided maze learning in man: Effects of bilateral hippocampal, bilateral frontal, & unilateral cerebral lesions. *Neuropsychologia, 3,* 317–338.

Newcombe, F. B., & Russel, W. R. (1969). Dissociated visual perceptual and spatial deficits in focal lesions of the right hemisphere. *Journal of Neurology, Neurosurgery and Psychiatry, 32,* 73–81.

Orgass, B., Poeck, K., Kerschensteiner, M. & Hartje, W. (1972). Visuo-cognitive performances in patients with unilateral hemispheric lesions. *Zeitschrift fur Neurologie, 202,* 177–195.

Paterson, A., & Zangwill, O. L. (1944). Disorders of visual space perception associated with lesions of the right cerebral hemisphere. *Brain, 67,* 331–358.

Petrovici, I. N. (1972). Schläfenlappen und Apraxie. *Fortschritte der Neurologie, Psychiatrie und Ihrer Grenzgebiete, 40,* 656–672.

Piercy, M., Hécaen, H., & Ajuriaguerra, J. (1960). Constructional apraxia associated with unilateral cerebral lesions—left and right sided cases compared. *Brain, 83,* 225–242.

Piercy, M. F., & Smyth, V. O. G. (1962). Right hemisphere dominance for certain nonverbal intellectual skills. *Brain, 85,* 775–789.

Poppelreuter, W. (1917). *Die psychischen Schädigungen durch Kopfschuss, im Kriege 1914–1916,* (Vol. 1). *Die Störungen der niederen und hoheren Sehleistungen durch Verletzungen des Occipitalhirns.* Leipzig: Voss.

Porteus, S. D. (1918). The measurement of intelligence: Six hundred and fifty-three children examined by the Binet and Porteus tests. *Journal of Educational Psychology, 9,* 13–31.

Semmes, J. (1968). Hemispheric specialization: A possible clue to mechanism. *Neuropsychology, 6,* 11–26.

Semmes, J., Weinstein, S., Ghent, L., & Teuber, H. L. (1963). Correlates of impaired orientation in personal and extrapersonal space. *Brain, 86,* 747–772.

Taylor, A. M., & Warrington, E. K. (1973). Visual discrimination in patients with localized cerebral lesions. *Cortex, 9,* 82–93.

Warrington, E. K., & James, M. (1967). An experimental investigation of facial recognition in patients with unilateral cerebral lesions. *Cortex, 3,* 317–326.

Warrington, E. K., & Rabin, P. (1970). Perceptual matching in patients with cerebral lesions. *Neuropsychology, 8,* 475–487.

Whitely, A. M., & Warrington, E. K. (1982). *Material specificity of right hemisphere perceptual skills.* Paper presented at the Fifth International Neuropsychological Society European Conference, Deauville, France, June.

Wolpert, I. (1924). Die Simultanagnosie: Storung der Gesamtauffassung. *Zeitschrift fuer die Gesamte Neurologie und Psychiatrie, 93,* 397–415.

20

Localization of Lesions in Neglect

Kenneth M. Heilman,
Robert T. Watson,
Edward Valenstein,
and Antonio R. Damasio

Introduction

Because the major intent of this book is to correlate behavioral abnormalities and their pathological substrates, this chapter concentrates on the anatomy of unilateral neglect. Before discussing anatomical aspects of the neglect syndrome, we define and discuss the associated symptoms and signs. The reader can find a detailed discussion of the pathophysiology of neglect in recent reviews (e.g., Heilman, 1979).

Definition

The patient with unilateral neglect fails to report, respond, or orient to stimuli presented to the side contralateral to a central lesion. A

471

patient is not considered to have neglect if he or she fails to respond to stimuli because of a primary motor or sensory defect. The symptoms of neglect may occur under a variety of stimulus and performance conditions. Different behavioral signs and symptoms may be seen during the evolution of, and recovery from, neglect. In addition, not all patients with neglect will have the complete spectrum of signs and symptoms associated with the neglect syndrome. In general, there are five major components of the neglect syndrome— (1) inattention; (2) hemispatial neglect; (3) hemiakinesia; (4) allesthesia; and (5) extinction. We discuss these signs and symptoms in the following section.

Signs and Symptoms

INATTENTION

Patients with the neglect syndrome often fail to respond to unilateral stimuli (hemineglect or hemi-inattention). It is difficult to distinguish between hemineglect and primary sensory disturbances in the visual and somesthetic modalities. Occasionally, a patient with visual or somesthetic hemi-inattention can report a stimulus when his attention is drawn to it; otherwise, one often must verify the locus of the lesion to exclude a primary sensory disturbance. Because the auditory system has bilateral projections, a unilateral hemispheric lesion cannot induce contralateral deafness. Therefore, an absent response to unilateral auditory stimuli suggests neglect.

HEMISPATIAL NEGLECT

Hemispatial neglect (visuospatial agnosia, hemispatial agnosia) may be shown by a variety of tasks. Hemispatial neglect can be demonstrated in drawings of a daisy or clock. Often, the patient with hemispatial neglect will draw only half of a daisy (Figure 1) or clock. The line-bisection and crossing-out tasks may be more sensitive for demonstrating hemispatial neglect. In the former task, a horizontal line is drawn and the patient is asked to bisect the line. The patient with hemispatial neglect tends to bisect the line toward the normal side (Figure 2). In the crossing-out task, a patient is presented a sheet

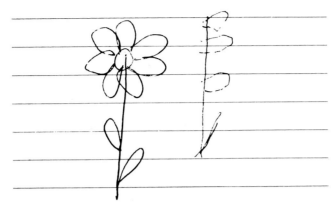

Figure 1. Examiner's drawing of daisy on left; patient's drawing on right.

of paper with short lines randomly distributed over the entire sheet. When a patient with hemispatial neglect is asked to mark out all lines, he will fail to mark out some of the ones in the neglected side of space.

Hemispatial neglect can also be identified in the activities of daily living. The patient may fail to eat food from one side of the plate, to groom one side of the face or body, or to dress half of the body. He may fail to read one side of a word or sentence (neglect-induced paralexia) or type on one side of the keyboard (neglect-induced paragraphia) (Valenstein & Heilman, 1979).

Hemispatial neglect can be shown by tasks not requiring afferent input (e.g., drawing a daisy) and is, therefore, not synonymous with

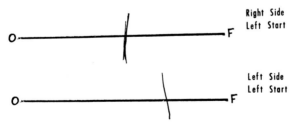

Figure 2. Line bisection tasks demonstrating the hemispatial effect on hemispatial neglect. On first trial, line is in right hemispace (right side); before bisecting the line the patient reads the letter O (left start). On second trial, the line is placed in left hemispace (left side), and the patient reads the letter O (left start) before bisecting line.

visual hemi-inattention. *Hemispace* is defined as the half of space to one side of the median plane of the head and body. Hemispace is not synonymous with a visual half field. Patients with neglect perform the line-bisection task better when the page is placed in the hemispace ipsilateral to the lesion than when it is placed in the neglected hemispace (Figure 2) (Heilman & Valenstein, 1979).

HEMIAKINESIA

Patients with the neglect syndrome may also be *hemiakinetic.* In the absence of gross motor defects, a patient may fail to raise the arm contralateral to the lesion unless encouraged to do so. Although these patients tend to be bilaterally bradykinetic, the arm contralateral to the lesion is often slower than the ipsilateral arm. These patients may fail to orient the head and eyes to a stimulus contralateral to the lesion. Responses such as following or passive head turning ("dolls eyes") can demonstrate that this hemispatial orienting defect is not being induced by a gaze or oculomotor paralysis. By asking the patient to orient to the side opposite that stimulated, it can be shown that these akinesias are not being induced by afferent defects or by hemi-inattention as the akinesias persist with these maneuvers. Occasionally, contralesional hypokinesia can be made worse when the ipsilesional extremity is simultaneously being used (motor extinction) (Valenstein & Heilman, 1981).

ALLESTHESIA

When a patient with neglect of left hemispace is touched on the left side, he may report or respond as if he were touched on the right side (Obersteiner, 1882). This phenomenon is *allesthesia.*

EXTINCTION

Patients with hemi-inattention or allesthesia often improve so that they can successfully detect, respond to, and lateralize unilateral stimuli. With frequent repetition of stimuli, some will again show inattention (fatigue phenomenon). Even when not fatigued, however, some patients, given bilateral simultaneous stimuli, will fail to report the stimulus presented contralateral to the damaged hemisphere. This phenomenon, extinction to double simultaneous stimulation, can be visual, tactile, and auditory. As the patient improves, the defect tends to persist longer in the visual and tactile modalities than in the auditory modality.

ASSOCIATED SIGNS AND SYMPTOMS

We have defined the neglect syndrome as a failure to report, respond, or orient to stimuli; but many clinicians and investigators include additional signs and symptoms. *Anosognosia* (denial of illness) is common in patients with neglect who deny the existence of their hemiparesis or even deny ownership of their paretic extremities. With anosodiaphoria, other patients admit that something is wrong but appear to be unconcerned (Critchley, 1966). Many have a *flattened affect* (Gainotti, 1972). They cannot comprehend or express affective intonations in speech (Heilman, Scholes, & Watson, 1975; Tucker, Watson, & Heilman, 1977) or recognize the emotional expression of a face (DeKosky, Heilman, Bowers, & Valenstein, 1980). Often, there is an associated decrease of autonomic responses to unpleasant and emotional stimuli (Heilman, Schwartz, & Watson, 1978). Patients with neglect often have visuoperceptive and visuoconstructive defects (construction apraxia) that cannot be completely explained by visual inattention or hemispatial neglect. They also may show motor impersistence, decreased vigilance, and decreased problem-solving ability.

Localization of Lesions That Induce Neglect

Ideally, one would like to correlate each of the signs and symptoms of neglect (discussed previously) with a specific lesion locus. However, many signs and symptoms coexist, and factors other than lesion locus influence the abnormal behavior, including: the speed of the ablative process, the nature of the ablation, the time between ablation and testing, premorbid processing strategies, and the ability of the unaffected brain to compensate. In general, therefore, we have not broken down the various signs and symptoms associated with neglect but discuss the anatomic localization of the entire syndrome.

Neglect has been associated with lesions in many parts of the central nervous system, including cortical polymodal sensory convergence areas, the cingulate gyrus and nearby supplementary motor area, basal ganglia, thalamus, and mesencephalic reticular formation (MRF). At first, it is difficult to see what these areas have in common. On the basis of clinical and physiological features of the neglect syndrome, we propose that neglect is a manifestation of a defect in systems mediating arousal and attention to meaningful stimuli. Although cortical sensory convergence areas may be necessary to analyze sensory input and determine its significance, subcortical systems, including the MRF and portions of the thalamus, probably are necessary for mediating arousal. Most of these areas either are limbic or receive heavy projections from the limbic system. Limbic input may also help determine biological significance. These corticolimbic and reticular areas, together with portions of the frontal lobes and basal ganglia, are important for initiating responses. It becomes apparent that the regions of the central nervous system associated with neglect are all highly interconnected and that they all can be construed, in part, as subserving attention–arousal–activation (intention) functions.

CORTICAL LESIONS

PARIETAL LOBE

In 1876, John Hughlings Jackson (Taylor, 1932) described a patient who neglected the left side of the page when reading. Autopsy disclosed a glioma of the right posterior temporal lobe. Subsequently, many investigators have noted that neglect is usually associated with a lesion in the area of the temporoparieto-occipital junction (posterior portion of Brodmann's Area 22) and the angular and supramarginal gyri (Brodmann's areas 39 and 40) (Hécaen, 1962).

We have examined 10 patients with hemispatial neglect and multimodal extinction who had cortical and subcortical lesions as determined by computerized tomography (CT). All the lesions were in the right hemisphere. The CT scans of one patient are shown in Figure 3. Figure 4 shows a lateral view of the right hemisphere. We have projected and superimposed the CT scans of these 10 patients on this lateral projection. Figure 5 illustrates that when damaged,

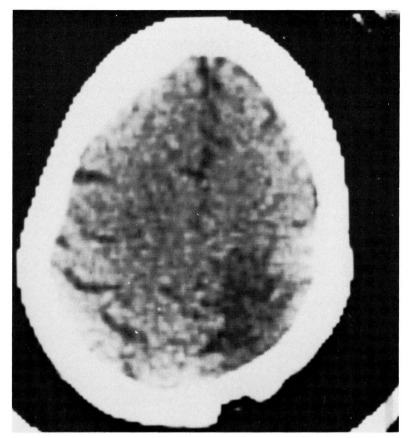

Figure 3. A section of a computerized tomographic scan (CT) demonstrating hypodense area in parieto-occipital region suggesting an infarction.

the inferior parietal lobule—together with the temporoparieto-occipital junction—is a critical area for inducing neglect.

The inferior parietal lobule is not as well developed in the monkey as in man. In the monkey, both banks of the superior temporal sulcus receive multimodal sensory input from visual, somesthetic, and auditory association areas (Pandya & Kuypers, 1969). The caudal portion of the monkey's inferior parietal lobe receives input from the posterior cingulate gyrus, the multimodal sensory association cortex (both banks of the superior temporal sulcus), and the dorsolateral frontal lobes (Mesulam, Van Hoesen, Pandya, & Geschwind, 1977).

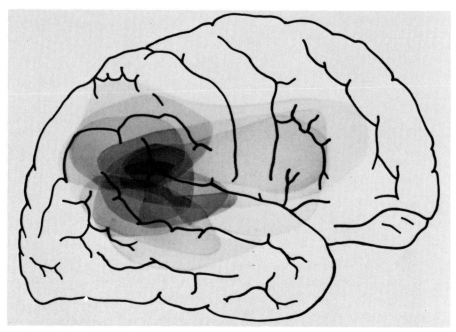

Figure 4. Lateral view of right hemisphere where we have projected and superimposed the CT scans of 10 patients with the neglect syndrome.

Lynch, Mountcastle, and Talbot (1977) have recorded electrical activity from cells in Brodmann's Area 7 of the monkey. These cells become active when an object is presented in a specific portion of the visual field. If the stimulus, such as food, is important to the animal, these cells increase the rate of firing. It has been proposed that the monkey's inferior parietal lobule (Area 7) and both banks of the superior temporal sulcus may be the precursor of man's inferior parietal lobule. In monkeys, lesions of Area 7 and both banks of the superior temporal sulcus have induced multimodal neglect (Heilman, Pandya, & Geschwind, 1970).

DORSOLATERAL FRONTAL LOBE

We describe three patients with extinction to simultaneous visual stimuli, two of whom also had somesthetic extinction and hemispatial neglect (Heilman & Valenstein, 1972). Radioisotope brain scan determined that these patients had lesions in the dorsolateral frontal lobe (Figure 5). The lesions appeared to involve Brodmann's

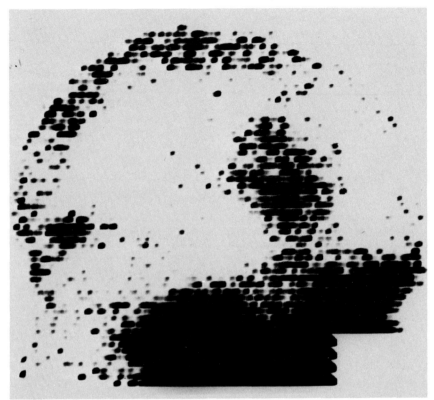

Figure 5. Radioisotope scan of patient with neglect syndrome demonstrating a large dorsolateral frontal lobe lesion.

Areas 8 and 9, as well as Area 46, which includes the frontal eye fields.

More recently Damasio, Damasio, and Chui (1980) reported a case of hemispatial neglect with inattention to auditory and visual stimuli induced by a dorsolateral frontal lesion as determined by CT scan (Figure 6).

Although the frontal lobe of a monkey is not as well developed as that of man, a lesion in the region of the arcuate gyrus, which is cytoarchitectonically similar to Area 8, also induces neglect (Welch & Stuteville, 1958). In man, however, it is not known whether lesions restricted to the inferior portion of Area 8 would induce neglect.

The dorsolateral frontal lobe, like the inferior parietal lobule, receives projections from visual, somesthetic, and auditory associa-

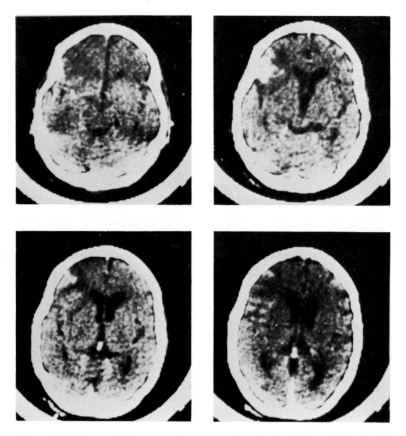

Figure 6. CT scan with contrast demonstrating a lesion (infarction) in the left lower frontal operculum with involvement of adjoining areas.

tion areas. The inferior parietal lobule and dorsolateral frontal lobe have strong corticocortical interconnections. Therefore, an anatomical substrate, similar to that proposed for the inferior parietal lobule, exists for the dorsolateral frontal lobe. However, a lesion of prefrontal structures may be more important for preparing the organism to respond than for selective attention to sensory stimuli.

MEDIAL FRONTAL LOBE

Heilman and Valenstein (1972) described three patients with the neglect syndrome from right medial frontal lobe lesions in the region of the cingulate gyrus and supplementary motor area. The lo-

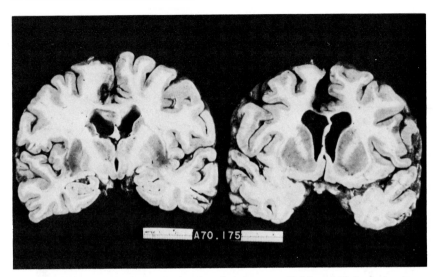

Figure 7. Postmortem examination showing a medial frontal lobe lesion in a patient with neglect syndrome.

cation was determined by postmortem examination (Figure 7) in one patient, and radioisotope scans in two. Damasio *et al.* (1980) described two patients with the neglect syndrome induced by left anterior cingulate–supplementary motor area lesions as demonstrated by CT (Figure 8).

The anterior cingulate of monkeys is similar to that of man. To confirm that focal lesions of the anterior cingulate gyrus can induce neglect, Watson, Heilman, Cauthen, and King (1973) made such lesions in monkeys and induced contralateral neglect. An anatomic substrate for this finding exists, since the dorsolateral frontal lobe and inferior parietal lobule have extensive reciprocal corticocortical connections with the cingulate gyrus (Pandya & Kuypers, 1969).

SUBCORTICAL LESIONS

MESENCEPHALIC RETICULAR FORMATION

In cats (Reeves & Hagamen, 1971) and in monkeys (Watson, Heilman, Miller, & King, 1974), MRF lesions induce profound and enduring contralateral multimodal sensory inattention and akinesia.

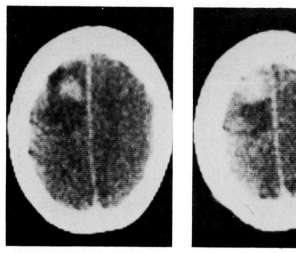

Figure 8. CT scan with enhancement demonstrating a medial frontal lobe lesion involving supplementary motor area, cingulate gyrus.

Watson *et al.* (1974) proposed that this lesion induced neglect by disrupting unilateral tonic arousal. The mechanism of this disruption may be from ablating direct MRF cortical connections or from interrupting the inhibitory influence of MRF on nucleus reticularis thalami (NR), a structure normally inhibiting thalamic transmission (Watson, Valenstein, & Heilman, 1981). Bilateral MRF lesions induce coma in man, and unilateral lesions would be likely to induce neglect, although a discrete unilateral MRF lesion in man, to our knowledge, has not been described.

THALAMUS

Watson and Heilman (1979) described three cases of the neglect syndrome induced by thalamic hemorrhage (Figure 9). Some of the patients had hemispatial neglect, a poor orienting response to the contralesional side, limb akinesia, multimodal extinction to simultaneous stimuli, anosognosia, and flattened affect. Postmortem examination of one patient showed that, although edema and mass effect compressed the ipsilateral internal capsule, there were no abnormalities of the cortex (Figure 10). The thalamic hemorrhages were too large to help determine which part of the thalamus may be critical for inducing neglect. Orem, Schlag–Rey, and Schlag (1973) induced unilateral visual neglect in cats by unilateral intralaminar thalamic lesions.

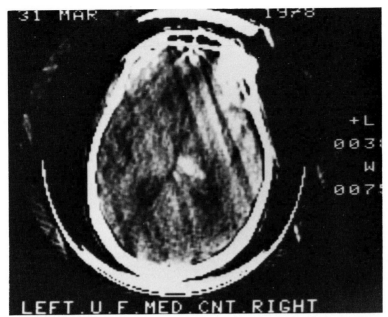

Figure 9. Hyperdense CT abnormality suggesting right thalamic hemorrhage.

Watson, Miller, and Heilman (1978) induced multimodal neglect in monkeys with centromedian parafascicularis (CM-PF) lesions. Neither anterior nor medial dorsal thalamic lesions induced neglect. Recently, we (Watson *et al.*, 1981) described a patient who had the neglect syndrome induced by a discrete thalamic infarction (Figure 11) that involved portions of the posterior ventral nucleus, most of the medial nuclear group including CM-PF, and possibly the anterior inferior aspect of the pulvinar. We proposed that medial thalamic lesions predominantly may induce motor neglect (akinesia) because the CM-PF is anatomically associated with motor systems such as the ventrolateral nucleus (VL) of the thalamus, frontal lobe, and neostriatum. Unilateral lesions of the CM-PF may, therefore, induce contralateral akinesia, whereas bilateral lesions of CM-PF or its connections induce akinetic mutism (Segarra & Angelo, 1970).

Velasco and Velasco (1979) demonstrated "motor inattention" in humans with VL lesions, and Hassler (1979) induced hemi-inattention in humans by pallidothalamic lesions, that is, by interrupting the pathway from the globus pallidus to the VL.

Watson *et al.* (1981) proposed also that lesions of the CM-PF or its

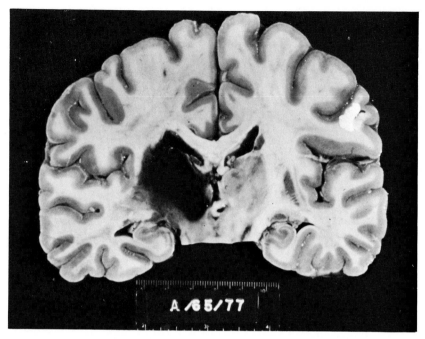

Figure 10. Right thalamic hemorrhages as determined by postmortem examination in patient with the neglect syndrome.

primary connections with the VL, prefrontal cortex, or neostriatum may disrupt preparation for a meaningful response to stimuli of behavioral significance. The CM-PF may mediate this preparation to respond primarily through a pathway from the CM-PF to prefrontal cortex to NR. The previously described corticocortical connections between the inferior parietal lobule and dorsolateral frontal lobes, as well as connections of the MRF (tonic arousal) and CM-PF to nucleus reticularis thalami (NR), serve as anatomic interfaces for sensorimotor integrations and aid in understanding why patients with neglect usually have both hemi-inattention and hemiakinesia.

BASAL GANGLIA

The caudate, putamen, globus pallidus, and substantia nigra comprise major portions of the basal ganglia. Hier, Davis, Richardson, and Mohr (1977) noted that patients with right putaminal hemorrhage often had unilateral neglect. We have noted also the associ-

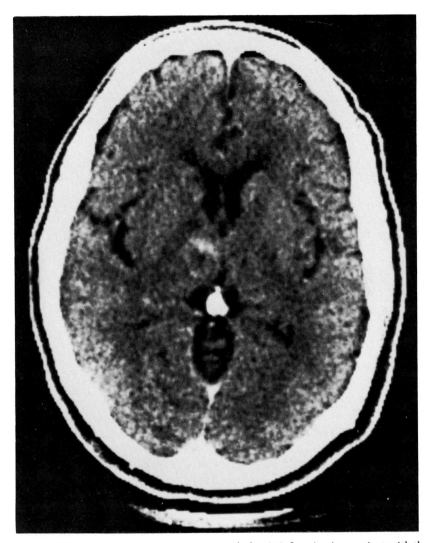

Figure 11. Hypodense CT scan suggesting thalamic infarction in a patient with the neglect syndrome.

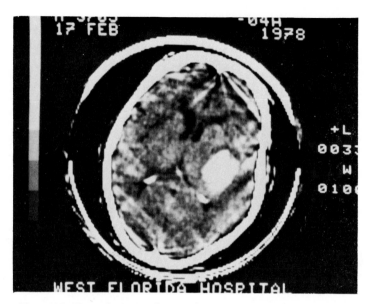

Figure 12. Hyperdense CT abnormality in lenticular region suggesting right ventricular (putaminal) hemorrage.

ation between unilateral neglect and putaminal hemorrhages (Figure 12). Because these lesions often compress the internal capsule—thereby inducing a contralateral hemiplegia and hemisensory loss—tests for inattention, akinesia, and extinction are invalid. However, we have examined several of these patients who were inattentive to auditory stimuli and who had a poor contralesional orienting response to the side opposite the lesion, or, less often, allesthesia.

Damasio *et al.* (1980) have described two patients with inattention and hemispatial neglect in association with infarction of the putamen and caudate (Figure 13). Valenstein and Heilman (1981) described a patient with a lesion mainly in the caudate nucleus (Figure 14). This patient did not show hemi-inattention, sensory extinction, or hemispatial neglect to simultaneous stimuli. He did, however, have a contralesional limb akinesia. This left-sided limb akinesia was dramatically increased by bilateral simultaneous movement (motor extinction). Marshall, Richardson, and Teitelbaum (1974) induced neglect by ablating the connections from the substantia nigra to the neostriatum (caudate and putamen).

Therefore, a neglect syndrome has followed lesions of all structures of the major basal ganglia. These structures are directly con-

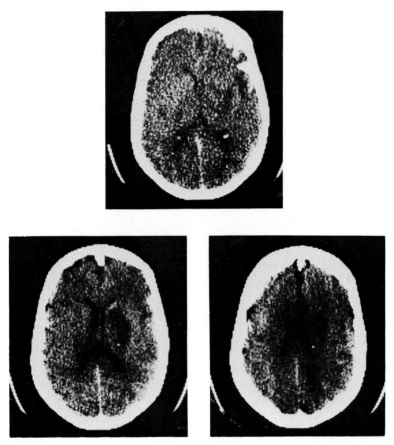

Figure 13. Hypodense CT abnormality suggesting infarction in region of ventricular nucleus.

nected to areas previously described as being important in the induction of neglect (e.g., CM-PF, VL, dorsolateral frontal lobe, and inferior parietal lobule).

SEIZURE-INDUCED NEGLECT

Multimodal sensory extinction present during a focal seizure and absent interictally has been reported (Heilman & Howell, 1980). This patient also had postictal hemispatial neglect. The seizure focus was in the right temporoparieto-occipital region (Figure 15).

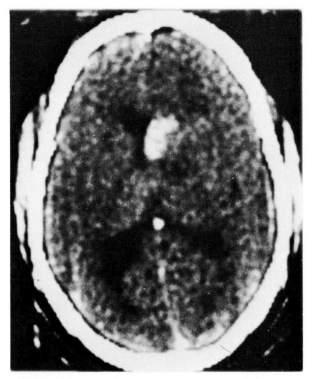

Figure 14. Hyperdense CT abnormality suggesting hemorrhage in region of right caudate.

RIGHT-LEFT HEMISPHERIC ASYMMETRIES OF NEGLECT

CORTICAL

Early investigators attributed neglect to right hemisphere lesions
(Brain, 1941; Critchley, 1966; McFie, Piercy, & Zangwill, 1950).

Denny–Brown and Banker (1954) showed that neglect (amorphosynthesis) could be induced by left hemisphere lesions. Battersby,
Bender, and Pollack (1956) found that neglect was more common
after right hemisphere lesions. Because there were many untestable
aphasic patients who may have had neglect, these authors attributed this asymmetry to a sampling artifact.

Albert (1973) used a line-crossing-out task to test for hemispatial
neglect. He did not eliminate aphasic subjects. He found that neglect was more severe with right than with left hemisphere lesions.

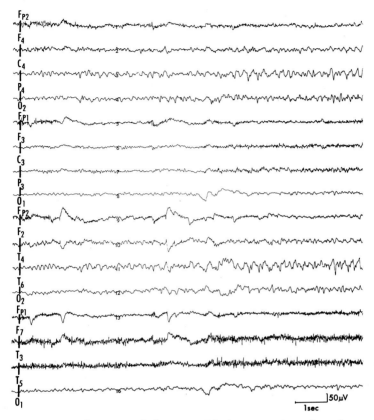

Figure 15. Electroencephalogram (EEG) demonstrating seizure focus in the right temporoparieto-occipital region.

Many other investigators have confirmed that the neglect syndrome is more common with right cortical lesions (Heilman, 1979).

SUBCORTICAL

All four of the patients described by Hier *et al.* (1977) had right hemisphere lesions in the basal ganglia. We have seen one case of putaminal hemorrhage and one case of caudate hemorrhage that induced the neglect syndrome; both were in the right hemisphere. Damasio *et al.* (1980) reported two cases of neostriatal infarction—one was of the left and one of the right. Thus, there is a total of seven cases induced by right-sided basal ganglia lesions and only one induced by a left-sided basal ganglia lesion.

In addition to the four cases of right thalamic neglect that we are reporting, we have seen another case of right thalamic infarction inducing neglect. This gives us a total of five right thalamic lesions that induced neglect and no left thalamic lesions.

It appears that the neglect syndrome is more common (or more severe) with right than with left hemisphere lesions, regardless of whether the lesion is cortical or subcortical.

To explain this hemispheric asymmetry, we have proposed that the right hemisphere in man may be dominant for mediating an attention–arousal–activation response. This hypothesis has been supported by psychophysiological studies in both patients and normal subjects (Heilman *et al.*, 1978; Heilman & Van Den Abell, 1979, 1980; Watson, Andriola, & Heilman, 1977).

Conclusions

The anatomy of neglect reveals connections of diverse cortical and subcortical structures that have one common feature: All are involved in arousal, attention, and activation. Each area interconnects with structures important for tonic arousal (MRF), selective multimodal sensory attention (parietotemporo-occipital junction), motivation (cingulate gyrus), and preparation to respond to a meaningful sensory stimulus (CM-PF, basal ganglia, and prefrontal cortex). These areas, in turn, may mediate this sensorimotor interaction through convergence on the NR and neostriatum.

References

Albert, M. L. (1973). A simple test of visual neglect. *Neurology, 23,* 658–664.

Battersby, W. S., Bender, M. B., & Pollack, M. (1956). Unilateral spatial agnosia (inattention) in patients with cerebral lesions. *Brain, 79,* 68–93.

Brain, W. R. (1941). Visual disorientation with special reference to lesions of the right cerebral hemisphere. *Brain, 64,* 224–272.

Critchley, M. (1966). *The parietal lobes.* New York: Hafner.

Damasio, R. R., Damasio, H., & Chui, H. G. (1980). Neglect following damage to frontal lobe or basal ganglia. *Neuropsychologia, 18,* 123–131.

DeKosky, S. T., Heilman, K. M., Bowers, D., & Valenstein, E. (1980). Recognition and discrimination of emotional faces and pictures. *Brain and Language, 9,* 206–330.

Denny-Brown, D., & Banker, B. Q. (1954). Amorphosynthesis from left parietal lesions. *Archives of Neurology and Psychiatry, 71,* 302–313.

Gainotti, G. (1972). Emotional behavior and hemispheric side of the lesion. *Cortex, 8*, 41–55.

Hassler, R. (1979). Striatal regulation of adverting and attention directing induced by pallidal stimulation. *Applied Neurophysiology, 42*, 98–102.

Hécaen, H. (1962). Clinical symtomology in right and left hemisphere lesions. In V. Mountcastle (Ed.), *Interhemispheric relations and cerebral dominance*. Baltimore: Johns Hopkins University Press, pp. 215–243.

Heilman, K. M. (1979). Neglect and related disorders. In K. M. Heilman & E. Valenstein: (Eds.), *Clinical neuropsychology*. London & New York Oxford University Press, pp. 268–308.

Heilman, K. M., & Howell, G. (1980). Seizure-induced neglect. *Journal of Neurology, Neurosurgery and Psychiatry, 43*, 1035–1040.

Heilman, K. M., Pandya, D. N., & Geschwind, N. (1970). Trimodal inattention following parietal lobe ablations. *Transactions of the American Neurological Association, 95*, 259–261.

Heilman, K. M., Scholes, R., & Watson, R. T. (1975). Auditory affective agnosia. *Journal of Neurology, Neurosurgery and Psychiatry, 38*, 69–72.

Heilman, K. M., Schwartz, H. D., & Watson, R. T. (1978). Hypoarousal in patients with a neglect syndrome and emotional indifference. *Neurology, 28*, 229–232.

Heilman, K. M., & Valenstein, E. (1972). Frontal lobe neglect in man. *Neurology, 22*, 660–664.

Heilman, K. M., & Valenstein, E. (1979). Mechanisms underlying hemispatial neglect. *Annals of Neurology, 5*, 166–170.

Heilman, K. M., & Van Den Abell, T. (1979). Right hemisphere dominance for mediating cerebral activation. *Neuropsychologia, 17*, 315–321.

Heilman, K. M., & Van Den Abell, T. (1980). Right hemisphere dominance for attention: The mechanism underlying hemispheric asymmetries of inattention. *Neurology, 30*, 327–330.

Hier, D. B., Davis, K. R., Richardson, E. P., Jr., & Mohr, J. P. (1977). Hypertensive putaminal hemorrhage. *Annals of Neurology, 1*, 152–159.

Lynch, J. C., Mountcastle, V. B., & Talbot, W. H. (1977). Parietal lobe mechanisms of directed visual attention. *Journal of Neurophys'ology, 40*, 362–389.

Marshall, J. F., Richardson, J. S., & Teitelbaum, P. (1974). Nigrostriatal bundle damage in the lateral hypothalamic syndrome. *Journal of Comparative and Physiological Psychology, 87*, 808–830.

McFie, J., Piercy, M. F., & Zangwill, O. L. (1950). Visual spatial agnosia associated with lesions of the right hemisphere. *Brain, 73*, 167–190.

Mesulam, M. M., Van Hoesen, G. W., Pandya, D. N., & Geschwind, N. (1977). Limbic and sensory connections of the inferior parietal lobule (area PG) in the Rhesus monkey: A study with a new method for horseradish peroxidase histochemistry. *Brain Research, 136*, 393–414.

Obersteiner, H. (1882). On allochiria—a peculiar sensory disorder. *Brain, 4*, 153–163.

Orem, J., Schlag-Rey, N., & Schlag, J. (1973). Unilateral visual neglect and thalamic intralaminar lesions in the cat. *Experimental Neurology, 40*, 784–797.

Pandya, D. N., & Kuypers, H. G. J. M. (1969). Cortico-cortical connections in the rhesus monkey. *Brain Research, 13*, 13–36.

Reeves, A. G., & Hagamen, W. D. (1971). Behavioral and EEG asymmetry following unilateral lesions of the forebrain and midbrain in cats. *Electroencephalography and Clinical Neurophysiology, 30*, 83–86.

Segarra, J. M., & Angelo, J. N. (1970). *Behavioral change in cerebral vascular disease*. New York: Harper & Row, pp. 7–14.

Taylor, J. (Ed.) (1932). *Selected writings of John Hughlings Jackson.* London: Hodder & Stoughton.

Tucker, D. M., Watson, R. T., & Heilman, K. M. (1977). Discrimination and evocation of affectively intoned speech in patients with right parietal disease. *Neurology, 27,* 947–950.

Valenstein, E., & Heilman, K. M. (1979). Apraxic agraphia with neglect-induced paragraphia. *Archives of Neurology (Chicago), 36,* 506–508.

Valenstein, E., & Heilman, K. M. (1981). Unilateral hypokinesia and motor extinction. *Neurology, 31,* 443–488.

Velasco, F., & Velasco, M. (1979). A reticulothalamic system mediating proprioceptive attention and tremor in man. *Neurosurgery, 4,* 30–36.

Watson, R. T., Andriola, M., & Heilman, K. M. (1977). The EEG and neglect. *Journal of the Neurological Sciences, 34,* 343–348.

Watson, R. T., & Heilman, K. M. (1979). Thalamic neglect. *Neurology, 29,* 690–694.

Watson, R. T., Heilman, K. M., Cauthen, J. C., & King, F. A. (1973). Neglect after cingulectomy. *Neurology, 23,* 1003–1007.

Watson, R. T., Heilman, K. M., Miller, B. D., & King, F. A. (1974). Neglect after mesencephalic reticular formation lesions. *Neurology, 24,* 294–298.

Watson, R. T., Miller, B. D., & Heilman, K. M. (1978). Nonsensory neglect. *Annals of Neurology, 3,* 505–508.

Watson, R. T., Valenstein, E., & Heilman, K. M. (1981). Thalamic neglect: The possible role of the medial thalamus and nucleus reticularis in behavior. *Archives of Neurology (Chicago), 38,* 501–506.

Welch, K., & Stuteville, P. (1958). Experimental production of neglect in monkeys. *Brain, 81,* 341–347.

21

Right-Hemisphere Lesions in Disorders of Affective Language

Elliott D. Ross

Introduction

Ever since the remarkable publications by Paul Broca (1861, 1865) and Carl Wernicke (1874), most clinical inquiries about language and the brain have been exclusively oriented to aphasic disorders secondary to left-hemisphere lesions, thus giving rise to the current belief that "left hemisphere dominance for language is a basic fact that must be accepted and remembered: for almost every right handed and for many left handed adults, the left hemisphere subserves all or most of the functions of language" (Benson, 1979). This chapter elaborates the idea and recent clinico-anatomical evidence that the right hemisphere has dominant language contributions that appear to involve the affective (or emotional) components of lan-

LOCALIZATION
IN NEUROPSYCHOLOGY

guage and behavior through the modulation of prosody and gesturing.

The first person to suggest that the right hemisphere might have language functions was Hughlings Jackson (1878, 1879). He observed that the emotional components of language seemed to be intact in patients who were aphasic and suggested that these components might be functions of the right hemisphere, whereas the propositional components of language, disturbed in aphasia, were functions of the left hemisphere. Despite these perceptive observations, almost 100 years elapsed before the first clinico-anatomical correlations were made supporting the idea that the right hemisphere had dominant language functions.

Beginning in the late 1940s, Monrad-Krohn (1947a, 1947b, 1957, 1963) published a series of articles dealing with the prosodic aspects of language. He divided speech into three parts: (1) *vocabulary*, comprising individual spoken words and articulation; (2) *grammar*, which sets the rules for word ordering, conjugation, and declination; and (3) *prosody* (the melodic line produced by the variation of pitch, rhythm, and stress of pronunciation) which conveys certain semantic and emotional meaning to speech beyond vocabulary and grammar. He went on to divide prosody into four categories.

Intrinsic prosody consists of common prosodic patterns found within a language that have specific semantic information. For example, if a person wishes to ask a question, the pitch of his voice rises on the last word. *Intellectual prosody* imparts subtle shades of meaning to language, such as sarcasm, skepticism, annoyance, or emphasis. For instance, if the sentence "He is clever" is stressed on the "is," it becomes an emphatic acknowledgment of a person's ability. If the stress resides on "clever," skepticism becomes apparent. If the word "he" is stressed, then the sentence acknowledges a person's ability but also implies that perhaps the person's associates are not clever. *Emotional prosody* represents the insertion of certain prosodic features into language that convey emotions: anger, pleasure, sorrow, joy, or surprise. *Inarticulate prosody*, the last category, is characterized by utterances such as grunts and other nonarticulate sounds that further communicate information to the listener.

If one were to categorize these components of prosody into whether they had propositional or emotional value—in keeping with Jackson's ideas—intrinsic and intellectual prosody and some components of inarticulate prosody appear to have propositional value whereas emotional prosody and some components of inarticulate prosody appear to have emotional value. However, certain aspects of intellectual prosody may also have emotional valence (Ross & Mesulam, 1979).

Monrad-Krohn (1963) also described certain disturbances of prosody encountered clinically. *Hyperprosody* is associated with maniacal states and "motor types of aphasia where the vocabulary is reduced to one or two words. The patients may make pathetic attempts at making themselves understood by pronouncing the one remaining word with varying prosody which is in itself quite correct—but often exaggerated" (Monrad-Krohn, 1963). *Dysprosody,* the result of incomplete recovery from motor aphasia, can be considered a form of "ataxic prosody." *Hypoprosody* or *aprosody* is the complete failure or absence of normal prosodic variation that is frequently encountered in Parkinson's disease as part of the masked facies, motor akinesia, and weak voice. Although Monrad-Krohn did not describe disorders of prosody secondary to right hemisphere damage, his inquiry was the first clinical attempt to look at nonaphasic language disturbances resulting from brain damage.

In a paper published in 1972, Gianotti described changes in emotional behavior associated with right versus left hemispheric lesions. He noted that left hemisphere brain-damaged patients overwhelmingly had a catastrophic–depressive reaction to their illness, whereas right hemisphere brain-damaged patients were euphoric, indifferent, and unconcerned (and thus unemotional about their illness). Although this particular difference has been well known since Babinski (1914, 1918) first described anosognosia, the impact of Gianotti's work was to refocus attention to the neurology of affective behavior and to help rekindle the idea that the modulation of emotions may be a function of the right hemisphere.

In 1975, Heilman, Scholes, and Watson described a new syndrome, *auditory affective agnosia,* in a series of right-handed nonaphasic patients with right temporoparietal lesions. These patients were markedly impaired in identifying the affective components of spoken language and, in fact, were far more impaired than controls with left hemisphere damage and aphasia. In a follow-up publication, Tucker, Watson, and Heilman (1977) further demonstrated that patients with right parietotemporal damage, when asked to repeat sentences with affective intonation, had marked difficulty in accomplishing the task.

Although previous work by Zurif (1974) and Blumstein and Copper (1974) (using dichotic listening tasks) demonstrated that the left ear–right hemisphere was superior in processing the prosodic elements of speech, the two pioneering papers by Heilman *et al.* (1975) and Tucker *et al.* (1977) represent the first observations to provide solid clinico-anatomical evidence that the right hemisphere has language functions—the modulation of the affective components of language.

In 1979, two patients were reported by Ross and Mesulam with left hemiplegia and sensory loss secondary to right supra-Sylvian infarctions involving the frontal and anterior parietal lobes (Figure 1). They had strikingly flattened affects with total inability to impart emotions into their language and behavior through prosody and gesturing. They appeared to retain, by their own introspections and by limited testing, the ability to comprehend and appreciate emotions in others and to feel emotions within themselves; both complained about their frustrating inability to express emotions that they felt inwardly. The right supra-Sylvian location of their lesions (causing a motor disturbance of affective language) coupled with Heilman *et al.* (1975) and Tucker *et al.* (1977) observations that right temporoparietal lesions produce comprehension and repetition disturbances of affective language gave rise to the proposal that the right hemisphere has a dominant role in modulating the affective com-

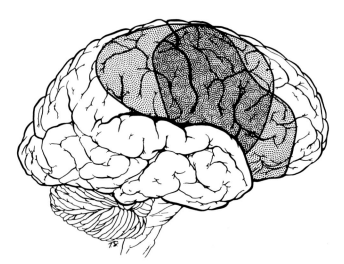

Figure 1. The lesion distributions in the two patients reported by Ross and Mesulam (1979) with inability to impart emotions into speech and gestures are displayed on a right lateral hemisphere template. The CT scans can be found in the original publication. The lesions were reconstructed from the CT scans, utilizing the atlas of Matsui and Hirano (1978).

ponents of language and that the anatomical organization of this contribution mirrors that of propositional language in the left hemisphere (Ross & Mesulam, 1979).

The Aprosodias

With the preceding points in mind, it occurred to Ross (1981) that it might be possible to examine the affective components of language using the same strategies as one does for propositional language. Because the eight known categories of aphasia—motor, sensory, conduction, global, transcortical motor, transcortical sensory, anomic, and mixed transcortical—can be classified by observations concerning (1) spontaneous speech (fluency versus nonfluency); (2) repetition ability; (3) comprehension of spoken language; and (4) visual language skills (naming and reading), patients with focal right hemisphere damage might be examined in a similar manner by evaluating (1) spontaneous prosody and emotional gesturing; (2) the ability to repeat sentences with prosodic-affective

TABLE 1

The Aprosodias[a]

	Spontaneous Prosody and Gesturing	Prosodic–Affective Repetition	Prosodic–Affective Comprehension	Comprehension of Emotional Gesturing
Motor[b]	**Poor**	**Poor**	**Good**	**Good**
Sensory[b]	Good	Poor	Poor	Poor
Global[b]	Poor	Poor	Poor	Poor
Conduction	**Good**	**Poor**	**Good**	**Good**
Transcortical motor	**Poor**	**Good**	**Good**	**Good**
Transcortical sensory[b]	Good	Good	Poor	Poor
Mixed transcortical	**Poor**	**Good**	**Poor**	**Poor**
Anomic[c]	**Good**	**Good**	**Good**	**Poor**

[a] The aprosodias set in bold type have already been described. The existence of the aprosodias set in italic type has been postulated but not demonstrated (Ross, 1981).

[b] Good anatomical correlation with lesions in the left hemisphere known to cause homologous aphasias.

[c] Although anomic aphasia is the least localizable of the aphasic disturbances, if it is accompanied by alexia with agraphia, then damage to the angular gyrus is invariably present (Benson, 1979). Anomic aprosodia should result from damage to the right angular gyrus if the postulated functional–anatomical approach to the affective components of language is correct.

TABLE 2

The Aphasias

	Fluency	Repetition	Comprehension	Reading Comprehension
Motor (Broca)	Poor	Poor	Good	Good
Sensory (Wernicke)	Good	Poor	Poor	Poor
Global	Poor	Poor	Poor	Poor
Conduction	Good	Poor	Good	Good
Transcortical motor	Poor	Good	Good	Good
Transcortical sensory	Good	Good	Poor	Poor
Mixed transcortical	Poor	Good	Poor	Poor
Anomic (alexia with agraphia)	Good	Good	Good	Poor

variation; (3) the ability to comprehend the prosodic-affective components of language; and (4) the ability to comprehend emotional gesturing.

Using this strategy, 10 patients with various disorders of affective language secondary to right brain lesions were collected over 1 year's time (Ross, 1981). As the disturbances of affective language were so similar to the various aphasias secondary to focal left hemisphere lesions, it seemed appropriate to call these disorders "aprosodias" (ā·pro·sō′di·a·s) and apply the same modifiers to classify them as one uses in the aphasias (Tables 1 and 2).

Bedside Evaluation of Affective Language

To clinically assess the affective components of language, some practice is required by the examiner. However, once the clinician becomes familiar with the examination, it readily can be incorporated into the routine neurologic examination much the same way one conventionally tests for propositional language. The tasks described here are easily and flawlessly done by normals and non-brain-damaged patients, regardless of educational level.

Spontaneous Prosody and Emotional Gesturing

During the interview, observations should be made about the prosodic variation of the patient's voice. The examiner should ask emotionally loaded questions such as "How do you feel about your neurological deficits? Have you experienced a loss of a loved one? or Have you had any close calls with death or maiming?" One should ignore overall loudness or softness of speech and pay strict attention to the finer aspects of prosodic variation to see if it conveys emotional information about the situation. Also, observations should be made about the patient's gesturing ability. In addition to judging whether speech is aprosodic or prosodic, there may be instances where prosodic variation (and gesturing) actually will mismatch the semantic content of speech much like posterior aphasics who are fluent even though their speech output is quite paraphasic.

PROSODIC–AFFECTIVE REPETITION

In this evaluation, a declarative sentence devoid of emotional words is used. The patient is then asked to repeat the sentence with exactly the same affective tone used by the examiner. Thus, the statement "I am going to the movies" is said in a happy, sad, tearful, disinterested, angry, and surprised voice. The patient is requested to repeat the statement in the same way. Again, repetition ability should be judged on how well the patient fine tunes his prosodic variation to that of the examiners. Merely raising or lowering the loudness of voice without other prosodic variation, or raising the voice at the end of a statement to indicate a question, should not be interpreted as constituting good prosodic repetition.

PROSODIC–AFFECTIVE COMPREHENSION

To examine prosodic-affective comprehension, a declarative statement devoid of emotional words is used in conjunction with differing affective tones (described previously). Standing behind the patient during this assessment will avoid giving the patient visual clues. The patient is then asked to identify the kind of affect that was injected into the statements. Sometimes a multiple-choice format is necessary to initially orient the patient to the requested task.

COMPREHENSION OF EMOTIONAL GESTURING

This is done by pantomiming—in front of the patient—emotional gestures involving the face and limbs to convey a particular affective state. As with prosodic comprehension, the patient is requested to identify the emotion by name or description. Occasionally, a multiple-choice format is needed during initial testing to help orient the patient to the task.

Functional–Anatomical Correlations

In collecting the series of 10 right-handed, nonaphasic patients (Ross, 1981), no patient was encountered with a lesion involving the right periSylvian region who did not also have an aprosodia. Thus, all patients examined, with lesions in the right hemisphere that were homologously located to the classical periSylvian speech areas in the left hemisphere, had some form of aprosodia. The CT lesions have been reconstructed on a right lateral hemisphere template (Figure 2), based on the anatomical relationships published in Matsui and Hirano's atlas (1978). The actual CT scans of the patients can be found in the original paper (Ross, 1981). In the time since this chapter was accepted for publication, eight more cases of aprosodia (four motor, two global, and two sensory) have been encountered. All have had similar lesion locations determined by CT, as described subsequently and in Figure 2.

MOTOR APROSODIA (Figure 2a)

Three patients sustained a motor aprosodia with moderate to severe left hemiplegia and variable left-sided sensory loss. All the patients had had a cerebrovascular accident involving the right frontal and anterior-parietal opercular region by CT, in a supra-Sylvian distribution that was homologous to lesions in the left hemisphere known to cause persistant Broca (motor) aphasia (Kertesz, 1979; Mohr, 1976). Some patients had transient anosognosia early in their course. Their language deficit was characterized by a flat monotone voice without prosodic variation and loss of spontaneous gesturing. Prosodic–affective repetition was severely compromised but pro-

---

Figure 2. The lesion distributions in 8 of the 10 patients reported by Ross (1981) with various aprosodias are displayed on a right lateral hemisphere template. The CT scans can be found in the original publication. The lesions were reconstructed from the CT scans utilizing the atlas of Matsui and Hirano (1978). (Copyright 1981, American Medical Association.)

MOTOR APROSODIA

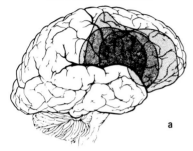

a

SENSORY APROSODIA

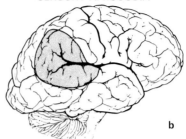

b

GLOBAL APROSODIA

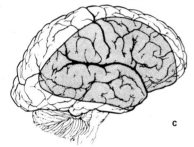

c

TRANSCORTICAL SENSORY
APROSODIA

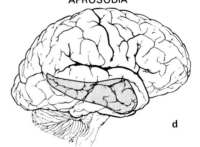

d

MIXED TRANSCORTICAL
APROSODIA

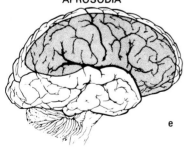

e

MOTOR APROSODIA +
PURE PROSODIC DEAFNESS

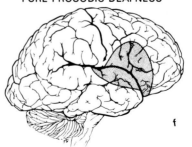

f

sodic–affective comprehension and visual comprehension of emotional gesturing were completely intact. One of the patients was followed for 8 months and showed remarkable improvement in his aprosodic–agestural state, but according to him and his wife, he never fully regained normal affective function. Another patient became suicidally depressed during his illness; however, he never displayed a depressive affect. In fact, his flattened affect remained unchanged even after his depression was treated. Thus, the flattened affect caused by the aprosodic–agestural state, characteristic of motor aprosodia, is a true neurological deficit that cannot be accounted for by psychiatric or psychological explanations (Ross & Rush, 1981).

SENSORY APROSODIA (Figure 2b)

One patient was reported with a sensory aprosodia, characterized by excellent prosodic variation in speech and active spontaneous gesturing. Comprehension of the prosodic–affective components of language, visual comprehension of emotional gesturing, and prosodic–affective repetition were severely impaired. During the interview, the patient appeared somewhat euphoric and overly happy even when he talked about his stroke and the possibility of losing his job, suggesting that he may have been mismatching his affective components of language to the semantic contents of his speech. He had moderate deficits in vibration, position, and stereognosis in his left hand and a dense left hemianopsia. The infarction was confined to the right posterior–superior temporal and inferior–posterior parietal lobes by CT. This distribution is consistent with left hemisphere lesions known to cause Wernicke (sensory) aphasia (Kertesz, 1979; Kertesz & Benson, 1970).

GLOBAL APROSODIA (Figure 2c)

One patient had a global aprosodia secondary to a large right peri-Sylvian cerebrovascular accident involving the frontal, parietal, and temporal lobes on CT. He had a severe left hemiplegia with left hemisensory loss and a left hemianopsia. The patient had a totally flattened affect without prosodic variation in his voice or spontaneous gesturing. Prosodic–affective repetition, comprehension of the prosodic–affective elements of language, and visual comprehension of emotional gesturing were severely compromised. Over time, his prosodic comprehension improved but remained abnormal. The distribution of his lesion on CT was consistent with the periSylvian distribution of left brain lesions known to produce global aphasia (Kertesz, 1979). His improvement in prosodic comprehension is consistent with Kertesz's (1979) observations that the most likely parameter to improve in global aphasics is comprehension.

TRANSCORTICAL MOTOR APROSODIA

Two patients were reported with the phenomenon of transcortical motor aprosodia, characterized by aprosodic-agestural speech with preserved prosodic-affective repetition and intact comprehension of affective prosody and emotional gesturing. Both patients had left hemipareses without sensory loss. The CT scans in these patients did not show lesion distributions that one would normally associate with transcortical motor aphasia arising from left hemisphere lesions (Alexander & Schmitt, 1980; Rubens, 1976). However, from a phenomonological point of view, the particular mix of deficits in affective language was consistent with the classification of transcortical motor aprosodia and the phenomenon of transcortical motor aphasia.

One patient had metastatic tumor with tracking edema involving the right frontal, parietal, and temporal lobes, negating any precise functional–anatomical correlations. The second patient sustained a right striatal infarction by CT. Interestingly enough, her transcortical motor aprosodia rapidly resolved over a 2-week period that would be consistent with some transient motor types of aphasia that have been observed following left striatal lesions (Benson, 1979; Hermann, Turner, Gillingham, & Gaze, 1966).

TRANSCORTICAL SENSORY APROSODIA (Figure 2d)

One patient was reported with transcortical sensory aprosodia, characterized by intact spontaneous prosody and emotional gesturing, excellent prosodic–affective repetition, and exceedingly poor prosodic–affective comprehension. Comprehension of emotional gesturing could not be tested because of severe cataracts. The CT scan showed a large intracerebral hemorrhage, involving the right anterior–inferior temporal lobe with sparing of the posterior–superior temporal lobe. This particular distribution with sparing of the posterior–superior temporal lobe is consistent with left hemisphere lesions that are associated with transcortical sensory aphasia (Benson, 1979; Kertesz, 1979). Except for transient coma and left hemiplegia which completely resolved within 6 hours, the patient did not sustain any elementary neurological deficits from the hemorrhage.

Mixed Transcortical Aprosodia (Figure 2e)

One patient was discovered to have a mixed transcortical aprosodia. The lesion, by CT scan, involved the right supra-Sylvian region and a small portion of the posterior–superior temporal lobe. She had a severe left hemiplegia with hemisensory loss. The patient's affective language was first evaluated 6 months after the stroke. At that time, she demonstrated a flattened affect, characterized by aprosodic-agestural speech. Prosodic–affective repetition was good, but not fully normal. Prosodic–affective comprehension and comprehension of emotional gesturing were very poor. Although prosodic–affective repetition was not perfectly normal, it was so much better than her spontaneous prosody that she was classified as having a mixed transcortical aprosodia even though her lesion seemed to be most consistent with a global aprosodia. Most likely, if she had been evaluated closer to her ictus, she would have demonstrated a global aprosodia.

Kertesz (1979) has reported that patients with large supra-Sylvian lesions with minimal involvement of the superior temporal lobe initially may present with a global aphasia that subsequently evolves into a mixed transcortical or transcortical motor aphasia. These observations are pertinent to the findings in this patient since her mixed transcortical aprosodia eventually evolved into a transcortical motor aprosodia.

Pure Prosodic Deafness Plus Motor Aprosodia
(Figure 2f)

The last patient reported was admitted to the hospital with a left hemiplegia without any sensory loss. His voice was flat and devoid of prosodic variation, and his gesturing was blunted. Prosodic–affective repetition and prosodic–affective comprehension were poor. However, comprehension of emotional gesturing was flawless, in distinct contrast to his prosodic–affective comprehension. The CT scan showed an enhancing lesion, involving the right frontal operculum, anterior insula, and the anterior–superior temporal lobe with sparing of the posterior–superior temporal lobe and parietal operculum. This case was interpreted as an example of motor aprosodia in combination with pure prosodic deafness. This constellation of deficits is similar to left brain-damaged patients who have been reported to have global aphasia without alexia (Heilman, Rothi, Campanella, & Wolfson, 1979). The right frontal opercular lesion can easily account for the patient's aprosodic–agestural speech and poor prosodic–affective repetition. The prosodic–affective comprehension difficulty could be accounted for by the anterior–superior temporal lesion if it isolated the right posterior–superior temporal lobe from ipsilateral and contralateral auditory inputs, much like the mechanism postulated to explain pure word deafness arising from a unilateral lesion in the left temporal lobe (Gazzaniga, Glass, Sarno, & Posner, 1973). If the visual connections to the right posterior–superior temporal lobe remain intact, as suggested by the CT scan, then it is not surprising that this patient was able to visually comprehend emotional gesturing but unable to auditorialy comprehend the prosodic-affective components of language.

Conclusion

Although the number of cases reported in the literature are limited at this time, the initial clinico–anatomical data suggest that the right hemisphere has dominant language functions involving the modulation of the affective components of language through prosody and emotional gesturing. Six different aprosodias have already been observed—motor, sensory, global, transcortical motor, transcortical sensory, and mixed transcortical. The corresponding lesions in the right hemisphere associated with these syndromes seem to be in good agreement, for the most part, with the published functional–anatomical data correlating the aphasias to left hemisphere lesions. In addition, the possibility of pure prosodic deafness has been raised. Thus, it would appear that affective language in the right hemisphere is anatomically and functionally organized in a similar manner to propositional language in the left hemisphere.

Additional evidence to support the above hypothesis is provided by recent observations published by Larsen, Skinhøj, and Lassen in 1978. Utilizing the technique (Lassen, Ingvar, & Skinhøj, 1978) of intracarotid injection of radioactive Xenon to measure changes in focal cerebral blood flow during an "automatic" speech task, these investigators found changes in focal cerebral blood flow in the right hemisphere that were homologous to those observed in the left hemisphere. Although a ready explanation for this startling finding was not offered because of the traditional belief that language was a dominant function of the left hemisphere, perhaps Larsen *et al.* had actually observed the functional–anatomical organization of the affective components of language in the right hemisphere (Ross, 1981).

Further research, both qualitative and quantitative, must be done to firmly establish these initial clinico-anatomical correlations concerning the dominant language and behavioral functions of the right hemisphere. Already these initial studies have led to inquiries about the neurology of depression (Ross and Rush, 1981), further linguistic studies of prosody in right-brain-damaged patients (Weintraub, Mesulam, and Kramer, 1981) and an anatomical hypothesis concerning how the brain integrates the right and left hemisphere contributions to language into a unified behavior (Ross, Harney, deLacoste and Purdy, 1981). Until the affective functions of the right hemisphere are unraveled, the neurological basis of human language never will be fully realized, especially since the affective components of language are probably, in the long run, far more influential in human discourse than the actual words one chooses.

References

Alexander, M. P., & Schmitt, M. A. (1980). The aphasia syndrome of stroke in the left anterior cerebral artery territory. *Archives of Neurology (Chicago)*, 37, 97–100.

Babinski, J. (1914). Contribution à l'étude des troubles mentaux dans l'hémiplégié organique cérébrale. *Revue Neurologique*, 1, 845–848.

Babinski, J. (1918). Anosognosie. *Revue Neurologique*, 25, 365–367.

Benson, D. F. (1979). *Aphasia, alexia, and agraphia*. Edinburgh & London: Churchill-Livingstone.

Blumstein, S., & Cooper, W. E. (1974). Hemispheric processing of intonation contours. *Cortex*, 10, 146–158.

Broca, P. (1861). *Bulletin de la Societe Anatomique de Paris, 2,* 330–357. In G. von Bonin (tráns.), *The cerebral cortex.* Springfield, Illinois: Thomas, 1960.

Broca, P. (1865). Sur le siège de la faculté du langage articulé. *Bulletin d'Anthropologie, 6,* 377–393.

Gazzaniga, M. S., Glass, A. V., Sarno, M. T., & Posner, J. B. (1973). Pure word deafness and hemispheric dynamics: A case history. *Cortex, 9,* 136–143.

Gianotti, G. (1972). Emotional behavior and hemispheric side of the lesion. *Cortex, 8,* 41–55.

Heilman, K. M., Rothi, L., Campanella, D., & Wolfson, S. (1979). Wernicke's and global aphasia without alexia. *Archives of Neurology (Chicago), 36,* 129–133.

Heilman, K. M., Scholes, R., & Watson, R. T. (1975). Auditory affective agnosia. Disturbed comprehension of affective speech. *Journal of Neurology, Neurosurgery and Psychiatry, 38,* 69–72.

Hermann, K., Turner, J. W., Gillingham, F. J., & Gaze, R. M. (1966). The effects of destructive lesions and stimulation of the basal ganglia on speech mechanisms. *Confinia Neurologica, 27,* 197–207.

Jackson, J. H. (1878). On affections of speech from disease of the brain. *Brain, 1,* 304–330.

Jackson, J. H. (1879). *2,* 203–222, 323–356.

Kertesz, A. (1979). *Aphasia and associated disorders.* New York: Grune & Stratton.

Kertesz, A., & Benson, D. F. (1970). Neologistic jargon. A clinicopathological study. *Cortex, 6,* 362–386.

Larsen, B., Skinhøj, E., & Lassen, N. A. (1978). Variations in regional cortical blood flow in the right and left hemispheres during automatic speech. *Brain, 101,* 193–209.

Lassen, N. A., Ingvar, D. H., & Skinhøj, E. (1978). Brain function and blood flow. *Scientific American, 239,* 62–71.

Matsui, T., & Hirano, A. (1978). *An atlas for the human brain for computerized tomography.* Tokyo: Igaku-Shoin Ltd.

Mohr, J. P. (1976). Broca's area and Broca's aphasia. In H. Whitaker & H. A. Whitaker (Eds.), *Studies in neurolinguistics* (Vol. 1). New York: Academic Press.

Monrad-Krohn, G. H. (1947). Dysprosody or altered "Melody of language." *Brain, 70,* 405–415. (a)

Monrad-Krohn, G. H. (1947). The prosodic quality of speech and its disorders. *Acta Psychiatrica Neurologica Scandinavica, 22,* 255–269. (b)

Monrad-Krohn, G. H. (1957). The third element of speech: Prosody in the neuropsychiatric clinic. *Journal of Mental Science, 103,* 326–331.

Monrad-Krohn, G. H. (1963). The third element of speech: Prosody and its disorders. In L. Halpern (Ed.), *Problems of dynamic neurology.* Jerusalem: Hebrew University Press, pp. 101–117.

Ross, E. D. (1981). The aprosodias. Functional-anatomic organization of the affective components of language in the right hemisphere. *Archives of Neurology (Chicago), 38,* 561–569.

Ross, E. D., Harney, J. H., deLacoste, C., and Purdy, P. (1981). How the brain integrates affective and propositional language into a unified brain function. Hypotheses based on clinicopathological correlations. *Archives of Neurology (Chicago), 38,* 745–748.

Ross, E. D., & Mesulam, M. M. (1979). Dominant language functions of the right hemisphere? Prosody and emotional gesturing. *Archives of Neurology (Chicago), 36,* 144–148.

Ross, E. D., and Rush, A. J. (1981). Diagnosis and neuroanatomical correlates of depression in brain-damaged patients: Implications for a neurology of depression. *Archives of Neurology (Chicago)*, *38*, 1344–1354.

Rubens, A. B. (1976). Transcortical motor aphasia. In H. Whitaker & H. A. Whitaker (Eds.), *Studies in neurolinguistics*. New York: Academic Press, pp. 293–303.

Tucker, D. M., Watson, R. T., & Heilman, K. M. (1977). Discrimination and evocation of affectively intoned speech in patients with right parietal disease. *Neurology*, *27*, 947–950.

Wernicke, C. (1874). [*Der aphasische Symptomencomplex. Eine psychologische Studie auf anatomischer Basis.*] Breslau: Cohn & Weigert. In G. H. Eggert (trans.), *Wernicke's works on aphasia. Sourcebook and review*. Paris: Mouton, 1977.

Weintraub, S., Mesulam, M-M. and Kramer, L. (1981). Disturbances in prosody. *Archives of Neurology (Chicago)*, *38*, 742–744.

Zurif, E. B. (1974). Auditory lateralization: Prosodic and syntactic factors. *Brain and Language*, *1*, 391–404.

22

An Overview

Andrew Kertesz

The preceding chapters attempt to summarize our current knowledge of the localization of lesions that produce clinically distinct cognitive deficits in man. The major language disturbances, syndromes of the right hemisphere, and deficits of the frontal, temporal, and parieto-occipital lobes are dealt with separately in addition to sections on the advances in neuroanatomy and cytoarchitectonics, cortical stimulation, quantitative computerized tomography (CT), positron emission tomography (PET), regional cerebral blood flow (CBF), and nuclear magnetic resonance (NMR). A regular summary would seem repetitious but a critical overview to highlight some of the topics discussed in the chapters appears to be warranted.

The anatomical method is summarized and updated by Galaburda and Mesulam in Chapter 2. Besides the latest techniques on the preservation and preparation of brains and the various staining techniques detailed in the Appendix, a review of anatomical asymme-

tries, surface landmarks, cytoarchitectonics, and connectivity studies is accomplished. The silver method of axonal degeneration after
lesions promises new information on connectivity in selected human
cases. The recently successful pigment architectonics in addition to
other methods of anatomical mapping may correspond better to
functional units in the cortex than sulci or gyri. The similarity of
lipofuscin-rich cells in both the inferior portion of the frontal lobe
and the temporoparietal area suggest a functional unity borne out
by clinical studies. Although many questions are raised, some answers are beginning to appear. The ingenuity and persistence of
these anatomical efforts are needed to overcome the handicap of
clinical scientists, who cannot control lesion size, location or the
time of anatomical examination.

The issue of terminology and classification in localization has been
dealt with in the introduction. The general chapter on the localization of the aphasias with CT scanning uses a terminology which is
becoming acceptable to most aphasiologists. However, a few entities, especially that of transcortical motor aphasia (TMA) as used by
Naeser in Chapter 3, remain debatable. Most aphasiologists would
prefer to restrict the use of this term to the well-defined entity characterized by nonfluent spontaneous speech, good repetition, and
good comprehension. It appears from the report of spontaneous
speech of Naeser's patients that at least some of them had full propositional sentences, even though their speech was hesitant. Some of
these patients were examined several months post-stroke and would
almost certainly be considered recovering Broca's aphasics in other
taxonomies. Naeser's terminology allows the many frontal convexity or subcortical lesions to be included under the TMA group, adding new sites to the more convincing and specific localization in the
superior mesial frontal cortex supplementary speech area usually
in the anterior cerebral artery distribution. This localization has
been dealt with extensively in Chapter 10.

Lassen and Roland (Chapter 5) undertake a unique approach to a
challenging question: Where are the sensory modalities integrated?
They use the physiological method of cerebral blood flow changes
in the intact normal person engaging in a specified cognitive activity. There seems to be a considerable task-specific activation in certain areas of the brain although the statistical and technical
limitations of the procedure should be kept in mind when considering the specificity of regional activation. The principle of increased cerebral blood flow accompanying cerebral function is

established, but the extent of the correspondence to specific physiological processes such as inhibition and activation is not known.

Interesting findings include the activation of prefrontal cortex
during visual, auditory, and tactile perception. Yet, the authors are
ambivalent about considering the frontal region as a unique supramodal association area. Neither do they accept the large posterior
regions as the area for functional integration because no area in the
posterior part of the brain showed a greater activation during multimodality conditions than during single modality tests. However,
the posterior parietal cortex qualified as a bimodal integrative area
for visual and tactile activation and the inferior posterior portion
for simultaneous visual and auditory tasks. They do not find a separate posterior area for supercomplex multimodality activity.
Rather they feel that sensory integration may occur in the frontal
regions to a greater degree than expected.

They also emphasize that the areas showing CBF increase were
rather large even when only a small component of a function was
carried out. In fact, even the anticipation of an action is sufficient
to activate the area concerned. The responses appear to be graded
in intensity but not in extension, indicating that entire cortical systems and not subcomponents are activated.

Benson, Phelps, Mettler, and Kuhl present data on a new and ex-
citing method of functional–anatomical localization. Positron emission tomography (PET) is an expensive and difficult technique with
relatively poor anatomical resolution but unique capacity to reflect
the actual location of functional changes, such as oxygen uptake or
high-energy phosphate metabolism. This is a major step beyond the
localization of structural lesions as discussed in most of the chapters. The technique can reveal functional changes where structural
lesions are not detectable. Some changes are specific for certain
cognitive functions and tell us more about the brain–behavior correlation than just lesion localization. The subcortical changes with
cortical lesions indicate the functional interdependence of these
structures. Benson's new data concerning the site of the metabolic
alterations in various forms of dementia are important advances in
the understanding of this prevalent medically and socially relevant
illness.

Localization through stimulation, like cerebral blood flow and
PET, enables us to look at the function of normal brain over and
above lesion localization. Unlike the other two, however, it entails
interference with physiological function by applying electric cur-

rent to the surface of brain tissue. The stimulating current inhibits and stimulates at the same time, and its properties concerning the local spread and physiological effect often are difficult to determine. Even more problematic is the reproducibility of the stimulating electrode placements. The often-voiced criticism of stimulation experiments—that they are carried out in brains operated on because of epilepsy and, therefore, not normal to begin with—is more than counterbalanced by the enormous amount of potentially useful information accumulated by the method. Our knowledge of the mechanisms of word finding, articulation, vocalization, grammaticality, and comprehension is greatly advanced by the work of Mateer and the others she reviewed (Chapter 6).

One of the most striking pieces of information we gain from the stimulation studies is the incredible dissociation of various language functions. When one site is stimulated compared to a neighboring square centimeter of cortex in the same patient, a different functional deficit is produced. There is a great deal of individual variability, some of which may be related to sex differences or to IQ. Males appear to use a broader overall area for naming. Patients with lower IQ also appear to have a wider distribution of changes in naming brought on by stimulation. The inferior frontal region appears to be the most constant locale where the various language functions can be disrupted by stimulation. Interference with grammar, semantics and phonology are widely distributed but only a few sites of stimulation produce neologisms. The dissociation of cortical sites for different languages is difficult to correlate with the bulk of experience concerning polyglot aphasics although there are a few reports of differential recovery in the literature. The results of the stimulation studies reported here indicate that the less competent language is affected from a greater number of cortical sites.

Various right hemisphere functions have also been studied through stimulation. Perceptual and memory errors for line orientation and face recognition were elicited from the posterior temporal gyrus, parietal lobe, and posterior frontal regions which corroborates some of the findings in the right hemisphere lesion studies reported in this book. However, the dissociation of the right hemisphere functions is also quite comparable to the dissociations between left hemisphere functions, leading Mateer to conclude that visuospatial functions in the nondominant hemisphere appear to be as discretely localized as verbal functions in the dominant hemisphere.

These studies of stimulation require much attention to detail because the method is crucial for the interpretation of the results. The extent of dissociation of functions and the individual variability obtained in these results are difficult to reconcile with traditional concepts of cerebral organization and open up a host of new possibilities. The surprising amount of dissociation of functions between neighboring sites of stimulation creates a mosaic that is even more finely detailed than the diagrams of the phrenologists. The author makes it clear that this is an empirical finding and the interpretation of the findings should be a challenge to all readers.

Levine and Sweet in Chapter 7 reintroduce a forgotten twist in the century-old argument about the localization of "Broca's aphasia." The usual controversy concerns whether Broca's aphasia occurs with lesions restricted to Broca's area. Recent reviews, summarized in the chapter, are in keeping with the clinical experience of others: persisting severe Broca's aphasia usually involves more than Broca's area, and, in fact, is usually produced by an extensive lesion that includes the precentral gyrus and the inferior parietal area. Levine and Sweet go beyond that and support the idea of Niessl von Mayendorf that it is the inferior portion of the precentral gyrus that is crucial for the syndrome of Broca's aphasia. The reader is to judge their well-developed argument, which also deals with other theories, current and past, in a detailed and logical manner. The crucial issue, in my view, is the persistence of the lesions versus the improving or recovering syndrome, an important but much neglected facet of this phenomenological issue. Even relatively large lesions may be associated with no deficit if examined in the chronic stage because recovery and compensation have taken place. On the other hand, smaller lesions may indicate the role of the area in the production of acute deficit.

Chapter 8 on Wernicke's aphasia approaches the classification of fluent sensory aphasia, characterized by poor comprehension and repetition, from the viewpoint of distinctive output patterns. Wernicke's aphasia is a large syndrome, and there have been several attempts to subdivide it. The questionably unitary nature of comprehension disturbance is complicated by the variety and extent of paraphasias and the degree of repetition disturbance. Reviewed also, in conjunction with the taxonomic issue, are the localization of word deafness, auditory agnosia and cortical deafness. Pure word deafness is rarely, if ever, pure as the presented case exemplifies, but it can be seen with unilateral, dominant temporal lesions. Cortical deafness, on the other hand, has usually been described in the literature with bilateral temporoparietal lesions. The unique localization of neologistic jargon aphasia is also reviewed, concluding that superior temporal and inferior parietal lesions are both necessary for the production of this striking language disturbance. Finally, the various syndromes of fluent or sensory aphasia are fitted to a model of auditory language process that is compatible with modern concepts of linguistics and lesion localization.

The localization of lesions in conduction aphasia has been traditionally linked with the arcuate fasciculus. This relatively large structure that connects the temporal with the frontal lobe and curves around the Sylvian fissure can be impaired at several levels. CT lesions are often central or more posterior in the parietal lobes. The Damasios (Chapter 9) show that insular lesions which would impair presumably cortical–cortical connections between the temporal and frontal lobes could also produce conduction aphasia. Wernicke then was not too far off the mark when he first suggested this.

The transcortical syndromes (Chapter 10) have been controversial from the time of their initial description. The schema of Lichtheim predicted these syndromes but it was met with skepticism. Large anatomical works on localization such as those of Moutier and Henschen indicated this skepticism by adding the qualifier "so-called" to these entities when they discussed them. Yet, clinicians have been impressed by the distinctive preservation of repetition even to the point of echolalia that allowed these patients to be grouped separately. The transcortical syndromes share certain anatomical peculiarities also. They are associated with lesions at the watershed or border zones of the middle cerebral artery supply. They are outside or adjacent to the traditional "language area" that is broadly defined as the peri-Sylvian region including Wernicke's (posterior–superior temporal) area and Broca's (posterior–inferior frontal) area and other cortical and subcortical areas in between. The location of lesions in transcortical sensory aphasia has not been studied well and many authors came to the conclusion in the past that this entity does not have a specific localization. This is partly related to the frequency with which Alzheimer's disease presents or develops symptoms compatible with this entity, and partly related to the frequent recovery of patients and relative paucity of autopsy material. However, since isotope and CT scanning have revealed many focal lesions causing the same syndrome, the temporo–occipital location (posterior cerebral artery or watershed infarct) of the lesions in transcortical sensory aphasia has become evident.

Thalamic hemorrhages occupy a special category in the study of language disturbances. We had some inclination about the significance of the thalamus in language production and reception in the past, but many of the language behaviors due to thalamic involvement were not clearly recognized or were categorized with the dysarthrias. Prior to CT scanning, some autopsied cases of thalamic hemorrhages revealed complex manifestations, most prominently anomia and dysarthria, but these were considered to be analogous to the extrapyramidal manifestations which were commonly observed after thalamotomy. Larger lesions involving the thalamus produced features similar to cortical syndromes but they were usually associated with cortical destruction as well.

Since the CT scanner has been available to us, we have seen many more small hemorrhages in the thalamic region. Mohr has previously collected several cases of thalamic hemorrhages; in Chapter 11, he reviews the evidence accumulated since. It would appear that the unique feature of thalamic hemorrhages is a fluctuating level of fluency, in which, at times, neologistic jargon and rather fluent speech is seen with partially impaired comprehension and relatively good repetition. This is intermittent, however; at other times, the fluent jargon disappears and a great deal of hesitation and word-finding difficulty is seen. The fluctuation in the symptomatology is an intriguing phenomenon, not fully explained in our present state of knowledge. Jargon production by thalamic lesions, in addition to the well-documented temporoparietal ones (see Chapter 8), indicates the important role that thalamocortical connections play in language.

Other subcortical lesions are dealt with by Naeser (Chapter 3), who describes several syndromes involving striatal structures. "Putaminal aphasia" may not be a term accepted by all nor may it reflect a specific enough behavior to correlate with lesion sites, but these descriptions, in addition to those of the thalamic syndromes, have regenerated interest in the role of subcortical structures in behavior and language. Further references to the activation of subcortical structures are found in Chapter 4 and are scattered throughout the rest of the volume. Subcortical–cortical integration is likely to remain a topic of active interest to investigators in the field.

Neurosurgical case material has been a classic method of localization of lesions in cognitive function. Varieties of lesions causing alexia are dealt with extensively by Greenblatt from this point of view (Chapter 13). Some of his evidence is derived from his own neurosurgical experience, but his review of various lesions causing alexia is comprehensive. In addition to the traditional concept of alexia without agraphia being caused by a dominant occipital and associated callosal lesion, Greenblatt discusses the notion of the subangular alexias, indicating that the lesion undercuts the connections to the angular gyrus which is the presumed locus of visual and auditory language and lexicographic integration. Greenblatt's classification of alexia is essentially pragmatic and clearly anatomically oriented although he pays attention to recent psycholinguistic advances in sorting out the mechanisms of reading. He further systematizes the anatomical classification of alexias enabling the reader to follow a clinicopathologic progression of the types of lesions that can produce alexia from the occipital to the frontal lobes.

Chapter 14 on the modality-specific disorders of written language by Vignolo complements the chapters on alexia and on Gerstmann syndrome, by presenting case reports on pure alexia and pure agraphia. The occipitocallosal lesions in alexia are similar despite the variation in the clinical picture. Superior parietal lesions in pure agraphia are quite uncommon, and localization in these cases is unique and intriguingly consistent.

Apraxia-producing lesions have not been clearly categorized in the past, and confusion continues not only about the definition of the various apraxias but also about the neural mechanisms that are disrupted when they occur. Most apraxia seen in clinical practice is associated with aphasia and the lesions are those that produce aphasia also. In other words, apraxia is seen after frontal, central, and parietal lesions of the left hemisphere and the extent and complexity of the structures interrupted are formidable. That buccofacial apraxia is seen more prominently with frontal and central lesions does not mean that it does not occur with purely parietal lesions. The lesions producing limb-kinetic apraxia are yet to be outlined with any clarity, perhaps because this poorly defined or even nonexistent higher-level syndrome is often considered clumsiness or mild hemiparesis. Heilman, Rothi and Kertesz (Chapter 15) outline the importance of callosal lesions especially in hemiapraxia. Ideational apraxia, another controversial entity, most often occurs with bilateral parietal infarcts or widespread cortical degenerations (common in Alzheimer's disease), occasionally with large lesions of the left hemisphere.

Visual agnosia is a striking cognitive disturbance that created much interest and controversy in the past and continues to do so. Alexander and Albert review much of the material including their own in Chapter 16. They take a positive side in the controversy pertaining to the existence of optic aphasia. Others feel that it is just another term used for associative visual agnosia. They also take a firm position based on evidence with focal lesions against those who consider visual agnosia only a perceptual deficit associated with dementia or some other general clouding of consciousness. They review the issue of the associated phenomena and the nature of the association, functional or structural.

A unique localization is available for two unusual but interesting conditions. One is prosopagnosia, or impaired recognition of familiar faces reviewed by Damasio and Damasio in Chapter 17. They point out that the autopsy-proven lesions which have been published so far in the literature have always been bilateral. This is discussed against the background of a right posterior hemisphere dominance for facial recognition tasks. Unilateral CT lesions, although not as certain as anatomical confirmations, have been seen with prosopagnosia and visual agnosia. Could it be that the patients who have bilateral lesions come to autopsy, while those with unilateral abnormality tend to survive? This is possible, but sooner or later, one should see the odd unilateral case postmortem if that was sufficient to produce the syndrome.

Achromatopsia is a color recognition defect that, as pointed out by the Damasios, can be restricted to a hemifield or even a homonymous quadrant. The inferior portions of the occipital lobes on either side seem to be the specialized structural areas responsible for this uniquely isolated function. This points to a close relationship of anatomy and behavior beyond the primary sensorimotor areas.

One of the best known controversies in localization in neuropsychology concerns the Gerstmann syndrome. Strub and Geschwind (Chapter 12) defend the localizationist's point of view against a barrage of criticism ably led by Arthur Benton. Both points of view highlight some fundamental issues in clinical neurology and neuropsychology such as the validity and usefulness of syndromes. Does the strength of association of certain symptoms justify the creation of syndromes, and are the syndromes of higher cortical function reliable to predict the location of lesions?

The frontal lobes have been traditionally regarded as the *terra incognita* of neuropsychology. Clinical observations have established their role in judgment, planning, and sustaining activity, shifting concepts, social and interpersonal adaptation, and affective behavior, but many of these turned out to be difficult to quantitate. Much of the classical experience was based on trauma and tumors, introducing a great deal of variability in the anatomical aspect of the correlation. Stuss and Benson in Chapter 18 contrast the unique experience of the Northampton Veterans Hospital followup of frontal leucotomies with the frontal lobe resections of the Montreal Neurological Institute. The results illuminate the issue of medial versus lateral lesions. The review also discusses unilateral versus bilateral lesions and hemispheric dominance for frontal lobe functions.

Localization in the right hemisphere has not been given equal time or space in the past but in this volume, we attempt to remedy this in chapters dealing with right hemisphere lesions in constructional apraxia and visuospatial deficit, the localization of lesions in neglect, and the lesions in dysprosody and emotional language. The reason the right hemisphere has not equally shared the interest of localizationists could be partly attributed to the finding that right hemisphere deficits are less likely to be caused by a unique focus of lesions than the left. Some of the evidence presented here in Chapter 19 for lesions in constructional apraxia and neglect support a more diffuse organization of the right hemisphere. Mateer, in Chapter 6, on localization by stimulation, came to a rather different conclusion. Although she also found that visuospatial deficit can be elicited from many areas outside the parietal area, she felt that the dissociation of function between the stimulated sites suggested as discrete localization in the right as in the left hemisphere. That frontal lesions can produce constructional apraxia, neglect and deficit on visuospatial tasks may come as a surprise given the traditional expectation of posterior lesions with such deficits.

Heilman, Watson, Valenstein, and Damasio (Chapter 20) contribute evidence that neglect can be associated with right-sided dorsofrontal, medial frontal, thalamic, caudate, and putaminal lesions, as well as left-sided lesions usually with a right hemispheric dominance for language. They attempt to link these sites in a system of attentional arousal supported by the animal evidence for a multimodality arousal system connecting limbic subcortical and cortical structures.

Ross, in Chapter 21, has created a systematic approach to the disturbances of the emotional aspects of communication on the analogy of the classical typing of language disorders. His "aprosodias," as he collectively labels these disturbances, seem to be distributed in the antero–posterior axis of the right hemisphere in much the same way as the motor–sensory dichotomy of language disturbance is distributed on the left. This attractive proposal, almost too logical and simple to accept without reservation, undoubtedly will challenge others to verify it by careful quantitation.

This book makes a case for the correlation of lesion localization and neuropsychological findings. Although the chapters are uneven in scope, length, and content as is inevitable with a multiauthored book, a certain integration is achieved by the common theme. That function is related to structure is intuitively acceptable but the complexity of the relationship is nowhere as prominent as in higher cerebral function. This volume hopefully presents contributions that are a step in solving some of the problems and ask further questions about these intriguing and important issues.

Index